AF597567

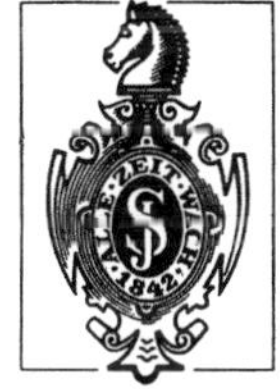

Heiko Traupe

The Ichthyoses

A Guide to Clinical Diagnosis, Genetic Counseling, and Therapy

Foreword by R. Happle

With a contribution by B. Melnik

With 81 Figurcs and 35 Tables

Springer-Verlag Berlin Heidelberg NewYork
London Paris Tokyo Hong Kong

Priv. Doz. Dr. HEIKO TRAUPE
Department of Human Genetics,
University of Nijmegen,
Geert Grooteplein zuid 20,
NL-6500 HB Nijmegen

ISBN 978-3-642-73652-0 ISBN 978-3-642-73650-6 (eBook)
DOI 10.1007/978-3-642-73650-6

Library of Congress Cataloging-in-Publication Data

Traupe, Heiko; The ichthyoses : a guide to diagnosis, genetic counseling, and therapy / Heiko Traupe ; foreword by R. Happle. p. cm. Includes bibliographies and index. ISBN-13:978-3-642-73652-0 (U.S.:alk.paper)1. Ichthyosis. 2.Genetic counseling.I. Title. [DNLM: 1. Genetic Counseling. 2. Ichthyosis–diagnosis. 3. Ichthyosis–therapy. WR 500 T77 i] RL435.T773 1989 616.5'44–dc20 89-19682 CIP

Softcover reprint of the hardcover 1st edition 1989

2127/3145-543210 Printed on acid-free paper

Foreword

It is a great pleasure for me to see this work in print. As outlined by Dr. Traupe, at least 20 different types of ichthyosis have been identified to date. This book will effectively help to establish a correct diagnosis, as a basis for genetic counseling. Dr. Traupe proposes a new classification of the ichthyoses, based on reasonable clinical criteria. He lets the reader share in his enormous knowledge and safely guides him through the difficult field of nomenclature. He describes the particular nature of these scaling disorders in a manner as simple as possible.

During the last few years, research on ichthyosis has become a fascinating scientific challenge due to the introduction of novel investigative approaches. The main advantage of this book lies in the fact that the author successfully combines recent achievements made in lipid analysis, enzymology, electron microscopy, and molecular genetics.

Heiko Traupe began his career in dermatology 11 years ago, as a resident in the Department of Dermatology in Münster. As we were both interested in the genetic aspects of skin diseases, this was the starting point of a most fruitful collaboration, which is still continuing. During our common work in Münster, Dr. Traupe was able, thanks to his unceasing clinical curiosity, to describe many novel aspects within the field of ichthyosis, and I took pride in coauthoring papers on new items such as cryptorchidism as a feature associated with X-linked recessive ichthyosis, autosomal dominant lamellar ichthyosis, and alopecia ichthyotica.

Both of us were impressed by the fact that even today it is still possible to detect new clinical entities, simply by use of a prepared mind. While rereading the first article we wrote together, which deals with the ichthyosis vulgaris group (reference 17 on page 53), I was surprised by the fact that we had already mentioned ichthyosis bullosa of Siemens then. I still remember the day, 5 years later, when Dr. Traupe presented to me a family affected with an uncommon type of ichthyosis, stating that this was most probably a skin disease which had been described 50 years before by Siemens and which had then fallen into oblivion. Dr. Traupe had immediately realized that we were dealing with a second family affected with ichthyosis bullosa of Siemens.

In this volume the author follows the tradition of the great morphologists by carefully presenting the historical aspects of given disease. Yet he is an iconoclast, rejecting time-honored misnomers such as "ichthyosiform erythroderma" or redefining the KID syndrome because he feels that the associated keratinization disorder is not an ichthyosis at all.

The author clearly distinguishes between confirmed data and his opinions, which are based, however, on ample clinical experience. The chapter on therapeutic modalities will be especially useful for any clinician dealing with patients affected with ichthyosis.

Although I had no part in the preparation of this book, I consider it a privilege to have had the opportunity to discuss many points beforehand with the author and to be the first to congratulate him on his outstanding work. I look forward to further fruitful discussions with him on clinical diagnosis, genetic counseling, and therapy of the ichthyoses.

I anticipate that this book will be considered a milestone in the literature on keratinization disorders. It will certainly be of great value to dermatologists, geneticists, and pediatricians and extensively used by them for the best of their patients.

Nijmegen, The Netherlands RUDOLF HAPPLE
June 1989

Preface

By convention, those cornification disorders that are genetic in nature and in which visible scaling involves the entire body surface are called *"ichthyoses"*. Though usually not life threatening, many of these diseases can be very disfiguring and can cause considerable distress to their sufferers throughout life.

To many colleagues, the field of the ichthyoses is a perplexing quagmire. Because of the enormous genetic heterogeneity and because of possible phenotypic variations even within the same genetic type, they often feel uneasy when confronted with an individual patient. I hope that having digested this book, the reader will tread on solid ground in such situations and will be able to entertain a definite diagnosis in more than 90% of his or her patients.

To help our patients, the next step should then be to offer genetic advice to them and their families. This should be done in cooperation with a clinical geneticist or a department specialized in genetic counseling. Throughout the book, special emphasis is given to this part of patient care, and problems relating to disease prevention by prenatal diagnosis are discussed in the individual chapters.

In contrast to many other genetic diseases, treatment is available for the ichthyoses. Because therapy is symptomatic, we can be "lumpers" in this respect. Most patients with ichthyosis can be managed irrespective of their genetic type in more or less the same ways, though some differences in response to retinoids exist. As the title states, it is the aim of this book to provide a guide for clinical diagnosis, genetic counseling, and therapy in this heterogeneous group of diseases.

It is obvious that the process of identifying new entities within the framework of ichthyosis has not yet been completed. There are two reasons for this. On the one hand, some of these diseases are very uncommon. Therefore, distinct, but so far unrecognized clinical syndromes such as the ichthyosis follicularis, atrichia, and photophobia (IFAP) syndrome still emerge. On the other hand, pedigree analysis and newly gained ultrastructural and biochemical insights result in splitting of long-recognized diseases thought to represent a single entity, such as lamellar ichthyosis.

I am sometimes asked by dermatologist colleagues: "Is it at all important to pin down new types of ichthyoses? Are the four 'major' types not enough? Why don't you work on a common disease like atopic dermatitis or psoriasis?" Questions like these reveal a lack of comprehension as to why research into genetic skin diseases is done. Establishing a correct diagnosis is not art for art's sake; it is the prerequisite for adequate genetic counseling and thus for adequate patient care. In some diseases like Refsum's syndrome, missing the proper diagnosis has far-reaching negative repercussions on the health of these patients. Moreover, before we can learn more about the biochemistry and molecular genetics of the ichthyoses it is necessary to establish a diagnosis that is as precise as possible. To put it in the words of Dr. Mary Williams, of San Francisco, one has to "sort out apples from oranges."

It was only 20 years ago that Dr. Wells and Dr. Kerr identified X-linked recessive ichthyosis as a new type of ichthyosis and separated it from the more common autosomal dominant ichthyosis vulgaris. Without their work, the fascinating recent advances with regard to steroid sulfatase deficiency would not have been possible. X-linked recessive ichthyosis has become a model disease for both disciplines, dermatology and genetics. It is now an open window, allowing deep insights into structure and function of the skin and regulation of X-linked genes. In the future, the other types of ichthyosis may likewise contribute to similar advances.

Last but not least, I want to acknowledge the help of many colleagues and friends in preparing this book. My own involvement in ichthyosis research began in 1978. Over many years, Dr. Rudolf Happle, now of Nijmegen, has been an enthusiastic counterpart and mentor. I owe a great deal to him, and I am glad he accepted the invitation to write the foreword.

I had the pleasure of working for almost 10 years in a department with a lively scientific and, at the same time, agreeable and friendly atmosphere. Much of the special spirit of the Münster Department of Dermatology is due to its head, Dr. Egon Macher. I want to specifically thank Dr. Gisela Bonsmann, Münster, and Dr. Henning Hamm, Münster, who helped a great deal with the clinical studies. Over many years, Dr. C. Müller, now of Würzburg, and Dr. H. H. Ropers, now of Nijmegen, performed steroid sulfatase tests for us. Dr. G. Kolde, Münster, studied the ultrastructure in some of our patients and kindly provided a number of electron micrographs. My warmest thanks also go to a number of nonacademic co-workers, especially to the two excellent photographers of the Münster Department of Dermatology, Mr. P. Wissel and Mrs. Jutta Bückmann. I am deeply indebted as well to Mrs. M. von Lovenberg, who typed the manuscript.

Dr. Bodo Melnik, Düsseldorf, kindly accepted the task of writing a chapter on epidermal lipid metabolism and its relationship to the ichthyoses. His important contribution shows how closely ichthyosis research is now interwoven with basic problems of skin metabolism and terminal epidermal differentiation. I am indebted to a great number of colleagues who provided me with photographic material. These are Dr. Ingrun Anton-Lamprecht and Dr. Marie-Luise Arnold, both of Heidelberg, Dr. T. Gedde-Dahl, Tromsø, Norway, Dr. R. Happle, Nijmegen, Dr. G. Kolde, Münster, Dr. W. Küster, Düsseldorf, Dr. F. Lawlor, London, Dr. B. Mevorah, Lausanne, Dr. H. Høyer, Rønne, Denmark, Dr. C. R. Müller, Würzburg, Dr. P. Unamuno, Salamanca, and Dr. Mary Williams, San Francisco.

I thank Hoffmann-La Roche Company, Federal Republic of Germany, for a financial contribution to lower the costs of printing. I am much indebted to the **Deutsche Forschungsgemeinschaft** which fully supports me (grant Tr 228/1-1).

Reactions, comments and suggestions on this book and on the subject of ichthyosis are most welcome. For correspondence, please note that I am now affiliated with the Department of Human Genetics at the University of Nijmegen, The Netherlands.

Nijmegen, The Netherlands HEIKO TRAUPE
June 1989

Table of Contents

1 Introduction

1.1 Definition of the Term “Ichthyosis”

“Ichthyosis” is a descriptive term used for a variety of hereditary keratinization disorders [3]. These disorders are grouped together because they always are genetic in nature and share a conspicuous scaling which is generalized and affects the whole integument. Localized keratinization disorders which confine themselves to certain parts of the body, such as the group of palmoplantar keratoses or the group of erythrokeratoderma, are excluded [2]. Though not explicitly stated, the term “ichthyosis” conveys the picture of a static disease process which may show some seasonal variation but does not exhibit the spontaneous coming and going of skin lesions that is typical, for example, of Darier’s disease. Ichthyosis may be accompanied by erythroderma, and for historical reasons these types of ichthyosis are usually referred to as *ichthyosiform erythroderma* rather than *ichthyotic erythroderma* [1], though *ichthyotic* would be grammatically more logical [4]. I suggest that usage of the attribute “ichthyosiform” be restricted to nongenetic cornification disorders. Following this definition, ichthyosiform skin changes are always acquired (e.g., the ichthyosis-like condition in Hodgkin’s disease). The word “ichthyosis” is derived from the Greek word “ichthys”, which means fish. It was already used in the eighteenth century by Willan [5] and was coined at a time when characteristics of human diseases were compared to those occurring in the animal kingdom.

The literal translation “scaly fish disease” should be avoided, since it is embarrassing for patients. When dealing with patients, I use the word “ichthyosis” and explain that this is one of many different disorders of cornification.

References

1. Brocq L (1902) Erythrodermie congénitale ichthyosiforme avec hyperépidermotrophie. Ann Dermatol Syph (Paris) 4 (3):1–31
2. Peukert M (1899) Über Ichthyosis. Eine Übersicht. Dermatologische Zeitschrift (Berlin) 6:171–204
3. Schnyder UW (1970) Inherited ichthyoses. Arch Dermatol 102:240–255
4. Voß M (1986) Neue Befunde bei Verhornungsstörungen. Dissertation B (Habilitationsschrift) an der Medizinischen Akademie Erfurt, East Germany
5. Willian R (1808) On cutaneous diseases, vol 1, chap 4: Ichthyosis. Barnard, London, pp 197–212

1.2 History of the Ichthyoses

The majority of the various types of ichthyoses do not affect general health, and therefore the reproductive fitness of these patients is not significantly impaired. Still, most types of ichthyosis are rare conditions. Hence, we may assume that the mutation rate for these diseases is very low and that these disorders must have been present many thousands of years ago. The recorded history of the ichthyoses, however, begins on March 16, 1731. On that day, the English astronomer John Machin presented to the Royal Society of London a 14-year-old boy who was suffering from a particular "cuticular distemper" [19]. This boy was Edward Lambert, who was born to healthy parents and suffered from a very severe type of ichthyosis hystrix. Despite his monstrous skin disease, he was able to find a wife and became the founding father of the famous Lambert family with six affected children. He reached the great age of 90 years and died in 1806 after an

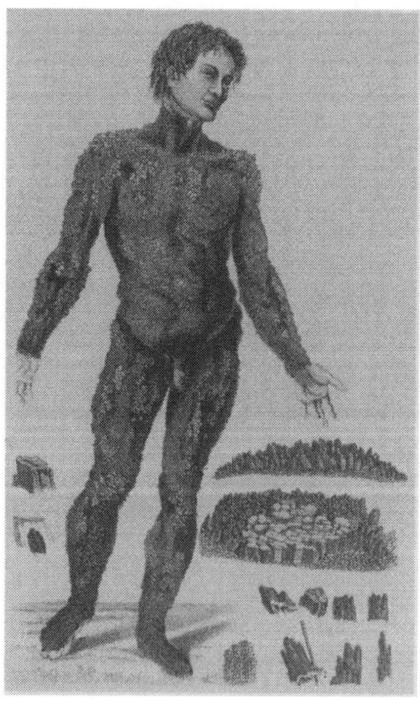

Fig. 1. Porcupine man. A member of the Lambert family drawn by Tilesius [29] in 1802

accident, which proves that this severe skin disease did not reduce his life span.

For many years Edward Lambert, his children, and grandchildren earned their living by exposing themselves publicly at fairs (Fig. 1). They traveled throughout Europe and were called "porcupine men" and considered a "new species of man" (Fig. 2). In 1801 two affected grandchildren of Edward Lambert went to Germany. To attract more attention, they claimed that only male family members were affected, and this false information was given in a report on the two brothers by Tilesius in 1802 [29]. Traveling through Europe, the two brothers spread the false information about the inheritance of their disease. Since they were studied by many medical authorities of their time, this misinformation was recorded in a number of medical reports. To complicate things further, in 1933 Cockayne [6] drew a pedigree of the family and even added two further generations showing male-to-male transmission only. These two generations did not really exist. Cockayne had misunderstood a paper of Gassman [11] in which

New SPECIES of MAN.
Among the Wonders of Nature, which have from time to time tempted the Curiosity of the Public, perhaps no object more worthy of attention has been offered to their notice, than a Singular Variety of the Human Species, now exhibiting at the
Great Room, 182, Fleet Street,
near St. Dunstan's Church.
covered with Scales, with the exception of the face, soles of the feet, and palms of the hand, which are like those of any other man. These Scales, nearly half an inch long, are so hard and firm, that with a touch of the finger they make a sound like stones striking together; those on the stomach are short, round, and distant; those on the arms, on the contrary, approach each other like the bristles of an hedge-hog. The great grandfather of the singular family to which this young man belongs, was found savage in the woods of North America. The peculiarity descends only in the male line. (For a description of this Species see the Works of Buffon.)

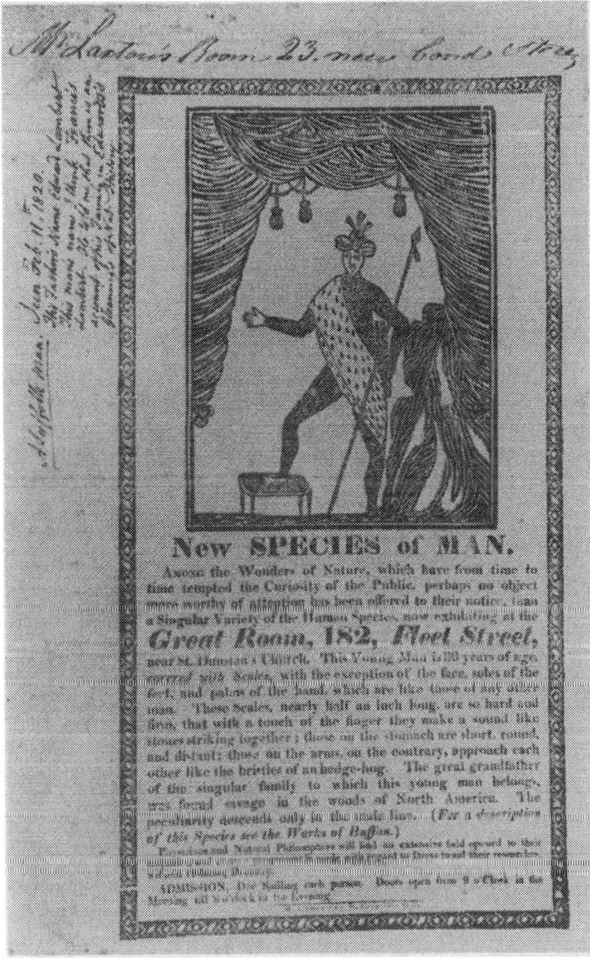

Fig. 2. Handbill from the year 1820 advertising the exposition of Francis Lambert in Fleet Street, London. (From Penrose and Stern [19])

these two generations were not mentioned at all. Cockayne interpreted the pedigree as evidence of Y-chromosomal (holandric) transmission in man. During the following years, the pedigree of this family, as drawn by Cockayne [6], was depicted in many textbooks of human genetics and was always taken as definite proof of the existence of Y-chromosomal transmission. It was not until 1958 that Penrose and Stern [19] were able to correct the myth of Y-chromosomal inheritance in this disorder by reconstructing the pedigree based on extensive study of parish registers of the county of Suffolk. The new pedigree elaborated by Penrose and Stern [19] is compatible with autosomal dominant inheritance only.

The exact nature of the ichthyosis of the Lambert family will remain a mystery, since the family died out and no histologic evaluation was ever made. Bullous episodes and erythroderma are not mentioned in the many clinical reports of the nineteenth century, thus exluding bullous ichthyotic erythroderma. On clinical grounds the disease would be classified nowadays as ichthyosis hystrix, and within the framework of this subset of ichthyoses it most closely resembles the rare ichthyosis hystrix of Curth-Macklin. The Lambert family's disease was very spectacular and focused considerable interest on the topic of ichthyosis at an early age. In one of the first textbooks of dermatology written in 1808, Robert Willan [32] devoted a whole chapter to the description of this family and introduced the term "ichthyosis" for their skin disease.

In the nineteenth century the harlequin fetus, a lethal variant of congenital ichthyosis, was described [12, 23], and autosomal dominant inheritance in ichthyosis vulgaris was mentioned by Alibert [1] in 1806. The occurrence of ichthyosis vulgaris in male members of a family was reported by Rayer [21] in 1835, and it is reasonable to assume that this may have been the first family found to have X-linked recessive ichthyosis. At the end of the nineteenth century Peukert [20] gave a stricter definition of the term "ichthyosis" and emphasized the general involvement of the skin, excluding by this definition, for example, unilateral keratotic nevi and the various palmoplantar keratoses. In 1900, Riecke [24] recognized that congenital ichthyosis was a heterogeneous disease and proposed classifying it according to the degree of severity into three subtypes:

Ichthyosis congenita I	(corresponding to harlequin fetus)
Ichthyosis congenita II	(corresponding to lamellar ichthyosis)
Ichthyosis congenita III	(noncongenital tarda type, most likely X-linked recessive ichthyosis)

The Riecke classification formed the basis for later modifications proposed by Siemens [27] and Schnyder [25]. As early as 1904, Gassmann [11] contributed largely to the histopathology of the ichthyoses and observed that the less severe type of ichthyosis vulgaris, designated "ichthyosis simplex" or "nitida," displayed a lack of the granular layer, whereas the more severe type, designated "ichthyosis serpentina," showed a prominent granular layer. This was the first histopathologic distinction between autosomal dominant ichthyosis vulgaris and the X-linked type of ichthyosis vulgaris, but without the concepts provided by genetics, these histopathologic differences could not be appreciated. Gassman [11] also developed the concept of retention and hyperproliferation hyperkeratosis and interpreted ichthyosis vulgaris as being a retention hyperkeratosis and congenital ichthyosis as being due to hyperproliferation of the epidermis. This modern pathophysiologic view of ichthyosis was confirmed many years later by biometric and autoradiographic studies [9, 10].

In 1902, Brocq [5] introduced the term "erythrodermie congénitale ichthyosiforme" for congenital ichthyosis and distinguished between a bullous form of congenital ichthyotic erythroderma and a nonbullous type. At that time the designation ichthyosis congenita was still identical with what is now called harlequin fetus. Therefore, it is quite understandable that Brocq described the skin changes of congenital ichthyosis as ichthyosiform (ichthyosis-like). The histologic features of the bullous type of congenital ichthyosis were fully described by Lapière [14, 15] in 1932 and 1953 as granular degeneration with acanthokeratolysis. This histologic pattern was later renamed "epidermolytic hyperkeratosis" by Frost and van Scott [9].

Since the classification of ichthyosis was based on clinical features only, gradual transitions between the various types of congenital and vulgar ichthyoses were thought possible for a long time. It was Siemens [27] who introduced modern genetic thinking into the field of ichthyosis and was able to demonstrate that such transitions cannot occur. He found that ichthyosis vulgaris is usually inherited as an autosomal dominant trait, whereas congenital ichthyosis is a recessive disease in most instances. At the same time, a number of papers appeared reporting X-linked recessive inheritance in families with ichthyosis vulgaris [8, 16]. In 1929, Orel [18] had already collected nine families with this type of inheritance from the literature. Dermatologists were not prepared, however, to use pedigree analysis as a tool for the classification of hereditary skin diseases in everyday practice.

The period from 1930 to 1965 was uneventful; only three types of ichthyosis were delineated in these three decades: Refsum's disease in 1946 [22], Sjögren-Larsson syndrome in 1957 [28], and Comèl-Netherton syndrome in the years 1949/1958 [7, 17].

The pathophysiologic studies by Frost et al. [9, 10], the ultrastructural characterization of specific defects in various ichthyoses by Anton-Lamprecht [2–4], and the rediscovery of X-linked recessive ichthyosis by Wells and Kerr [30, 31] renewed interest in the field. In the late 1970s, steroid sulfatase deficiency was established as the underlying biochemical defect in X-linked recessive ichthyosis [13, 26]. This discovery was an enormous impetus for biochemical and genetic research in the field and has attracted workers from various disciplines to investigate the mechanisms of cornification disorders. Keratinization disorders are no longer considered oddities, but are now viewed as model diseases and experiments of nature that, once deciphered, will provide us with new insights into the normal functions of the skin.

References

1. Alibert L (1806) Descriptions des maladies de la peau, observés à l'hópital Saint-Louis et exposition des meilleurs méthodes suivives pour le traitement. Paris
2. Anton-Lamprecht I (1973) Zur Ultrastruktur hereditärer Verhornungsstörungen. III. Autosomal-dominante Ichthyosis vulgaris. Arch Dermatol Forsch 248:149–172

3. Anton-Lamprecht I, Hofbauer M (1972) Ultrastructural distinction of autosomal dominant ichthyosis vulgaris and X-linked recessive ichthyosis. Hum Genet 15:261–264
4. Anton-Lamprecht I, Schnyder UW (1974) Ultrastructure of inborn errors of keratinization. VI. Inherited ichthyoses - a model system for heterogeneities in keratinization disturbances. Arch Dermatol Forsch 250:207–227
5. Brocq L (1902) Erythrodermie congénitale ichthyosiforme avec hyperépidermotrophie. Ann Dermatol Syph, Serie 4,3:1–31
6. Cockayne EA (1933) Inherited abnormalities of the skin and its appendages. Oxford University Press, London
7. Comèl M (1949) Ichthyosis linearis circumflexa. Dermatologica 98:133–136
8. Csörsz K (1929) Recessiv geschlechtsgebundene Vererbung bei Ichthyosis. Mschr Ung Mediziner 2:180–187
9. Frost P, van Scott EJ (1966) Ichthyosiform dermatoses. Classification based on anatomic and biometric observations. Arch Dermatol 94:113–126
10. Frost P, Weinstein G, van Scott EJ (1966) The ichtyosiform dermatoses. II. Autoradiographic studies of epidermal proliferation. J Invest Dermatol 47:561–567
11. Gassmann A (1904) Histologische und klinische Untersuchungen über Ichthyosis und ichthyosisähnliche Krankheiten. Arch Dermatol Syph [Suppl]
12. Jahn JF (1869) Über Ichthyosis congenita. Dissertation, Leipzig
13. Jöbsis AC, van Duuren CY, de Vries GP, Koppe JG, Rijken Y, van Kempen GMJ, de Groot WP (1976)Trophoblast sulfatase deficiency associated with X-chromosomal ichthyosis. Ned Tijdsch Geneeskd 120:1980
14. Lapière S (1932) Epidermolyse ichthyosiforme congénitale (erythrodermie ichthyosiforme congénitale forme bulleuse de Brocq). Ann Dermatol Syph 3:401–415
15. Lapière S (1953) Les génodermatoses hyperkératosiques de type bulleux. Ann Dermatol Syph 80:597–614
16. Lundborg H (1927) Geschlechtsgebundene Vererbung von Ichthyosis simplex (vulgaris) in einer schwedischen Bauernsippe. Hereditas 9:45–48
17. Netherton EW (1958) A unique case of trichorrhexis nodosa - "bamboo hairs". Arch Dermatol 78:483–487
18. Orel H (1929) Die Vererbung der Ichthyosis congenita und der Ichthyosis vulgaris. Kleine Beiträge zur Vererbungswissenschaft. V. Mitteilung. Z Kinderheilkd 47:312–340
19. Penrose LS, Stern C (1958) Reconsideration of the Lambert pedigree (ichthyosis hystrix gravior). Ann Hum Genet 22:258–283
20. Peukert M (1899) Über Ichthyosis. Eine Übersicht. Dermatol Z (Berlin) 6:171–204
21. Rayer P (1835) Traite théorique et pratique des maladies de la peau, vol 3. Baillière, Paris, pp 614–650
22. Refsum S (1946) Heredopathia atactica polyneuritiformis. Acta Psychiatr Scand [Suppl] 38:1–303
23. Richter CF (1792) Dissertatio medica de infanticidio in artis obstetriciae exercitio non semper evitabili. Richter, Leipzig
24. Riecke E (1900) Über Ichthyosis congenita. Arch Dermatol Syph (Wien) 54:289–340
25. Schnyder UW (1970) Inherited ichthyoses. Arch Dermatol 102:240–255
26. Shapiro LJ, Weiss R, Webster D, France JT (1978) X-linked ichthyosis due to steroid sulfatase deficiency. Lancet 2:70–72
27. Siemens HW (1929) Die Vererbung in der Ätiologie der Hautkrankheiten. In: Jadassohn J (ed) Handbuch der Haut- und Geschlechtskrankheiten, vol 3. Springer, Berlin, pp 1–165
28. Sjögren T, Larsson T (1957) Oligophrenia in combination with congenital ichthyosis and spastic disorders. A clinical and genetic study. Acta Psychiatr Scand [Suppl] 32 (113):1–112
29. Tilesius WG (1802) Ausführliche Beschreibung und Abbildung der beiden sogenannten Stachelschweinmenschen aus der bekannten englischen Familie Lambert oder the porcupine man. Altenburg: im Literarischen Comtoir, and J. H. Voigt's Mag f.d. neuesten Instanz d. Naturk. 4:422–432
30. Wells RS, Kerr CB (1966) Clinical features of autosomal dominant and sex-linked ichthyosis in an English population. Br Med J 1:947–950
31. Wells RS, Kerr CB (1966) The histology of ichthyosis. J Invest Dermatol 46:530–535
32. Willan R (1808) On cutaneous diseases, Vol 1. Barnard, London

1.3 New Classification and Tables for Differential Diagnosis of the Ichthyoses

The ichthyoses comprise about twenty different **well-established** genetic entities. The purpose of this classification is to give the clinician a framework and guidelines for rapid, yet accurate diagnosis appreciating the clinical and genetic diversity of this kind of disease. With this classification I have attempted to be didactic, and, admittedly, it is in some respects oversimplified. Recently it was suggested that terms like "ichthyosis", "palmoplantar keratosis", or "erythrokeratoderma" be abandoned and that all these types of diseases be classified as disorders of cornification and numbered [9]. Though the distinction between the ichthyoses and the palmoplantar keratoses is, of course, a historical one and in a way a bit arbitrary, it allows us to keep these two groups of skin diseases apart and to classify within each of the two groups. Simply numbering all disorders of cornification makes this task more difficult and to me seems undidactic.

Based mainly on histologic and cell kinetic studies, Frost and co-workers [1-3] proposed classifying the ichthyoses according to whether they were hyperproliferation hyperkeratoses or retention hyperkeratoses. Later it was shown that some of the diseases they grouped together, such as lamellar ichthyosis, are in fact heterogeneous. Furthermore, for many diseases this type of investigation has not yet been made. Using routine histology it is not possible to make a definite diagnosis of hyperproliferation or retention hyperkeratosis. Thus, X-linked recessive ichthyosis was initially considered a hyperproliferation hyperkeratosis because of its histologic features [6] but later was shown to be a retention hyperkeratosis [1]. The classification proposed in detail here [8] is in the tradition of previous classifications by Riecke [5], Siemens [7], and Schnyder [6] and, like the Schnyder classification, it is hierarchically structured. I suggest distinguishing between four major groups of ichthyoses at a clinical level: **isolated vulgar ichthyoses, associated vulgar ichthyoses, isolated congenital ichthyoses,** and **associated congenital ichthyoses**. Group diagnosis of an ichthyosis can be made by asking two questions:

1. Is the ichthyosis present at birth and can it be regarded as a congenital ichthyosis due to its clinical features (involvement of the flexures, possibly involvement of palms and soles), or was the diseases not present at birth but developed during the first year of life and would be classified as belonging to the vulgaris group on clinical grounds (sparing of the big flexures, no involvement of palms and soles except for accentuated palmoplantar creases)?
2. Is the skin disorder an isolated ichthyosis, i.e., is the ichthyosis the only disease present in the patient, or are we dealing with an associated or syndromic

ichthyosis in which the skin disease is only a cutaneous manifestation of a more general syndrome?

Having answered these two questions, we arrive at four different major groups of ichthyosis, and within each of these general groups it is now possible to classify according to genetic, clinical, histologic/ultrastructural, and biochemical features. This kind of subclassification within each of the four major groups should render a definite diagnosis (Table 1). Over the years to come, new types of ichthyosis will probably emerge. One advantage of this approach to classification is that all of these future ichthyoses will easily fit into one of the major groups. I hope that this classification [8] will stand the test of time and be of

Table 1. Classification of the ichthyoses into four major groups

Group	Diseases	Mode of inheritance
Isolated vulgar ichthyoses	Autosomal dominant ichthyosis vulgaris (ADI)	Autosomal dominant
	X-linked recessive ichthyosis (XRI)	X-linked recessive
Isolated congenital ichthyoses	**Lamellar ichthyoses**	Autosomal dominant
	Autosomal dominant lamellar ichthyosis	
	Erythrodermic lamellar ichthyosis	Autosomal recessive
	Nonerythrodermic lamellar ichthyosis	Autosomal recessive
	Bullous ichthyoses	
	Bullous ichthyotic erythroderma	Autosomal dominant
	Ichthyosis bullosa of Siemens	Autosomal dominant
	Special variants	
	Ichthyosis hystrix of Curth-Macklin	Autosomal dominant
	Harlequin fetus	Autosomal recessive
Associated vulgar ichthyoses	Refsum's disease	Autosomal recessive
	Multiple sulfatase deficiency	Autosomal recessive
	Associated steroid sulfatase deficiency (deletion mutation on the X-chromosome)	X-linked
	Atypical ichthyosis vulgaris with hypogonadism	Unknown
Associated congenital ichthyoses	KID syndrome (erythrokeratoderma of Burns) (keratitis, "ichthyosis", deafness)	Autosomal dominant
	X-linked dominant ichthyosis	X-linked, lethal for affected male embryos
	Comèl-Netherton syndrome	Autosomal recessive
	Neutral lipid storage disease	Autosomal recessive
	Sjögren-Larsson syndrome	Autosomal recessive
	Tay syndrome (IBIDS syndrome)	Autosomal recessive
	HID syndrome	Unknown
	IFAP syndrome	Unknown

value to clinicians even when the biochemical basis of most of these disorders has been established. A number of tables which will hopefully facilitate differential diagnosis for the clinician confronted with an individual patient are provided (Tables 2–7). I am aware of the fact that the listings under the headings may not be complete and that the headings do not cover all the signs and symptoms that may be found in ichthyosis, but rather represent a selection of these.

Table 2. Differential diagnosis: cutaneous signs and symptoms

Sign	Disease
Accentuated palmoplantar creases	Autosomal dominant ichthyosis vulgaris Refsum's disease Nonerythrodermic lamellar ichthyosis
Alopecia ichthyotica	Erythrodermic lamellar ichthyosis Nonerythrodermic lamellar ichthyosis Congenital ichthyosis (other types) KID syndrome X-linked dominant ichthyosis
Brittle hair	Comèl-Netherton syndrome Tay syndrome
Bullous eruptions	Bullous ichthyotic erythroderma of Brocq Ichthyosis bullosa of Siemens Comèl-Netherton syndrome (possible)
Collodion baby[a]	Erythrodermic lamellar ichthyosis Nonerythrodermic lamellar ichthyosis Comèl-Netherton syndrome Sjögren-Larsson syndrome Tay syndrome Autosomal dominant lamellar ichthyosis
Congenital ichthyotic erythroderma	Erythrodermic lamellar ichthyosis Bullous ichthyotic erythroderma of Brocq Comèl-Netherton syndrome KID syndrome Neutral lipid storage disease Tay syndrome X-linked dominant ichthyosis
Hystrix-like hyperkeratoses	Bullous ichthyotic erythroderma of Brocq Ichthyosis hystrix of Curth-Macklin HID syndrome KID syndrome (possible)
Nail changes	Tay syndrome Comèl-Netherton syndrome (possible)

[a] According to Larrègue et al. [4]

Table 3. Differential diagnosis: noncutaneous disease manifestations

Manifestation	Disease
Ataxia	Refsum's disease Neutral lipid storage disease
Anosmia	Refsum's disease Associated steroid sulfatase deficiency
Cataract	X-linked dominant ichthyosis Refsum's disease Tay syndrome
Cryptorchidism/hypogonadism	Autosomal dominant ichthyosis vulgaris (coincidental?) X-linked recessive ichthyosis Associated steroid sulfatase deficiency Atypical ichthyosis vulgaris Tay syndrome
Deafness/impaired hearing	Refsum's disease Neutral lipid storage disease KID syndrome HID syndrome
Growth retardation	X-linked dominant ichthyosis Comèl-Netherton syndrome (possible) Tay syndrome Associated steroid sulfatase deficiency (possible)
Mental retardation	Sjögren-Larsson syndrome Tay syndrome Associated steroid sulfatase deficiency Multiple sulfatase deficiency
Proneness to infections	Comèl-Netherton syndrome Tay syndrome KID syndrome

Table 4. Differential diagnosis: modes of inheritance

Mode of inheritance	Disease
Autosomal dominant	Autosomal dominant ichthyosis vulgaris Autosomal dominant lamellar ichthyosis Bullous ichthyotic erythroderma Ichthyosis bullosa of Siemens Ichthyosis hystrix of Curth-Macklin KID syndrome (erythrokeratodermia of Burns)
Autosomal recessive	Comèl-Netherton syndrome Erythrodermic lamellar ichthyosis Harlequin fetus Multiple sulfatase deficiency Nonerythrodermic lamellar ichthyosis Neutral lipid storage disease Sjögren-Larsson syndrome Tay syndrome

Table 4. (continued)

Mode of inheritance	Disease
X-linked	Associated steroid sulfatase deficiency X-linked recessive ichthyosis X-linked dominant ichthyosis
Unknown	Atypical ichthyosis vulgaris with hypogonadism HID syndrome IFAP syndrome

Table 5. Differential diagnosis: histologic patterns

Histologic pattern	Disease
Reduced or absent granular layer	Autosomal dominant ichthyosis vulgaris Comèl-Netherton syndrome (can vary within the biopsy) Refsum's disease Tay syndrome X-linked dominant ichthyosis
Prominent granular layer	Autosomal dominant lamellar ichthyosis Erythrodermic lamellar ichthyosis Nonerythrodermic lamellar ichthyosis Neutral lipid storage disease KID syndrome Sjögren-Larsson syndrome
Parakeratosis	Autosomal dominant Lamellar ichthyosis (possible) Comèl-Netherton syndrome (prominent) Lamellar ichthyosis (usually slight, occasionally very prominent, third recessive type?)
Epidermolytic hyperkeratosis	Bullous ichthyotic erythroderma Ichthyosis bullosa of Siemens Other keratinization disorders (palmoplantar keratosis of Vörner, keratotic nevi)
Positive PAS staining of the stratum corneum	Bullous ichthyotic erythroderma Ichthyosis bullosa of Siemens Comèl-Netherton syndrome Nonerythrodermic lamellar ichthyosis (faint, at variance with other reports)

PAS, Periodic-acid-Schiff

Table 6. Differential diagnosis: diagnostic clues — clinical features

Clinical features	Disease
Atopic dermatitis	Autosomal dominant ichthyosis vulgaris
Follicular atrophoderma	X-linked dominant ichthyosis
Linear skin lesions	X-linked dominant ichthyosis
Loss of dark vision (retinitis pigmentosa)	Refsum's disease
Macula degeneration ("glistening dots")	Sjögren-Larsson syndrome
Photosensitivity	Tay syndrome (possible) IFAP syndrome
Spastic paralysis of the Little type	Sjögren-Larsson syndrome
Vascularizing keratitis	KID syndrome

Table 7. Differential diagnosis: diagnostic clues — microscopic and laboratory findings

Microscopic/laboratory findings	Disease
Arylsulfatase C deficiency	X-linked recessive ichthyosis
Banding pattern of hair in polarizing microscopy	Tay syndrome
Elevated **n**-alkanes	Erythrodermic lamellar ichthyosis Autosomal dominant lamellar ichthyosis
Excessive IgE levels	Comèl-Netherton syndrome
Fast-moving β-lipoproteins	X-linked recessive ichthyosis
Increased creatinine kinase	Neutral lipid storage disease
Steroid sulfatase deficiency	X-linked recessive ichthyosis
Trichorrhexis invaginata	Comèl-Netherton syndrome
Vacuolated granulocytes	Multiple sulfatase deficiency Neutral lipid storage disease

References

1. Frost P (1973) Ichthyosiform dermatoses. J Invest Dermatol 60:541–552
2. Frost P, van Scott EJ (1966) Ichthyosiform dermatoses. Classification based on anatomic and biometric observations. Arch Dermatol 94:113–126
3. Frost P, Weinstein GD, van Scott EJ (1966) The ichthyosiform dermatoses, II. Autoradiographic studies of epidermal proliferation. J Invest Dermatol 47:561–567
4. Larrègue M, Ottovy N, Bressieux JM, Lorette J (1986) Bébé collodion. Trente-deux nouvelles observations. Ann Dermatol Venereol 113:773–785
5. Riecke E (1900) Über Ichthyosis congenita. Arch Dermatol Syph (Wien) 54:289–340
6. Schnyder UW (1970) Inherited ichthyoses. Arch Dermatol 102:240–255
7. Siemens HW (1929) Studien über Vererbung von Hautkrankheiten. XI. Ichthyosis congenita. Arch Dermatol Syph (Berlin) 158:111–127
8. Traupe H (1986) Die Ichthyosen: auf dem Weg vom Phän zum Gen. In: Macher E, Czarnetzki BM, Knop J (eds) Jahrbuch der Dermatologie 1986. Regensburg and Biermann, Münster, pp 35–48
9. Williams ML (1986) A new look at the ichthyoses: disorders of lipid metabolism. Pediatr Dermatol 3:476–497

1.4 Epidermal Lipids and the Biochemistry of Keratinization

B. MELNIK* M. D.

1.4.1 Introduction

Epidermal lipids constitute approximately 10%–14% of the dry weight of mammalian epidermis. During keratinization, the composition and quantities of epidermal lipids dramatically change from the basal to the granular layer with further striking modulations occuring within the stratum corneum. These compositional changes of epidermal lipids are closely linked to the functional requirements of the differentiating epithelium. The important role of the epidermal lipid metabolism in the homeostasis of the stratum corneum, the end product of epidermal differentiation, has been established by the pioneering work of Yardley (1983), Gray and White (1978), Yardley and Summerly (1981), Elias (1981) and Williams and Elias (1986). On the basis of light microscopy, transmission electron microscopy, freeze fracture studies, cell fractionation, and histochemical analyses, a two-compartment model ("brick and mortar model") of the stratum corneum consisting of protein-enriched corneocytes ("bricks") embedded in lipid-enriched intercellular material ("mortar") has been proposed (Elias 1983; Elias et al. 1983a).

With regard to the biochemical process of cornification the keratin matrix constituents of corneocytes have been the subject of intense research for the past few decades. However, until recently, the intercellular lipid-enriched compartment, which accounts for 10%–30% of the volume of the stratum corneum (Elias and Leventhal 1979) has received little attention. Now, evidence is growing that, besides the well-accepted barrier function of epidermal lipids (Elias et al. 1977; Elias and Brown 1978), the intercellular lipids are important for stratum corneum cohesion and desquamation. Alterations in epidermal lipids were detected in a number of inherited metabolic disorders of lipid metabolism such as X-linked recessive ichthyosis (XRI) (Elias et al. 1984; Shapiro 1983), Refsum's disease (Davies et al. 1978; Steinberg 1983), and neutral lipid storage disease (Chanarin et al. 1975; Elias and Williams 1985), all which exhibit ichthyotic skin changes. Further evidence comes from observations of altered epidermal lipids in various hyperkeratotic skin changes following the administration of several hypocholesterolemic drugs (Anderson and Martt 1965; Elias et al. 1986; Ruiter and Mexler 1960; Simpson et al 1964; Williams et al. 1987a; Winkelmann et al. 1963). In the near future, it will be possible to classify many circumscribed and

* With support by a grant from Deutsche Forschungsgemeinschaft (Me 760/3-2)

generalized disorders of keratinization as epidermal disturbances of either lipid and/or protein metabolism.

1.4.2 Changes in Lipid Composition of Epidermal Layers during Keratinization

Figures 3 and 4 show the chemical structures of some unique epidermal lipids. The epidermal lipid composition markedly changes in the successive layers of epidermal cells. In 1932, Kooyman was the first to recognize that phospholipids present in the viable epidermal layers were strikingly diminished in the stratum corneum. *Phospholipids,* which are essential for the maintenance of the cellular membrane bilayers, predominate in the lower layers of the epidermis as in other epithelia (Yardley and Summerly 1981). In human stratum corneum, phospholipids account for less than 5% of total stratum corneum lipids (Lampe et al. 1983b). The process of cornification or, more precisely, the biotransformation of the stratum granulosum into the stratum corneum is not only accompanied by the dramatic depletion of phospholipids, but also by an increase in the concentration of neutral lipids (free fatty acids, triglycerides, free and esterified sterols) as well as a large increase in the concentration of sphingolipids, especially ceramides (Fig. 5). With advancing differentiation there is an enrichment of sphingolipids composed of longer chain, more saturated fatty acids than are present in lipids of the subjacent viable layers (Ansari et al. 1970; Elias et al. 1977; Gray and White 1978). The relative amount of sphingolipids increases in human epidermis from 7.3% in the basal layers (stratum basale and spinosum) to 18.1% in the whole stratum corneum, reaching 26.6% in the outer stratum corneum (Lampe et al 1983b).

The *Ceramides* represent a unique heterogeneous group of lipids (Gray and White 1978; Wertz and Downing 1983). Recently, in human stratum corneum, six structurally distinct series of ceramides were identified (Long et al. 1985; Wertz et al. 1985), as demonstrated by high-performance thin-layer chromatography (Fig. 6). They are composed of the long-chain bases *sphingosine* of *phytosphingosine* with amide-linked nonhydroxy and α-hydroxy fatty acids. The most unusual of the epidermal ceramides, designated *ceramide 1,* consists of a sphingosine base with an amide-linked long-chain ω-hydroxy acid and an ester-linked nonhydroxy acid, 41% of which proved to be linoleic acid. It has been proposed that this ceramide ester may serve as a molecular rivet in locking together the multiple intercellular lipid membranes in the stratum corneum (Wertz and Downing 1982).

Glucosylceramides are glucosylated versions of the ceramides in which the β-D-glycopyranosyl moiety is glycosidically linked to the 1-hydroxyl group of the long-chain base (Fig. 4). Most intriguing among the epidermal glycosphingolipids is a compound called *glucosylceramide A,* an acylglucosylceramide, which accounts for nearly 50% of the total glycolipids. It consists of a sphingosine base with a long-chain ω-hydroxy acid in amide linkage. The ω-hydroxyl group of the hydroxy acid bears the ester-linked linoleic acid moiety (Abraham et al. 1985).

Glycerophosphatides Phosphatidylcholine Phosphatidylethanolamine Phosphatidylserine	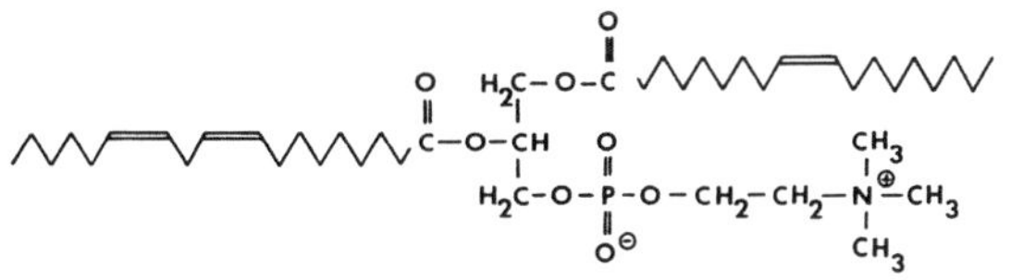 Phosphatidylcholine (Lecithin)
Triglycerides Tripalmitoyl Glycerol Triolein	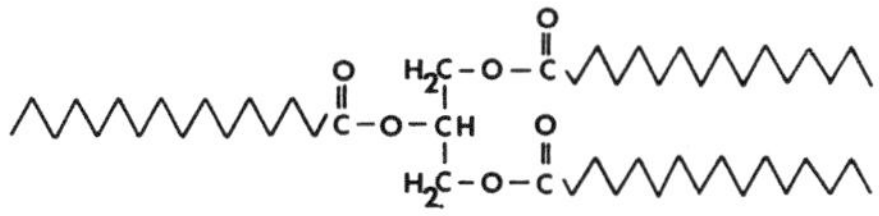 Tripalmitoyl Glycerol
Free Fatty Acids Oleic Acid (18:1) Palmitic Acid (16:0) Palmitoleic Acid (16:1) Linoleic Acid (18 2)	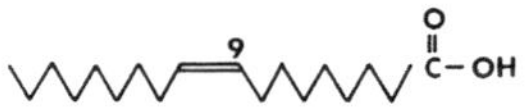 Oleic Acid 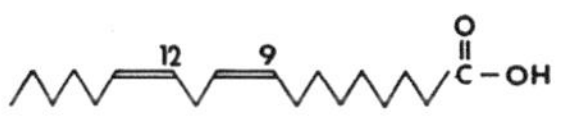 Linoleic Acid
Sterols (Isoprenoids) Cholesterol Cholesteryl Ester Cholesteryl Sulfate Squalene	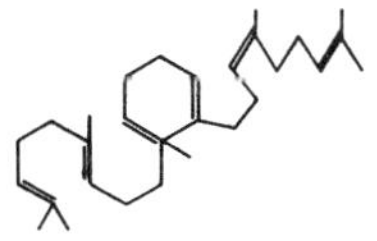 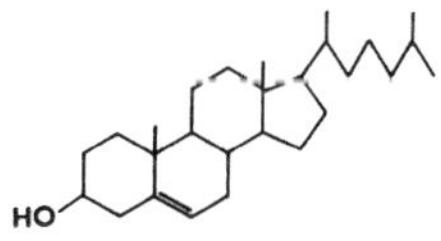 Squalene Cholesterol 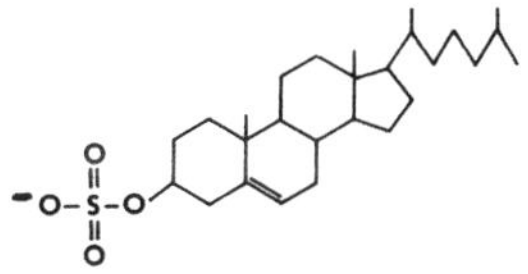 Cholesteryl Sulfate 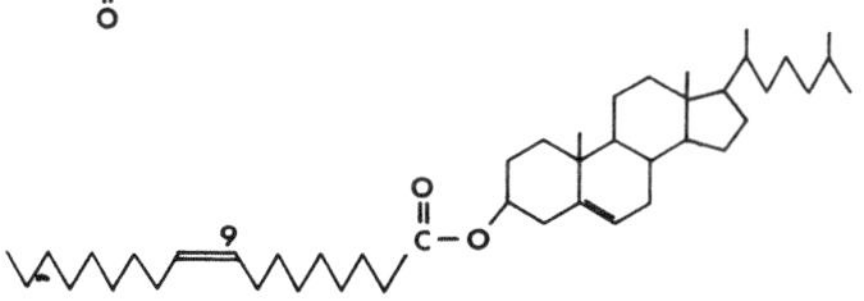 Cholesteryl Ester
n-Alkanes C19–35	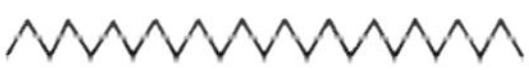 n-Pentacosane

Fig. 3. Chemical structures of important epidermal non sphingolipids. *n*-alkanes are straight-chain fully saturated hydrocarbons from $n = 19$ to $n = 35$

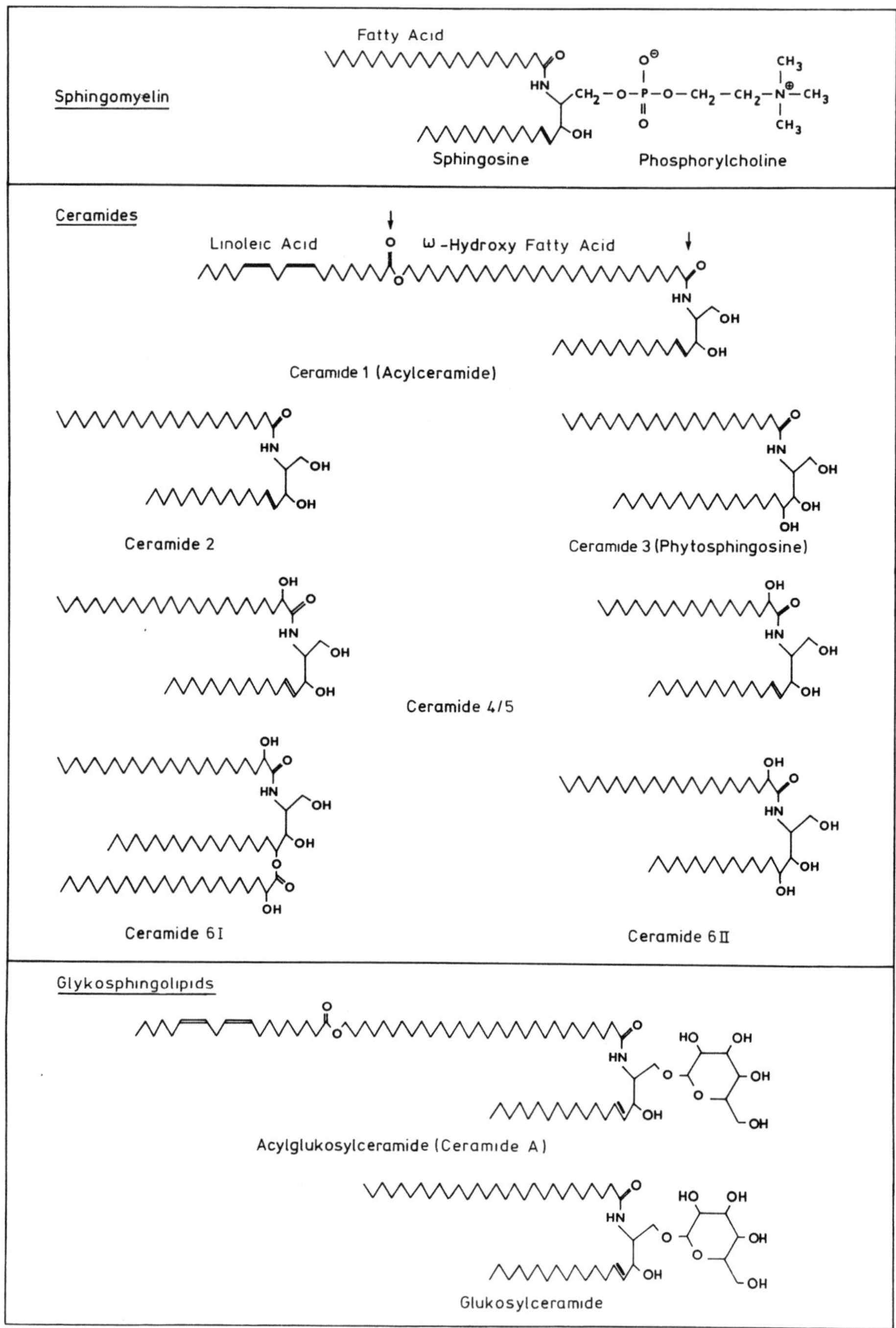

Fig. 4. Chemical structures of some important epidermal sphingolipids: In the ceramide fraction the majority of amide-linked fatty acids are nonhydroxy and α-hydroxy fatty acids. If the amide-linked fatty acid is an ω-hydroxy fatty acid the ω-hydroxyl group can be esterified to linoleic acid leading to the formation of an acylceramide (linoleylceramide = ceramide 1). In glucosylceramides the glucose moiety is glycosidically linked to the 1-hydroxyl group of the long-chain amino alcohol sphingosine or phytosphingosine

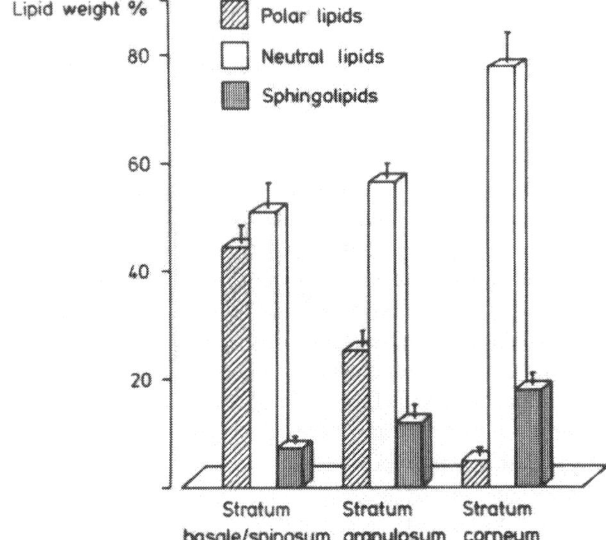

Fig. 5. Compositional changes of the major epidermal lipid classes from the basal to the horny layer. Data from Lampe et al. 1983b

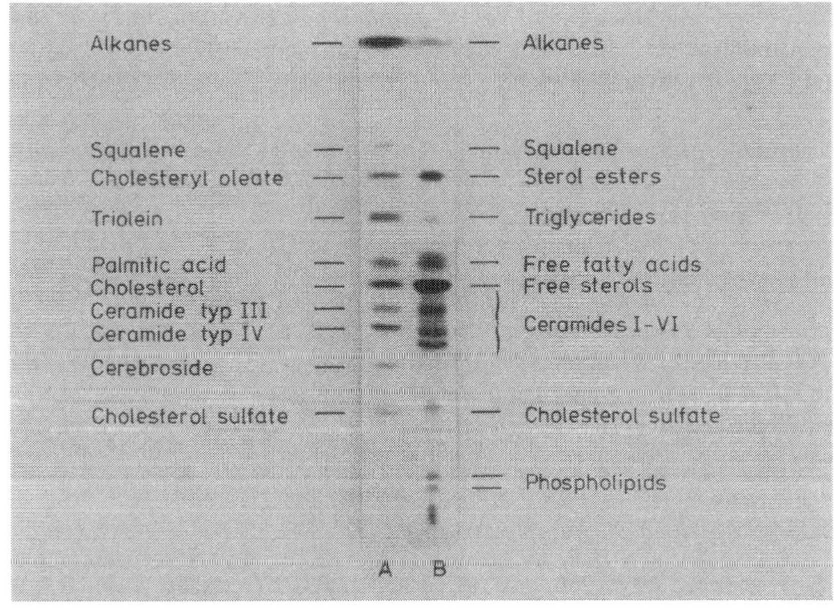

Fig. 6. Stratum corneum lipid separation by sequential high-performance thin-layer chromatography according to Melnik et al. 1989b. Lipid standards (*lane A*), plantar stratum corneum lipids (*lane B*)

The major ω-hydroxy acids found in this structure are the straight-chained C_{30} saturated and C_{32} monoenoic species. Acylglucosylceramides are enriched in lamellar bodies (Odland bodies) (Wertz et al. 1984), as will be discussed later. In the keratinizing epidermis the ceramides increase proportionately in the stratum corneum while glucosylceramides decrease. Under physiological conditions glucosylceramides are found only in the viable epidermis, but not in the stratum corneum (Yardley and Summerly 1981), whereas in differentiation disorders glycolipids are detectable in the stratum corneum. Yet, it is not clear whether ceramides are predominantly synthesized *de novo* or represent products of hydrolysis of both glucosylceramides and sphingomyelin.

Sterols, together with ceramides and free fatty acids, account for nearly all the lipid of the stratum corneum. In human epidermis most sterol is present as *cholesterol.* In the human stratum corneum the fraction of free sterols accounts for 14% of total lipids (Lampe et al 1983). *Sterol esters* are more prominent in the stratum corneum than in the Malpighian layers. Both free and esterified cholesterol slightly increase during epidermal differentiation (Lampe et al. 1983b). *Cholesterol sulfate,* a minor polar lipid of the stratum corneum comprising 1.5% of the total stratum corneum lipids deserves a special mention. It is one of the few remaining polar lipids in the stratum corneum and probably of critical importance in maintaining the intercorneocyte lipid bilayers (Williams 1983; Williams and Elias 1986). Cholesterol sulfate reaches its highest level in the stratum granulosum, diminishing in the stratum corneum and nearly disappearing from the outer stratum corneum. The lower layers of epidermis actively synthesize cholesterol for their own growth and membrane requirements. In the stratum basale and spinosum a minor cholesterol moiety is sulfated by action of the enzyme cholesterol sulfotransferase, which transfers a sulfate group from an active sulfate (3'-phosphoadenosine-5'-phosphosulfate) to cholesterol (Epstein et al. 1984a).

Steroid sulfatase (sterol sulfate sulfohydrolase, EC 3.1.6.2) hydrolyzes sulfate esters of 3-β-hydroxysterols, including cholesterol sulfate (Shapiro 1983). Steroid sulfatase activity leaves its microsomal location in the stratum granulosum to accumulate in the outer membrane region of corneocytes (Elias et al. 1984). Continual and controlled hydrolysis of cholesterol sulfate by steroid sulfatase may be the critical factor for destabilization of the intercorneocyte lipid lamellae leading to corneocyte desquamation (Williams 1983; Williams and Elias 1986). This hypothesis is supported by the fourfold decrease of cholesterol sulfate from cohesive to desquamated human stratum corneum (Long et al. 1985) and by the experiment of nature, i.e., XRI associated with steroid sulfatase deficiency, resulting in elevated levels of cholesterol sulfate in the stratum corneum (Elias et al. 1984; Shapiro 1983). Other functionally important sterols present in small amounts in the epidermis are *7-dehydrocholesterol* and *previtamin* D_3.

The *triglyceride* and *free fatty acid* levels also increase as the epidermis keratinizes. In the whole stratum corneum, trigylcerides account for 25% and free fatty acids for 19% of the total concentration of lipids (Lampe et al. 1983a). Whether the increasing level of free fatty acids is derived from hydrolysis of phospholipids and acylglucosylceramides or predominantly from *de novo* synthesis is not known.

Squalene and *n-alkanes* can be demonstrated in human epidermis under physiological as well as pathological conditions (Williams 1983; Williams and Elias 1986). It was thought that the former represent a contamination by sebaceous lipids and the latter a contamination from the environment. However, both hydrocarbons have been detected in plantar stratum corneum, where sebaceous glands are absent (Lampe et al. 1983a), as well as isolated populations of human epidermal cells (Lampe et al. 1983b). The straight-chain fully saturated *n*-alkanes form a homologous series with a bell-shaped distribution from C_{19} to C_{35} revealing a peak at $C_{25/26}$ with an equal representation of both odd and even chains (Williams and Elias 1982). Moreover, it has been recognized that mammals are able to catabolize hydrocabons, whereby the enzymatic activity most likely resides in the cytochrome P-450 system (Bickers 1983).

The composition of stratum corneum lipids displays remarkable regional variations reflecting differences in stratum corneum thickness as well as skin permeability (Lampe et al 1983a). Thus, the lipid pattern obtained from palmoplantar stratum corneum is quite different from that found in the extensor surfaces of the extremities.

1.4.3 Organization and Metabolism of Epidermal Lipids

1.4.3.1 The Role of Lamellar Bodies

The process of normal desquamation is systematic and invisible (desquamatio insensibilis). The edges of individual corneocytes detach from each other and are

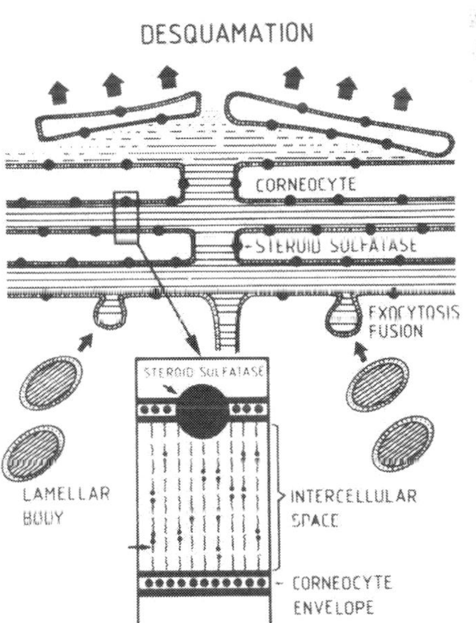

Fig. 7. Two-compartment model ("brick and mortar model") of stratum corneum with protein-rich corneocytes ("bricks") and intercellular multilamellar lipid sheets ("mortar") representing the water permeability barrier. Exocytosis of lamellar bodies at the stratum granulosum-stratum corneum interface

shed as intact cells (Heilmann et al. 1983; Kligman 1964; Plewig and Marples 1969; Plewig 1970). The most important lipid biochemical events for the dynamics of desquamation occur at the interface of the stratum granulosum and stratum corneum (Fig. 7). At this histological level the majority of the intracellular lipids of the granular cells are extruded into the intercorneocyte space. In the granular cells as well as in the intercellular space of the stratum corneum, the lipids are highly ordered and arranged into multilamellar structures, which most likely represent flattened liposomes (Landmann 1980). Liposomes are lipid vesicles containing an inner aqueous compartment enclosed by a bimolecular lipid sheet.

In the granular layer most of the lipid being destined for the intercorneocyte space is packed and transported in unique, 0.2–0.3 μm diameter, ovoid, secretory organelles, the *lamellar bodies* (also known as lamellar granules, keratinosomes, Odland bodies, membrane-coating granules, and cementsomes). They are filled with stacks of lipid-rich disks exhibiting alternately electron-lucent and electron-dense structures. The lamellar bodies are synthesized primarily in the spinous cells and originate ultrastructurally from the Golgi apparatus (Landmann 1980). After being displaced to the apex of the granular cells, these organelles fuse with the plasma membrane thereby secreting their contents into the intercellular space of the stratum corneum (Elias 1983; Hashimoto 1971; Wolff-Schreiner 1977).

Recent lipid biochemical characterization of the content of lamellar bodies confirmed the electron microscopical observations that the intercellular lipids of the stratum corneum are derived from exocytosis of these organelles. It could be shown that subcellular lamellar body-enriched fractions contain lipids nearly identical to those found in the stratum corneum (Freinkel and Traczyk 1985; Grayson et al. 1985; Wertz er al. 1984). Thus, the process of intercellular lipid sequestration imparts to the stratum corneum a unique two-compartment configuration of lipid-depleted cells embedded in multilamellar lipid sheets (Fig. 7).

Wertz and Downing (1982) proposed that the acylglucosylceramides serve in the assembly of the stacks of membranous disks seen within lamellar bodies. It seems possible that the ω-hydroxyacyl chain of an acylglucosylceramide extends through one bilayer of a liposome while the linoleyl group extends into an adjacent liposome, thus locking the two together. A similar flattening effect of liposomes is expected from ceramide 1 (Wertz 1986). This hypothesis is supported by the experimental formation of flattened, discoid liposomes by adding 5% of an acylgucosylceramide to spherical phosphatidylcholine/cholesterol liposomes (Landmann et al. 1984). Further evidence comes from the observation that in essential fatty acid deficiency, lamellar bodies lack lamellae (Elias and Brown 1978), most likely due to the absence of linoleic acid from acylglucosylceramides (Wertz et al. 1983).

Upon extrusion into the intercorneocyte space, the tightly packed disks of lamellar bodies are reorganized and coalesce into broad bilayer sheets of 40–60 Å in thickness. (Elias et al. 1977) providing the epidermal barrier to water diffusion. The unstacking of the disks and the formation of the broad intercellular multilamellar lipid sheets of stratum corneum may result from glycolipid catabolism (Wertz 1986).

1.4.3.2 *The Role of the Cholesterol/Cholesterol Sulfate Pathway for Epidermal Differentiation and Desquamation*

Cholesterol is an important component of cellular membranes and serves as a bioregulator of membrane fluidity and cell functions (Cooper 1977; Demel and Dekruijff 1976). Mammalian epidermis, which on a tissue weight basis exhibits the highest sterol biosynthesis, possesses the enzymatic capacity for *de novo* cholesterol synthesis (Feingold et al. 1982; Feingold et al. 1983; Menon et al. 1985; Schroepfer 1981). Whereas cholesterol synthesis in most peripheral tissues depends on the availability of serum low-density lipoprotein cholesterol (LDL cholesterol), epidermal cholesterol synthesis appears to be independent of the serum cholesterol supply as it has been recognized that confluent cultured keratinocytes lack LDL receptors (Ponec et al. 1983b, 1984, 1985). By use of LDL-gold labeling it has been shown that only basal cells of normal human epidermis exhibit binding and uptake of LDL-gold complexes (Mommaas-Kienhuis et al. 1987). Furthermore, LDL cholesterol has no regulative effects on sterol metabolism in hair bulbs (Brannon et al. 1975). These observations strongly imply that mammalian epidermis must possess its own mechanisms for the regulation of cholesterol biosynthesis.

Indeed, it has been shown that cholesterol sulfate, an important polar sterol of the stratum corneum intercellular space, is a potent inhibitor of the rate-limiting enzyme of cholesterol biosynthesis, 3-hydroxy-3-methylglutaryl coenzyme A reductase, in cultured human keratinocytes and fibroblasts (Williams et al. 1985, 1987b). In contrast to LDL cholesterol, cholesterol sultate readily enters cells in the absence of lipoprotein carriers or receptors (Williams et al. 1985). Besides the inhibition of sterol synthesis, cholesterol sulfate exerts inhibitory effects on sterol esterification but stimulatory effects on fatty acid synthesis (Williams et al. 1987b). It is generally accepted that the stratum corneum cholesterol content is critical for normal desquamation. Therefore, it seems reasonable that epidermal cholesterol biosynthesis depends on cholesterol requirements of the stratum corneum, rather than on the availability of exogenous cholesterol. Evidence for this comes from the observation of a two- to threefold stimulation of epidermal sterologenesis after solvent or detergent disruption of the cutaneous barrier function (Menon et al. 1985). These experiments have demonstrated that the water content of the stratum corneum plays a role in the regulation of epidermal cholesterol biosynthesis. In mice deficient in essential fatty acids and with disrupted epidermal barrier function the increased transepidermal water loss is accompanied by a twofold increase in epidermal cholesterol synthesis (Feingold et al. 1986). Taken together these observation indicate that epidermal sterologenesis responds to water barrier requirements (Grubauer et al. 1987).

Stratum corneum cholesterol is presumably derived from exocytosis of lamellar bodies (Elias 1983). By ultrastructural analysis with the sterol marker *filipin*, substantial amounts of sterols were detected in the external membranes of lamellar bodies whereas the internal lamellar structures were poorly labeled (Kitajima et al. 1985). In the stratum corneum the intercellular lamellar structures were well labeled, while the plasma membranes of the corneocytes were rarely labeled with filipin (Kitajima et al. 1985).

Scales from autosomal recessive lamellar ichthyosis exhibit increased levels of free cholesterol (Williams and Elias 1985), whereas in scales of XRI, decreased free cholesterol but increased cholesterol sulfate levels were found (Elias et al. 1984; Williams and Elias 1981). This suggests that the stratum corneum cholesterol content has to be regulated within rather narrow limits in order to maintain the specific physiochemical requirements for normal desquamation.

In summary, cholesterol sulfate seems to be a very important constituent for the maintenance of the stratum corneum intercellular lipid lamellae due to (a) its presence within the intercorneocyte space (Elias et al. 1984), (b) its amphipathic character (Williams and Elias 1985), and (c) the influence it has on the interactions and physicochemical properties of the intercellular lipids (Rehfeld et al. 1986). In normal stratum corneum a constant ratio of free cholesterol to cholesterol sulfate of about 10:1 is reported (Williams and Elias 1981). There is an enzymatically controlled decrease of cholesterol sulfate with high cholesterol sulfate levels in the stratum granulosum and the lowest levels in the outer stratum corneum (Elias et al. 1984; Lampe et al. 1983b; Long et al. 1985). Cholesterol sulfate has been shown to stabilize cell membranes. Further evidence comes from *in vitro* studies on squamous differentiation of rabbit tracheal epithelial cells, indicating that cholesterol sulfate accumulated upon squamous differentiation and could be used as an effective marker of the differentiation equivalent to cross-linked envelope formation, transglutaminase induction, or keratin synthesis (Rearick and Jetten 1986). Together, these observations are in excellent accordance with the hypothesis that the stabilization-destabilization of membranes mediated by the level of cholesterol sulfate regulates normal desquamation (Epstein et al. 1984b).

1.4.3.3 Role of Lipolytic Enzymes for Epidermal Keratinization

The catabolism of epidermal lipids is closely related to the late stages of epidermal differentiation. Catabolic enzymes must be involved in the dramatic modulations in lipid composition during terminal differentiation, especially in the reduction of phospholipids, the increase of free fatty acid and ceramide levels as well as in the hydrolysis of cholesterol sulfate. Both acid and neutral lipase, sphingomyelinase, phospholipase A and glucosidase have been localized to lamellar bodies (Freinkel and Traczyk 1985; Grayson et al. 1985; Menon et al. 1986; Mier et al. 1974), whereas in stratum corneum, lipases were found within the intercellular space (Menon et al. 1986). The presence of lipid catabolic enzymes among extruded lamellar bodies correlates with the conversion of predominantly polar contents of lamellar bodies into neutral lipids and sphingolipids finally accumulating in the intercellular lipid sheets. The lipid catabolic enzymes are most likely in an inactive *proenzyme* state prior to fusion and secretion of lamellar bodies at the stratum granulosum-stratum corneum interface (Menon et al. 1986).

During cornification, the degradation of phospholipids is probably mediated by *phospholipases*. Phospholipase A may also be of importance in the fusion of lamellar bodies with the plasma membrane mediating the exocytosis of these organelles (Freinkel 1987).

Lipases are needed for the hydrolysis of triglycerides in free fatty acids, which are vital for the formation of coenzyme A esters, and are needed for the maintenance of cellular energy in the differentiating cells, these being further removed from the substrate gradient of the subepidermal vasculature.

Sphingomyelinase may have a role in the generation of ceramides by hydrolysis of sphingomyelin to ceramides and phosphorylcholine (Bowser and Gray 1978; Grayson et al. 1985). Additionally, *de novo* synthesis of ceramides must be assumed in order to explain the great quantities of ceramides present in stratum corneum (Kondoh et al. 1983).

Since lysosomal *acid lipase* exhibits activity for triglycerides as well as for cholesteryl esters, acid lipase has been considered identical to *cholesterol acylhydrolase* in some tissues (Assmann and Frederickson 1983). If this holds true for epidermis, acid lipase might regulate the stratum corneum cholesterol content by release of free cholesterol and fatty acids from cholesteryl esters.

Little is known about lipase-dependent generation of *diglycerides*. Diglycerides are functionally important as second messengers in the regulation of protein kinases, which are closely involved in cell differentiation processes (Berridge 1984).

Alterations of membrane glycoconjugates are associated with differentiation and growth control in many mammalian tissues, including epidermis. By lectin staining it was demonstrated that keratinocytes lose membrane sugars at the level of the stratum corneum, an effect that seems to be a direct consequence of a specific *sugar-glycosidase* activity in the outer epidermis (Nemanic et al. 1983). Coincidently with the loss of lectin staining, glycosphingolipids were found to be degraded to ceramides during the final stages of epidermal differentiation (Nemanic et al. 1983).

That sterol sulfatase-mediated hydrolysis of cholesterol sulfate plays an important role in the destabilization of intercorneocyte lipid lamellae has already been extensively discussed. Freinkel and Traczyk (1985) were unable to demonstrate localization of *steroid sulfatase activity* among the hydrolases of lamellar bodies, although it was much greater in outer stratum corneum membranes. Despite the apparent lack of enzymatic activity, the possibility cannot be excluded that the enzyme is transported in lamellar bodies in an inactive proenzyme state and is activated only after extrusion into the intercellular space. Thus, the present data do not shed any light on the mechanisms by which steroid sulfatase finds its way from the intracellular microsomal compartment to the membrane regions of stratum corneum.

1.4.4 Epidermal Lipids and the Permeability Barrier

Besides the dynamics of desquamation, the cutaneous permeability barrier is a very important functional product of epidermal differentiation, protecting the organism from loss of essential body fluids and restricting the penetration of chemicals, allergens, water, and microorganisms. The principal structural element providing the barrier function are the intercorneocyte lipid lamellae (Elias and Friend 1975; Elias et al. 1977; Elias and Brown 1978; Landmann 1986 and 1988). Indirect evidence is derived from studies on essential fatty acid-deficient animals, in which oleic acid replaces the essential linoleic acid in the O-acylated sphingolipids (Wertz et al. 1983). Under those conditions, lamellar bodies reveal an amorphous appearance rather than discrete stacks of lammellae, and the intercellular membranes of the stratum corneum are markedly disturbed, a condition which leads to excessive transepidermal water loss (Elias and Brown 1978).

Recently it has been discovered that besides the presence of intercorneocyte lipid lamellae, each corneocyte appears to possess a lipid envelope consisting of a monomolecular layer of N-(ω-hydroxyacyl) sphingosines that are ester-linked to proteins of the outer corneocyte membrane (Swartzendruber et al. 1987). This corneocyte lipid envelope may also play a role in the barrier function and in corneocyte cohesion.

The structural lipids of the intercorneocyte lamellae are not only involved in the regulation of skin permeability, but are also critical for the water-holding property of the stratum corneum, providing a reservoir function for stratum corneum hydration (Imokawa and Hattori 1985; Imokawa et al. 1986). It was recognized from solvent challenge of human stratum corneum that the water-holding property of the stratum corneum depends predominantly on the presence of ceramides. This concept is supported by studies on stratum corneum lipids of atopic patients with dry skin, who revealed significant reduction in the ceramide fraction (Melnik et al. 1988).

1.4.5 Effect of Retinoids on Epidermal Lipid Metabolism

Retinoids profoundly influence epidermal differentiation, but neither the nature of their antikeratinizing activity nor their precise biochemical mechanisms are known. The antikeratinizing effect of retinoids is associated with alterations in transepidermal water loss and with loosening of the stratum corneum (Elias et al. 1981). Therefore, it seems likely that retinoids affect the composition of stratum corneum intercellular lipids.

In fact, in confluent human keratinocyte cultures 13-*cis*-retinoic acid (isotretinoin), etretinate (aromatic retinoid), and its major metabolite acitretin, (Ro 10-1670 proprietary name formely used was *etretin*) suppress cholesterol synthesis in a dose-dependent manner (Ponec et al. 1983a). Moreover, in cultured rabbit tracheal epithelial cells several synthetic retinoids are able to suppress the formation of cholesterol sulfate by inhibition of cholesterol sulfotransferase (Rearick and Jetten 1986). The effect of retinoids on glycolipid synthesis seems to depend on the degree of epithelial differentiation. Whereas in monolayered keratinocyte cultures a depression of glycolipid synthesis was observed, a marked increase in this of 200%–400% was found in organ-cultured epidermis (Orozco-Topete et al. 1983).

Although the retinoid-induced changes of epidermal lipid metabolism and the resulting effects on the water permeability barrier are not completely understood at present, studies on artificial membrane systems indicate that *all-trans*-retinoic acid as well as retinol increase the water permeability of phospholipid liposomes and lower their phase-transition temperature (Stillwell at al. 1982). From these experiments it can be concluded that retinoids exert some of their effects by increasing membrane fluidity. Similar liposome pertubations may affect the epidermal lamellar lipid sheets which are regarded as flattened liposomes. Therefore, retinoid-induced alterations of lipid bilayer systems could be involved in desquamation, the barrier function, and the water-holding properties of the stratum corneum.

1.4.6 Disorders of Cornification Associated with Abnormalities in Epidermal Lipid Metabolism

As might be anticipated from the foregoing, several disorders of cornification have been linked to disturbances of epidermal lipid metabolism. It has been shown that alterations in the composition of intercorneocyte lipids can induce excessive corneocyte adhesion and disturbances of normal barrier function (Elias 1981, 1983; Elias et al. 1983a; Williams 1983; Williams and Elias 1986). So far, the majority of disorders associated with disturbances of the epidermal lipid metabolism exhibit the clinical picture of ichthyosis, although there is increasing evidence to indicate that regional disorders of cornification, like palmoplantar keratoderma (Nicollier et al. 1986; Prost et al. 1985), and disorders of follicular keratinization, such as acne vulgaris (Downing et al. 1986; Melnik et al. 1988) are also linked to alterations of the epidermal lipid metabolism (Tables 8 and 9). Up to now, there are only a few diseases in which a defective lipid metabolism is believed to be directly responsible for the pathomechanism of a

Table 8. Inherited disorders of differentiation closely linked to disturbances of epidermal lipid metabolism

Disease	Lipid abnormality
Defined	
X-linked recessive ichthyosis	Cholesterol sulfate $\uparrow$, free sterols $\downarrow$
Multiple sulfatase deficiency	Cholesterol sulfate $\uparrow$, free sterols $\downarrow$
Refsum's disease	Phytanic acid $\uparrow$, linoleate $\downarrow$
Probable	
Non-erythrodermic lamellar ichthyosis	Cholesterol $\uparrow$
Autosomal dominant lamellar ichthyosis	Free fatty acids $\uparrow$, triglycerides $\uparrow$, free sterols $\downarrow$, ceramides $\downarrow$
Erythrodermic lamellar ichthyosis	n-Alkanes $\uparrow$
Neutral lipid storage disease	n-Alkanes $\uparrow$
Harlequin fetus	Triglycerides $\uparrow$, abnormal sterol metabolism?
Sjögren-Larsson syndrome	Disturbed linoleate metabolism and impaired fatty alcohol oxidation; products of $\Delta 6$ desaturation $\downarrow$
Continual skin peeling syndrome	Intercorneocyte lipid-like deposits

Table 9. Acquired disorders of differentiation associated with disturbances of epidermal lipid metabolism

Disease	Lipid abnormality
Triparanol-induced ichthyosis Butyrophenone-induced ichthyosis 20,25-Diazacholestenol-induced palmoplantar keratoderma Nicotinic acid-induced pseudoacanthosis nigricans	Cholesterol ↓
Human essential fatty acid deficiency	Linoleate ↓, arachidonate ↓, oleate in O-acylsphingolipids ↑
Acrodermatitis enteropathica	Linoleate ↓, arachidonate ↓
Atopic dermatitis	**Plasma phospholipids:** γ-linolenic acid ↓, dihomo-γ-linolenic acid ↓, arachidonate ↓ **Stratum corneum:** ceramides ↓
Palmoplantar keratoderma	Short-chain and monoene fatty acids ↑
Acne vulgaris	**Comedo:** Free sterols ↓, ceramides ↓, linoleate in O-acylceramides ↓
Scaling in hypothyroidism	Free sterols ↓, sterol esters ↓
Sodium dodecyl sulfate-induced scaling	Changes in the relative composition of ceramides and neutral lipids

particular scaling disorder, i.e., XRI, multiple sulfatase deficiency, and Refsum's disease. Whether the various lipid abnormalities observed in other inherited and acquired disorders of cornification are related to the pathogenesis of these disorders or represent an epiphenomenon of disturbed epidermal differentiation requires further investigation.

In the following sections lipid biochemical changes in a number of ichthyoses and in some other keratinization disorders will be discussed in more detail. Cross-references to the corresponding chapters in this volume are given for clinical and genetic features.

1.4.6.1 Ichthyoses Caused by Disturbances of Epidermal Lipid Metabolism

X-Linked Recessive Ichthyosis

Steroid sulfatase deficiency is the underlying genetic basis of XRI (Epstein and Bonifas 1985; Sect. 2.2). Steroid sulfatase deficiency is a single nosological entity manifested prenatally as *placental sulfatase deficiency disease* and postnatally as XRI (Williams 1983; Williams and Elias 1986). Whereas placental sulfatase deficiency is characterized by the prenatal accumulation of sulfated steroid hormones, especially dehydroepiandrosterone sulfate, postnatally cholesterol sulfate, another substrate of the missing enzyme, accumulates in serum (Epstein et al. 1981a), erythrocyte membranes (Bergner and Shapiro 1981) and ichthyotic scales (Elias et al. 1984; Williams and Elias 1981). The increased cholesterol sulfate content of serum LDL confers on them increased electrophoretic mobility in comparison with normal LDL. Thus, the simple technique of lipoprotein electrophoresis permits an indirect laboratory diagnosis (Epstein et al. 1981a; Ibsen et al. 1986; Traupe et al. 1983) without quantification of the accumulating substrate or determination of the missing enzyme activity (Epstein and Leventhal 1981; Meyer and Gilardi 1986; Okano et al. 1985).

The biochemical mechanisms relating the increased cholesterol sulfate content of the stratum corneum to pathological scale formation have been extensively discussed elsewhere (Elias et al. 1984; Epstein et al. 1981b; Williams and Elias 1981, 1986; Williams 1983; Williams et al. 1983). The pathophysiological role of steroid sulfatase deficiency in the development of the retention hyperkeratosis of XRI is supported by the fact that the application of partially purified steroid sulfatase to the skin of patients with XRI results in a significant release of stratum corneum fragments (Yoshiike et al. 1985). The importance of cholesterol sulfate for the pathogenesis of XRI is further underlined experimentally by the observation that the topical application of cholesterol sulfate to hairless mice induces scaling (Maloney et al. 1984), whereas the topical cholesterol treatment of patients with XRI seems to improve the scaling disorder (Lykkesfeldt and Høyer 1983). Further evidence for the cohesive effect of increased levels of cholesterol sulfate is derived from lipid analysis of horse hoof, a fully keratinized tissue, in which cholesterol sulfate accounts for 15%–20% of total lipids (Wertz and Downing 1984).

However, there is also support for an alternative hypothesis, proposing that abnormal desquamation in XRI is primarily caused by a decreased level of free cholesterol in the stratum corneum. This opinion is based on the concept that cholesterol is important for the regulation of membrane fluidity. Furthermore, ichthyotic skin changes have been observed in conditions with either cholesterol excess (Williams and Elias 1985) or cholesterol deficiency (Elias et al. 1983b, 1986). The two hypotheses of abnormal desquamation in XRI are compatible if one assumes that the ratio of free cholesterol to cholesterol sulfate in the stratum corneum is the critical determinant for desquamation.

Multiple Sulfatase Deficiency

Multiple sulfatase deficiency (MSD) is a rare autosomal recessive disorder involving all known sulfatases (Austin et al. 1965; Dulanez and Moser 1978). The biochemical phenotype reveals deficiencies of at least seven sulfatases, including the lysosomal arylsulfatases A and B of the glycolipid and mucopolysaccharide metabolism, as well as the activity of microsomal arylsulfatase C and sterold sulfatase (Basner et al. 1979; Dulanez and Moser 1978). MSD causes accumulation of a variety of sulfated compounds, including steroids, certain mucopolysaccharides, and sphingolipids (Dulanez and Moser 1978).

The clinical pattern of scaling in MSD resembles that in XRI and it has been recognized that scales contain increased amounts of cholesterol sulfate (Williams 1983). This supports the hypothesis that the pathogenesis of ichthyosis in MSD is identical to that in XRI (Williams and Elias 1986).

Refsum's Disease (Heredopathia Atactica Polyneuritiformis)

Refsum's disease is an autosomal recessive trait associated with the accumulation of an unusual C_{20} branched-chain fatty acid, *phytanic acid* (3,7,11,15-tetramethylhexadecanoic acid), in blood and in many tissues including epidermis (Anton-Lamprecht and Kahlke 1974; Davies et al. 1978; Dykes et al. 1978). Phytanic acid is exclusively of dietary origin. Its major mechanism of degradation via the α-oxidative pathway involves an initial α-hydroxylation followed by decarboxylation to generate *pristanic acid*, the C_{19} lower homologue, which is consecutively degraded by β-oxidation. In patients with Refsum's disease the rate of oxidation of phytanic acid is less than 5% of that in normal subjects. The metabolic defect has been localized to the initial step of phytanic acid degradation, catalyzed by *phytanic acid α-hydroxylase* (Herndon et al. 1969; Steinberg 1983).

The ichthyotic changes in Refsum's disease resemble those in ichthyosis vulvaris (Sect. 3.1). The presence of neutral lipid-containing droplets within the lower epidermal strata clearly distinguishes the ichthyosis in Refsum's disease from autosomal dominant ichthosis vulgaris and XRI (Anton-Lamprecht and Kahlke 1974; Davies et al. 1977, 1978). Due to the progressive accumulation of phytanic acid within the epidermis, normal fatty acids are replaced by phytanic acid, which becomes the major constituent in all epidermal lipids composed of fatty acids (Dykes et al. 1978). It appears that epidermal linoleic acid is also disproportionately decreased by phytanic acid (Davies et al. 1978; Dykes et al. 1978). It can be speculated that the substitution of linoleic acid might also affect the composition of linoleic acid-containing sphingolipids, especially acylglucosylceramide and ceramide 1, which are important for the formation and integrity of the multilamellar lipid sheets of stratum corneum (Wertz et al. 1987). Although it is still uncertain whether linoleic acid and its metabolites are absolutely or relatively diminished, Refsum's disease and *essential fatty acid deficiency,* another hyperproliferative scaling disorder associated with linoleic acid deficiency, may share a common pathomechanism.

1.4.6.2 Ichthyoses Associated with Disturbances of Epidermal Lipid Metabolism

In the past few years an increasing *genetic heterogeneity* of lamellar ichthyoses has been recognized in which lipid biochemical analyses have been very helpful. Currently, at least three different types of lamellar ichthyosis can be differentiated. There are two autosomal recessive types of lamellar ichthyosis: *nonerythrodermic lamellar ichthyosis* (NELI) and *erythrodermic lamellar ichthyosis* (ELI) (Sect. 4.2). For ELI, the older descriptive term *nonbullous congenital ichthyosiform erythroderma* is still used in the literature. The third type of lamellar ichthyosis is inherited as a dominant trait and therefore has been designated *autosomal dominant lamellar ichtyosis* (ADLI) (Sect. 4.2.2).

Nonerythrodermic lamellar ichthyosis

The composition of scale lipids in NELI closely resembles that of normal palmoplantar stratum corneum (Williams and Elias 1984). It is noteworthy, however, that scale lipids in NELI reveal significantly increased amounts of *free sterols* (23.6% total lipid weight) in comparison with normal stratum corneum (15.6% total lipid weight (Williams and Elias 1985). The presence of elevated free sterols in scales of NELI patients may be related to pathological desquamation (Williams and Elias 1986).

Erythrodermic Lamellar Ichthyosis

A very important biochemical discriminator for the differentiation of ELI from NELI is the marked increase of *n-alkanes*, accounting for 24.8% total scale lipid weight versus 7.2% in scales of NELI, and 5.5% in normal stratum corneum (Williams and Elias 1985). Because *n*-alkane levels were not found to be elevated in the serum of ELI patients, Williams and Elias concluded that *n*-alkanes might be generated *de novo* in the epidermis of such patients (Williams and Elias 1986). Alternatively, ELI scales might possess an increased capability to absorb exogenous hydrocarbons. Furthermore, the finding of increased *n*-alkanes is also detectable in other hyperproliferative scaling disorders like psoriasis and epidermolytic hyperkeratosis (Williams and Elias 1982).

The accumulating *n*-alkanes in ELI exhibit a bell-shaped distribution from C_{19} to C_{35} representing both odd and even chains with a peak at $C_{25/26}$ (Williams and Elias 1982, 1984, 1985). *n*-Alkanes impair the membrane fluidity of lipid bilayers (McIntosh and Costello 1981; Snyder et al. 1981). It is conceivable that the abundant amounts of hydrophobic-*n*-alkanes in ELI intermingle with the multilamellar lipid sheets of the stratum corneum, thereby impairing the access of lipid catabolic enzymes to their natural substrates, resulting in delayed corneocyte shedding. Definitive biochemical evidence on whether elevated *n*-alkanes are related to the pathogenesis of ELI or represent an epiphenomenon of disturbed differentiation is still lacking.

Autosomal Dominant Lamellar Ichthyosis

At the ultrastructural level ADLI is characterized by a unique *transforming zone* between the granular and horny layers (Kolde et al. 1985; Traupe et al. 1984). Furthermore, a limited number of *lipid inclusions* have been observed in the stratum corneum. Recently, Melnik and coworkers (1989) differentiated ADLI from NELI and ELI by determination of excessive amounts of *free fatty acids, triglycerides,* and *reduced free sterols* with a nearly identical pattern in two untreated ADLI patients belonging to two generations. The scale lipid profile of ADLI clearly differed from that of NELI (increased cholesterol) and ELI (excessively increased *n*-alkanes), although slightly raised *n*-alkanes were identified in both ADLI patients. It is most likely that the significantly increased levels of free fatty acids and triglycerides in ADLI scales reflect the ultrastructurally recognized lipid inclusions in the stratum corneum.

Neutral Lipid Storage Disease (Dorfman's Syndrome)

Neutral lipid storage disease (NLSD) is a rare autosomal recessive multisystem disorder of an altered lipid metabolism, ichthyosis, myopathy, fatty liver, deafness, cataracts, and deposition of fat droplets in multiple tissues (Chanarin et al. 1975; Dorfman et al. 1974; Sect. 6.1). The syndrome is characterized by accumulation of *triglycerides* in cytoplasmatic non-membrane-coated lipid droplets detected in leukocytes, muslce cells, hepatocytes, and fibroblasts (Angelini et al.

1980; Chanarin et al. 1975; Dorfman et al. 1974; Miranda et al. 1979; Rozenszajin et al. 1966; Slavin et al. 1975).

Studies of the lipid metabolism of cultured fibroblasts and keratinocytes of patients with NLSD indicate that the impaired catabolism of fatty acids and their subsequent storage in triglycerides is the primary defect of NLSD (Williams and Elias 1986), most likely due to a deficiency of intracellular triacylglycerol lipase, an enzyme that is closely linked to phosphoacylglyceride biosynthesis. The lower strata of epidermis contain non-membrane-enclosed lipid droplets within the cytoplasm and lamellar bodies (Elias and Williams 1985). Further ultrastructural analysis of lamellar bodies has revealed *multilaminated spherules* that distort and displace the normal internal disk structure of these organelles (Elias and Williams 1985). Within the intercellular spaces of the outer epidermis these spherules remain interspersed with secreted lamellar body contents. However, when they have reached the stratum granulosum-stratum corneum interface, they apparently disperse into electron-lucent slits (Elias and Williams 1985). Therefore, NLSD can be regarded as a prototype of disturbed lamellar body function, providing further support for the concept that lamellar body-derived lipids have a direct impact on stratum corneum desquamation.

Unexpectedly, Elias and Williams (1985) did not observe increased levels of either triglycerides or free fatty acids in the scale lipids of a patient with NLSD, but an increase in *n-alkanes* of 18% total lipid weight. This lipid pattern closely resembles that of ELI scales, whereas in all other tissues triglycerides are known to accumulate. The observed similarity in lipid biochemistry is most intriguing in view of the clinical similarities between the ichthyosis of NLSD and ELI and the reciprocal relationship of the content of fatty acids and *n*-alkanes in ELI scale lipids (Williams and Elias 1985). Delineation of the metabolic defect in NLSD may contribute to the understanding of the origin of epidermal *n*-alkanes accumulating in some erythrodermic keratinization disorders.

Sjögren-Larsson Syndrome

The autosomal recessive Sjögren-Larsson syndrome (SLS) is a progressive neurodegenerative disease with parallels to other neuroichthyoses (Sect. 5.1). Hernell and coworkers (1982) found that metabolites derived from the linoleic acid of plasma phospholipids were significantly decreased in comparison with healthy controls. All individuals with SLS exhibited decreased products of Δ6 desaturation which also affected further metabolites in the metabolic sequence. Therefore, it was hypothesized that SLS is an *inborn error of essential fatty acid metabolism*. In three patients the administration of a diet in which all lipid was given in the form of medium-chain triglycerides resulted in a complete clearing of the scaling skin and an improvment in behavior (Guilleminault et al. 1973; Hooft et al. 1967). Recently, Rizzo and coworkers (1988) demonstrated an impaired oxidation of radioactive hexadecanol to fatty acid in cultured SLS fibroblasts. Fatty alcohol: nicotinamide adenine dinucleotide oxidoreductase, the enzyme catalyzing fatty alcohol oxidation, was deficient in SLS fibroblasts. Mean total enzyme activity was 13% of that in normal fibroblasts. Fibroblasts from two obligate SLS heterozygotes had enzyme activities intermediate between that in normal fibroblasts and individuals with SLS. These data indicate that the primary defect in SLS might be deficiency of fatty alcohol: NAD^+ oxidoreductase leading to an abnormality in fatty alcohol metabolism. The beneficial effect of a low fat diet supplemented with medium-chain triglycerides might result from a decrease of long-chain fatty alcohol synthesis and accumulation. Thus lipid biochemical investigations of epidermal cells in SLS are necessary in order to prove the assumed link between faulty fatty alcohol and fatty acid metabolism and the development of ichthyosis.

Harlequin Fetus
Clinical features of the harlequin fetus, a rare recessive scaling disorder, are described in Sect. 4.1. Buxman and associates (1979) reported a harlequin fetus that survived for 9 months, had an unusual histologic appearance, and showed elevated stratum corneum lipid levels. Whereas lamellar bodies were absent, lipid-containing vacuoles filled the keratinocytes of all epidermal layers, exhibiting an increased triglyceride content (Buxman et al. 1979; Williams 1983). Although other harlequin fetuses revealed protein abnormalities this phenotype may be linked to disturbances of both lipid and protein metabolism (Baden et al. 1982).

Peeling Skin Syndrome
Peeling skin syndrome (PSS) is a rare disorder in which generalized noninflammatory exfoliation of the stratum corneum occurs (Sec. 6.5). To date, only few reports of PSS have appeared in the literature (Abdel-Hafez et al. 1983; Fox 1921; Kurban and Azar 1969; Silverman et al. 1986). PSS is a retention hyperkeratosis and may represent a new form of ichthyosis (Silverman et al. 1986). Ultrastructural examination revealed that in PSS the stratum corneum is considerably thickened. Throughout the stratum corneum, globular deposits of an electron-dense, lipid-like material fill the intercellular spaces. The *intercellular lipid-like deposits* resemble a string of beads, and were only detectable within the stratum corneum. The lamellar bodies appeared normal. Histologically, the separation of corneocytes was localized above the granular cell layer. A striking ultrastructural feature of PSS was the observation of intracellular cleavage, in which the plasma membrane of the peeling cell remained firmly attached to the underlying cell while the upper part of the cell exfoliated (Silverman et al. 1986). Silverman and coworkers (1986) speculate that PSS may represent a retention hyperkeratosis due to a specific lipid abnormality accompanied by a unique type of intracellular cleavage.

1.4.6.3 Acquired Disorders of Cornification Associated with Disturbances of Epidermal Lipid Metabolism

There are a large number of acquired disorders of keratinization that are associated with disturbances of the epidermal lipid metabolism. Among others, these disorders include essential fatty acid deficiency, palmoplantar keratoderma climactericum and several drug-induced scaling-skin disorders (Table 9). If the term *disorder of cornification* is defined in a broader sense, even the follicular hyperkeratoses of acne vulgaris and xerosis of atopic individuals may be added to the list. Indeed, the normalization of disturbed intercorneocyte comedonal lipids seems to be a major mode of action of oral isotretinoin therapy (Melnik et al., 1988). In atopic patients, a marked reduction of ceramides has been detected, which may account for the dry skin in this condition (Melnik et al., 1988).

In the following section discussion of acquired disorders of cornification is confined to essential fatty acid deficiency and drug-induced scaling disorders. These conditions are of considerable conceptional value and shed light on the basic mechanisms involved in the process of cornification.

Essential Fatty Acid Deficiency

The symptoms of essential fatty acid deficiency (EFAD) in mammals were first described by Burr and Burr (1929). Experimental EFAD produces an ichthyosiform dermatitis characterized by scaling and impaired barrier function with increased transepidermal water loss (Elias and Brown 1978; Prottey 1976). After surgical or dietary intervention, especially with prolonged parenteral nutrition, alcoholism, the clinical syndrome of EFAD develops in humans (Paulsrud et al. 1972; Prottey 1976; Truchetet et al. 1988).

The essential fatty acids are long-chain unsaturated lipids, so named as they are essential to the diet of mammals because they cannot be synthesized *de novo*. Mammalian cells are unable to desaturate fatty acids at the ω-6 position. There are two major essential fatty acids, both of the ω-6 configuration (denoting the position of the first methylene-interrupted double bond, numbered from the methyl end of the chains): *linoleic acid* (C18:2), the most common essential fatty acid, and *arachidonic acid* (C20:4), its chain elongation product and precursor for prostanoid synthesis.

The excessively increased transepidermal water loss is a special feature of EFAD. As the water barrier is known to reside in the multiple intercellular lipid sheets of the stratum corneum, it is conceivable that a deficiency of essential fatty acids may affect the structure and function of these lipid bilayers (Grubauer et al. 1987). Arachidonic acid given intraperitoneally will heal the skin scaliness rapidly, without repairing the disturbed barrier function. Conversely, topical applied or intraperitoneally administered linoleate has been reported to restore the barrier function of essential fatty acid-deficient rats, independent of its role in the prostaglandin metabolism (Elias et al. 1980; Prottey et al. 1976; Prottey 1977). These findings suggest that linoleate or molecules containing linoleate are involved in the maintenance of the epidermal water barrier. These functionally extremely important molecules are *linoleate-rich O-acylsphingolipids*, which were first identified by Gray and White (1978) and were characterized in detail in various mammalian species by the outstanding work of Wertz and colleagues (Wertz and Downing 1982; Wertz et al. 1983; Wertz 1986; Wertz et al. 1987). It was demonstrated that O-acylsphingolipids are unique constituents of all keratinizing epithelia. They reflect the presence of lamellar bodies (Wertz 1986). The linoleate-rich acylglucosylceramides are the driving force behind the formation and integrity of the lamellar bodies (Wertz and Downing 1982). In EFAD, linoleate is replaced by oleate in O-acylsphingolipids (Wertz and Downing 1986). Due to this substitution the physical properties of these particular sphingolipids are markedly altered, resulting in failure to form lamellar bodies and leading to severe disturbances of the intercorneocyte lipids, where only occasional *fragments of lipid lamellae* are detectable (Elias and Brown 1978). Consequently, the water barrier breaks down, leading to increased transepidermal water loss.

Drug-Induced Scaling Skin Disorders

In 1961, the first suggestion of a relationship between ichthyosis and disturbances of epidermal lipid metabolism was made by Achor and coworkers and by Winkelmann and associates (Achor et al. 1961; Winkelmann et al. 1963) who reported the development of ichthyosis in patients treated with the cholesterol-lowering agent *triparanol* (MER-29). Some time ago, Parson and Flinn (1959) recognized that dryness of the skin and a picture of pseudoacanthosis nigricans were produced by *nicotinic acid* administered in large quantities to patients with hypercholesterolemia. This observation was later confirmed by Ruiter and Meyler (1960). Moreover, ichthyosiform skin changes were induced by the antipsychotic and hypocholesterolemic compound WY-3457, a *butyrophenone* (Simpson et al. 1964), whereas the hypocholesterolemic agent *20,25-diazacholestenol* produced myotonia and keratoderma, resembling karatoderma climactericum (Anderson and Martt 1965). These authors emphasized the importance of normal lipid synthesis in orderly cornification.

All of the hypocholesterolemic drugs mentioned inhibit the late stages of cholesterol biosynthesis (Williams et al. 1987a). The epidermis appears to be very vulnerable to the *inhibition of sterol biosynthesis*, a fact which can now be explained by the independence of epidermal sterologenesis from the serum LDL-cholesterol supply (Ponec et al. 1983b, 1984).

Experimentally, it has been possible to induce a scaling skin disorder in hairless mice by oral administration of *20,25-diazacholestenol*, an inhibitor of the *Δ24-reductase*, the converting enzyme of desmosterol to cholesterol (Elias et al. 1983b). Thus, oral 20,25-diazacholestenol administration leads to a marked decrease in the stratum corneum cholesterol content in conjunction with an accumulation of desmosterol. It is noteworthy that scaling could be corrected by topical application of cholesterol and 7-dehydrocholesterol (Elias et al. 1986) as well as by systemic coadministration of either etretinate or isotretinoin (Geiger and Hartmann 1986). These findings clearly point to the close relationship of epidermal sterologenesis with epidermal differentiation as well as to the pharmacological interference by synthetic retinoids.

1.4.7 Conclusion

It becomes apparent that the epidermal lipid metabolism is of critical importance for the maintenance of orderly epidermal differentiation and cornification. The stratum corneum can be represented by a two-compartment model which can be compared to a brick wall. The corneocytes filled with proteinaceous material resemble the bricks and the lipid-enriched intercorneocyte material the mortar. This intercorneocyte-lipid matrix is arranged in multilamellar lipid sheets with unique physicochemical features. Intriguingly, the multilamellar lipid bilayers are not composed of phospholipids as in other organs, but are enriched in sphingolipids. These lipid sheets play an important role in the cohesion of the stratum corneum and provide the permeability barrier and water-holding capacity of the stratum corneum. The intercorneocyte lipids sheets are formed by the intercellular deposition of the contents of an organelle unique to the epidermis of terrestrial vertebrates, the lamellar body. Further biochemical modulations occur by the action of lipid catabolic enzymes which are extruded into the intercellular space of the stratum corneum after fusion of the lamellar bodies at the stratum granulosum-stratum corneum interface.

The independent epidermal cholesterol biosynthesis, which is in part regulated by the degree of stratum corneum hydration, is another striking feature of epidermal lipid metabolism. The homeostasis of the ratio of free sterols to cholesterol sulfate is closely involved in the process of desquamation.

There remains much to be learned about the physiology of cornification by clinical experience with drugs inhibiting cholesterol biosynthesis, with nutritional animal models, such as essential fatty acid-deficient rodents or the diazacholestenol animal model of ichthyosis and XRI, the experiment of nature. It can be expected that the biochemical basis of other ichthyoses such as the group of lamellar ichthyoses will be unraveled in the near future. As has already been shown, the analysis of epidermal lipids can be used as a diagnostic tool for the classification of lamellar ichthyoses.

Thus, epidermal lipid research will offer new insights into the pathogenesis of inherited and acquired disorders of keratinization and may provide the pathophysiologic basis for innovative therapeutic modalities of systemic and topical treatment regimens.

References

Abdel-Hafez K, Safer AM, Selim MM, Rehak A (1983) Familial continual skin peeling. Dermatologica 166:23-31

Abraham W, Wertz PW, Downing DT (1985) Linoleate-rich polar lipids of epidermis: structure determination by proton magnetic resonance. Clin Res 33:621 A

Achor RWP, Winkelmann RK, Perry HO (1961) Cutaneous side effects from use of triparanol (MER-29): preliminary data on ichthyosis and loss of hair. Proc Staff Meet Mayo Clin 36:217-228

Anderson PC, Martt JM (1965) Myotonia and keratoderma induced by 20,25-diazacholestenol. Arch Dermatol 92:181-183

Angelini C, Phillipart M, Borrone EC, Bresolin N, Cantini M, Lucke S (1980) Multisystem triglyceride storage disease with impaired long-chain fatty acid oxidation. Ann Neurol 7:5-10

Ansari MNA, Nicolaides N, Fu HC (1970) Fatty acid composition of the living layer and stratum corneum lipids of human sole skin epidermis. Lipids 5:838-845

Anton-Lamprecht I, Kahlke W (1974) Zur Ultrastruktur hereditärer Verhornungsstörungen. V. Ichthyosis beim Refsum-Syndrom (heredopathia atactica polyneuritiformis) Arch Derm Forsch 250:185-206

Assmann G, Fredrickson DS (1983) Acid lipase deficiency: Wolman's disease and cholesteryl ester storage disease. In: Stanbury JB, Wyngaarden JB, Fredrickson DS (eds) The metabolic basis of inherited disease, 5th edn. McGraw-Hill, New York, pp 803-819

Austin J, Armstrong D, Shearer L (1965) Metachromatic form of diffuse cerebral sclerosis. V. The nature and significance of low sulfatase activity: a controlled study of brain, liver, and kidney in four patients with metachromatic leukodystrophy. Arch Neurol 13:593-614

Baden HP, Kubilus J, Rosenbaum K, Fletcher A (1982) Keratinization in the harlequin fetus. Arch Dermatol 118:14-18

Basner R, von Figura K, Glössl J, Klein U, Kresse H, Mlekusch W (1979) Multiple deficiency of mucopolysaccharide sulfatases in mucosulfatidosis. Pediatr Res 13:1316-1318

Bergner EA, Shapiro LJ (1981) Increased cholesterol sulfate in plasma and red blood cell membranes of steroid sulfatase deficient patients. J Clin Endocrinol Metab 53:221-223

Berridge M (1984) Inositol triphosphate and diacylglycerol as second messengers. Biochem J 220:345-360

Bickers DR (1983) Drug, carcinogen, and steroid hormone metabolism in the skin. In: Goldsmith LA (ed) Biochemistry and physiology of the skin, vol II. Oxford University Press, New York, pp 1169-1186

Bowser PA, Gray GM (1978) Sphingomyelinase in pig and human epidermis. J Invest Dermatol 70:331-335

Brannon PG, Goldstein JL, Brown MS (1975) 3-hydroxy-3-methylglutaryl coenzyme A reductase activity in human hair roots. J Lipid Res 16:7-11

Burr GO, Burr MM (1929) A new deficiency disease produced by the rigid exclusion of fat from the diet. J Biol Chem 82:345-367

Buxman MM, Goodkin PE, Fahrenbach WH, Dimond RL (1979) Harlequin ichthyosis with epidermal lipid abnormality. Arch Dermatol 115:189-193

Chanarin I, Patel A, Slavin G, Wills EJ, Andrews TM, Stewart G (1975) Neutral-lipid storage disease: a new disorder of lipid metabolism. Br Med J 1:553-555

Cooper RA (1977) Abnormalities of cell-membrane fluidity in the pathogenesis of disease. N Engl J Med 297:371-377

Davies MG, Marks R, Dykes PJ, Reynolds DJ (1977) Epidermal abnormalities in Refsum's disease. Br J Dermatol 97:401-406

Davies MG, Reynolds DJ, Marks R, Dykes PJ (1978) The epidermis in Refsum's disease (heredopathis atactica polyneuritiformis) In: Marks R, Dykes PJ (eds) The ichthyoses. MTP, Lancaster, pp 51-64

Demel RA, Dekruijff (1976) The function of sterols in membranes. Biochim Biophys Acta 457:109-132

Dorfman ML, Hershko C, Eisenberg S, Sagher R (1974) Ichthyosiform dermatosis with systemic lipidosis. Arch Dermatol 110:261-266

Downing DT, Stewart ME, Wertz PW, Strauss JS (1986) Essential fatty acids and acne. J Am Acad Dermatol 14:221-225

Dulanez JT, Moser HW (1978) Sulfatide lipidoses: metachromatic leukodystrophy. In: Stanbury JB, Wyngaarden JB, Frederickson DS (eds) The metabolic basis of inherited disease, 4th edn. McGraw-Hill, New York, pp 770-809

Dykes PJ, Marks R, Davies MG, Reynolds DJ (1978) Epidermal metabolism in heredopathia atactica polyneuritiformis. J Invest Dermatol 70:126-129

Elias PM (1981) Epidermal lipids, membranes, and keratinization. Int J Dermatol 20:1-19

Elias PM (1983) Epidermal lipids, barrier function, and desquamation. J Invest Dermatol 80:44s-49s

Elias PM (1987) Plastic wrap revisited. The stratum corneum two-compartment model and its clinical implications. Arch Dermatol 123:1405-1406

Elias PM, Brown BE (1978) The mammalian cutaneous permeability barrier. Defective barrier function in essential fatty acid deficiency correlates with abnormal intercellular lipid deposition. Lab Invest 39:574-583

Elias PM, Friend DS (1975) The permeability barrier in mammalian epidermis. J Cell Biol 65:180-191

Elias PM, Leventhal ME (1979) Intercellular volume changes and cell surface expansion during cornification. Clin Res 27:525

Elias PM, Williams ML (1985) Neutral lipid storage disease with ichthyosis. Arch Dermatol 121:1000-1008

Elias PM, Goerke J, Friend DS (1977) Mammalian epidermal barrier layer lipids: composition and influence on structure. J Invest Dermatol 69:535–546

Elias PM, Brown BE, Ziboh VA (1980) Permeability barrier in essential fatty acid deficiency: evidence for a direct role for linoleic acid in epidermal barrier function. J Invest Dermatol 74:230–233

Elias PM, Fritsch PO, Lampe M, Williams ML, Brown BE, Nemanic M, Grayson S (1981) Retinoid effects on epidermal structure, differentiation, and permeability. Lab Invest 44:531–540

Elias PM, Grayson S, Lampe MA, Williams ML, Brown BE (1983a) The intercorneocyte space. In: Marks R, Plewig G (eds) Stratum corneum. Springer, Berlin Heidelberg New York, pp 53–67

Elias PM, Lampe MA, Chung J-C, Williams ML (1983b) Diazacholesterol-induced ichthyosis in the hairless mouse. I. Morphologic, histochemical, and lipid biochemical characterization of a new animal model. Lab Invest 48:565–577

Elias PM, Williams ML, Maloney ME, Bonifas JA, Brown BE, Grayson S, Epstein Jr. EH (1984) Stratum corneum lipids in disorders of cornification: steroid sulfatase and cholesterol sulfate in normal desquamation and the pathogenesis of recessive X-linked ichthyosis. J Clin Invest 74:1414–1421

Elias PM, Williams ML, Maloney ME, Fritsch PO, Chung J-C (1986) Applications of the diazacholesterol animal model of ichthyosis. In: Marks R, Plewig G (eds) Skin models. Springer, Berlin Heidelberg New York, pp 122–135

Epstein Jr. EH, Bonifas JM (1985) Recessive X-linked ichthyosis: lack of immunologically detectable steroid sulfatase enzyme protein. Hum Genet 71:201–205

Epstein Jr. EH, Leventhal ME (1981) Steroid sulfatase of human leukocytes and epidermis and the diagnosis of recessive X-linked ichthyosis. J Clin Invest 67:1257–1262

Epstein Jr. EH, Krauss RM, Shackleton CHL (1981a) X-linked ichthyosis: increased blood cholesterol sulfate and electrophoretic mobility of low-density lipoprotein. Science 214:659–660

Epstein Jr. EH, Williams ML, Elias PM (1981b) Steroid sulfatase, X-linked ichthyosis, and stratum corneum cell cohesion. Arch Dermatol 117:761–763

Epstein Jr. EH, Bonifas JM, Barber TC, Haynes M (1984a) Cholesterol sulfotransferase of newborn mouse epidermis. J Invest Dermatol 83:332–335

Epstein Jr. EH, Williams ML, Elias PM (1984 b) The epidermal cholesterol sulfate cycle. J Am Acad Dermatol 10:866–868

Feingold KR, Wiley MH, Moser AH, Lau DT, Lear SR, Siperstein MD (1982) De novo sterologenesis in intact primate. J Lab Clin Med 100:405–410

Feingold KR, Brown BE, Lear SR, Moser AH, Elias PM (1983) Localization of de novo sterologenesis in mammalian skin. J Invest Dermatol 81:365–369

Feingold KR, Brown BE, Lear SR, Moser AH, Elias PM (1986) Effect of essential fatty acid deficiency on cutaneous sterol synthesis. J Invest Dermatol 87:588–591

Freinkel RK, Traczyk TN (1985) Lipid composition and acid hydrolase content of lamellar granules of fetal rat epidermis. J Invest Dermatol 85:295–298

Freinkel RK (1987) Lipids of the epidermis. In: Fitzpatrick TB, Eisen AZ, Wolff K, Freedberg IM, Austen KF (eds) Dermatology in general medicine, 3rd edn McGraw-Hill, New York, pp 191–194

Fox H (1921) Skin shedding (keratosis exfoliativa congenita): report of a case. Arch Dermatol 3:202

Geiger J-M, Hartmann H-R (1986) Diazacholesterol-induced ichthyosiform changes in hairless mice: effects of oral etretinate and isotretinoin. Arch Dermatol Res 278:426–428

Gray GM, White RJ (1978) Glycosphingolipids and ceramides in human and pig epidermis. J Invest Dermatol 70:336–341

Grayson S, Johnson-Winegar AG, Wintroub BV, Isseroff RR, Epstein Jr. EH, Elias PM (1985) Lamellar body-enriched fractions from neonatal mice: preparative techniques and partial characterization. J Invest Dermatol 85:289–294

Grubauer G, Feingold KR, Elias PM (1987) Relationship of epidermal lipogenesis to cutaneous barrier function. J Lipid Res 28:746–752

Guilleminault C, Harpey JP, Lafourcade J (1973) Sjögren-Larsson syndrome. Report of two cases in twins. Neurology 23:367–373

Hashimoto K (1971) Cementsomes, a new interpretation of the membrane-coating granule. Arch Derm Forsch 240:349–364

Heilmann BB, Ryckmanns F, Plewig G (1983) Scanning electron microscopy of human corneocytes. In: Marks R, Plewig G (eds) Stratum corneum. Springer, Berlin Heidelberg New York, pp 186–190

Herndon JH, Steinberg D, Uhlendorft BW (1969) Refsum's disease. Defective oxidation of phytanic acid in tissue cultures derived from homozygotes and heterozygotes. N Engl J Med 281:1034–1038

Hernell O, Holmgren G, Jagell SF, Johnson SB, Holman RT (1982) Suspected faulty essential fatty acid metabolism in Sjögren-Larsson syndrome. Pediatr Res 16:45–49

Hooft C, Kriekemans J, Van Acker K, Devos E, Traen S, Verdonk G (1967) Sjögren-Larsson syndrome with exudative enteropathy. Influence of medium-chain triglycerides on the symptomatology. Helv Paediatr Acta 5:447–458

Ibsen HH, Brandrup F, Blaabjerg O, Lykkesfeldt G (1986) Lipoprotein electrophoresis in recessive X-linked ichthyosis. Acta Derm Venereol (Stockh) 66:59–62

Imokawa G, Hattori M (1985) A possible function of structural lipids in the water-holding properties of the stratum corneum. J Invest Dermatol 84:282–284

Imokawa G, Akasaki S, Hattori M, Yoshizuka N (1986) Selective recovery of deranged water-holding properties by stratum corneum lipids. J Invest Dermatol 87:758–761

Kitajima Y, Sekiya T, Mori S, Nozawa Y, Yaoita H (1985) Freeze-fracture cytochemical study of membrane systems in human epidermis using filipin as a probe for cholesterol. J Invest Dermatol 84:149–153

Kligman AM (1964) The biology of the stratum corneum. In: Montagna W, Lobitz Jr. WC (eds) The epidermis. Academic, New York, pp 387–433

Kolde G, Happle R, Traupe H (1985) Autosomal-dominant lamellar ichthyosis: ultrastructural characteristics of a new type of congenital ichthyosis. Arch Dermatol Res 278:1–5

Kondoh H, Kanoh H, Ono T (1983) Deacylation of ceramide, triacylglycerol and phospholipids in guinea pig epidermal cells. Biochim Biophys Acta 753:97–106

Kooyman DJ (1932) Lipids of the skin. Some changes in the lipids of the epidermis during the process of keratinization. Arch Derm Syph 25:444–450

Kurban AK, Azar HA (1969) Familial continual skin peeling. Br J Dermatol 81:191–195

Lampe MA, Burlingame AL, Whitney J, Williams ML, Brown BE, Roitman E, Elias PM (1983a) Human stratum corneum lipids: characterization and regional variations. J Lipid Res 24:120–130

Lampe MA, Williams ML, Elias PM (1983b) Human epidermal lipids: characterization and modulations during differentiation. J Lipid Res 24:131–140

Landmann L (1980) Lamellar granules in mammalian, avian and reptilian epidermis. J Ultrastruct Res 72:245–263

Landmann L (1986) Epidermal permeability barrier: transformation of lamellar granule-disks into intercellular sheets by a membrane fusion process, a freeze-fracture study. J Invest Dermatol 87:202–209

Landmann L (1988) The epidermal permeability barrier. Anat Embryol 178:1–13

Landmann L, Wertz PW, Downing DT (1984) Acylglucosylceramide causes flattening and stacking of liposomes. An analogy for assembly of the epidermal permeability barrier. Biochim Biophys Acta 778:412–418

Long SA, Wertz PW, Strauss JS, Downing DT (1985) Human stratum corneum polar lipids and desquamation. Arch Dermatol Res 277:284–287

Lykkesfeldt G, Hoyer H (1983) Topical cholesterol treatment of recessive X-linked ichthyosis. Lancet ii:1337–1338

Maloney ME, Williams ML, Epstein Jr. EH, Law MYL, Fritsch PO, Elias PM (1984) Lipids in the pathogenesis of ichthyosis: topical cholesterol sulfate-induced scaling in hairless mice. J Invest Dermatol 83:252–256

McIntosh TJ, Costello MJ (1981) Effects of n-alkanes on the morphology of lipid bilayers: a freeze-fracture and negative stain analysis. Biochim Biophys Acta 645:318–326

Melnik B, Hollmann J, Plewig G (1988) Decreased stratum corneum ceramides in atopic individuals - a pathobiochemical factor for xerosis? Br J Dermatol 119:547-549

Melnik BC, Hollmann J, Erler E, Verhoeven B, Plewig G (1989a) Microanalytical screening of all major stratum corneum lipids by sequential high-performance thin-layer chromatography. J Invest Dermatol 92:231-234

Melnik B, Kinner T, Plewig G (1988) Influence of oral isotretinoin treatment on the composition of comedonal lipids. Implications for comedogenesis in acne vulgaris. Arch Dermatol Res 280:97-102

Melnik B, Küster W, Hollmann J, Plewig G, Traupe H (1989b) Autosomal dominant lamellar ichthyosis exhibits an abnormal scale lipid pattern. Clin Gen 35:152-156

Menon GK, Feingold KR, Moser AH, Brown BE, Elias PM (1985) De novo sterologenesis in the skin. II. Regulation by cutaneous barrier requirements. J Lipid Res 26:418-427

Menon GK, Grayson S, Elias PM (1986) Cytochemical and biochemical localization of lipase and sphingomyelinase activity in mammalian epidermis. J Invest Dermatol 86:591-597

Meyer JC, Gilardi S (1986) Biochemische Diagnose der X-chromosomalen Ichthyose. Hautarzt 37:205-209

Mier PD, Jose JMA, van den Hurk A (1974) Direct biochemical assay of the lipase activity of epidermis. Dermatologica 149:284-288

Miranda A, DiMauro S, Eastwood A, Hays A, Johnson WG, Olarte M, Whitlock R, Mayeux R, Rowland LP (1979) Lipid storage, myopathy, ichthyosis, and steatorrhea. Muscle Nerve 2:1-13

Mommaas-Kienhuis A-M, Grayson S, Wijsman MC, Vermeer BJ, Elias PM (1987) Low density lipoprotein receptor expression on keratinocytes in normal and psoriatic epidermis. J Invest Dermatol 89:513-517

Nemanic MK, Whitehead JS, Elias PM (1983) Alterations in membrane sugars during epidermal differentiation. Visualization with lectins and role of glycosidases. J Histochem Cytochem 31:887-897

Nicollier M, Massengo T, Remy-Martin J-P, Laurent R, Adessi G-L (1986) Free fatty acids and fatty acids of triacylglycerols in normal and hyperkeratotic human stratum corneum. J Invest Dermatol 87:68-71

Okano M, Kitano Y, Nakamura T, Matsuzawa Y (1985) Detection of heterozygotes of X-linked ichthyosis by measuring steroid sulfatase activity of lymphocytes. Mode of inheritance in three families. Br J Dermatol 113:645-649

Orozco-Topete R, Chung J-C, Elias PM (1983) Epidermal glycoconjugate biosynthesis in organ and cell culture: effect of retinoids. J Invest Dermatol 80:316

Parsons Jr. WB, Flinn JH (1959) Reduction of serum cholesterol levels and β-lipoprotein cholesterol levels by nicotinic acid. AMA Arch Intern Med 103:783-790

Paulsrud JR, Pensler L, Whitten CF, Stewart S, Holman RT (1972) Essential fatty acid deficiency in infants induced by fat-free intravenous feeding. Am J Clin Nutr 25:897-904

Plewig G (1970) Regional differences in cell sizes in the human stratum corneum. Part II. Effect of sex and age. J Invest Dermatol 54:19-23

Plewig G, Marples RR (1969) Regional differences of cell sizes in the human stratum corneum. Part I. J Invest Dermatol 54:13-18

Ponec M, Kempenaar J, Vermeer BJ (1083 a) Retinoids suppress cholesterol synthesis in cultured human epidermal keratinocytes. J Invest Dermatol 80:352

Ponec M, Havekes L, Kempenaar J, Vermeer BJ (1983 b) Cultured human skin fibroblasts and keratinocytes: differences in the regulation of cholesterol synthesis. J Invest Dermatol 81:125-130

Ponec M, Havekes L, Kempenaar J, Lavrijsen S, Vermeer BJ (1984) Defective low-density lipoprotein metabolism in cultured, normal, transformed, and malignant keratinocytes. J Invest Dermatol 83:436-440

Ponec M, Havekes L, Kempenaar J, Lavrijsen S, Wijsman M, Boonstra J, Vermeer BJ (1985) Calcium-mediated regulation of the low density lipoprotein receptor and intracellular cholesterol synthesis in human epidermal keratinocytes. J Cell Physiol 125:98-106

Prost O, Nicollier M, Laurent R, Adessi GL (1985) Estrone- and dehydroepiandrosterone sulfatase activities in human female epidermis. Arch Dermatol Res 277:195-200

Prottey C (1976) Essential fatty acids and the skin. Br J Dermatol 94:579-587

Prottey C (1977) Investigation of functions of essential fatty acids in the skin. Br J Dermatol 97:29–38

Prottey C, Hartop PJ, Black JG, McCormack JI (1976) The repair of impaired epidermal barrier function in rats by the cutaneous application of linoleic acid. Br J Dermatol 94:13–21

Rearick JI, Jetten AM (1986) Accumulation of cholesterol 3-sulfate during in vitro squamous differentiation of rabbit tracheal epithelial cells and its regulation by retinoids. J Biol Chem 261:13898–13904

Rehfeld SJ, Williams ML, Elias PM (1986) Interactions of cholesterol and cholesterol sulfate with free fatty acids: possible relevance for the pathogenesis of recessive X-linked ichthyosis. Arch Dermatol Res 278:259–263

Rizzo WB, Dammann AL, Craft DA (1988) Sjögren-Larsson syndrome. Impaired fatty alcohol oxidation in cultured fibroblasts due to deficient fatty alcohol: nicotinamide adenine dinucleotide oxidoreductase activity. J Clin Invest 81:738–744

Rozenszajin L, Klajman A, Yaffe D, Efrati P (1966) Jordan's anomaly in white blood cells. Report of a case. Blood 28:258–265

Ruiter M, Meyler L (1960) Skin changes after therapeutic administration of nicotinic acid in large doses. Dermatologica 120:139–144

Schroepfer Jr. GL (1981) Sterol biosynthesis. Ann Rev Biochem 50:585–621

Silverman AK, Ellis CN, Beals TF, Woo TY (1986) Continual skin peeling syndrome. An electron microscopic study. Arch Dermatol 122:71–75

Simpson GM, Blair JH, Cranswick EH (1964) Cutaneous effects of a new butyrophenone drug. Clin Pharmacol Ther 5:310–321

Shapiro LJ (1983) Steroid sulfatase deficiency and X-linked ichthyosis. In: Stanbury JB, Wyngaarden JB, Frederickson DS, Goldstein JL, Brown MS (eds) Metabolic basis of inherited disease. McGraw-Hill, New York, pp 1027–1039

Slavin G, Wills EJ, Richmond JE, Chanarin I, Andrews T, Stewart G (1975) Morphologic features in a neutral lipid storage disease. J Clin Pathol 28:701–710

Snyder RG, Maroncelli M, Qi SP, Strauss HL (1981) Phase transitions and nonplanar conformers in crystalline n-alkanes. Science 214:188–190

Srebrnik A, Tur E, Perluk C, Elman M, Messer G, Ilie B, Krakowski A (1987) Dorfman-Chanarin syndrome. J Am Acad Dermatol 17:801–808

Steinberg S (1983) Phytanic acid storage disease (Refsum's disease). In: Stanbury JB, Wyngaarden JB, Frederickson DS, Goldstein JL, Brown MS (eds) The metabolic basis of inherited disease. McGraw-Hill, New York, pp 731–747

Stillwell W, Ricketts M, Hudson H, Nahmias S (1982) Effect of retinol and retinoic acid on permeability, electrical resistance and phase transition of lipid bilayers. Biochim Biophys Acta 688:653–659

Swartzendruber DC, Wertz PW, Madison KC, Downing DT (1987) Evidence that the corneocyte has a chemically bound lipid envelope. J Invest Dermatol 88:709–713

Traupe H, Kövary PM, Schriewer H (1983) X-linked recessive ichthyosis vulgaris: rapid identification by lipoprotein electropheresis. Arch Dermatol Res 275:63–65

Traupe H, Kolde G, Happle R (1984) Autosomal dominant lamellar ichthyosis: a new skin disorder. Clin Gen 26:457–461

Truchetet E, Brändle I, Grosshans E (1988) Hautveränderungen, Pathophysiologie und Therapie bei Mangel an essentiellen Fettsäuren. Z Hautkr 63:290–301

Wertz PW (1986) Lipids of keratinizing tissues. In: Bereiter-Hahn J, Matoltsy AG, Richards KS (eds) Biology of the integument, vol 2. Vertebrates. Springer, Berlin Heidelberg New York, pp 815–823

Wertz PW, Downing DT (1982) Glycolipids in mammalian epidermis: structure and function in the water barrier. Science 217:1261–1262

Wertz PW, Downing DT (1983) Ceramides of pig epidermis: structure determination. J Lipid Res 24:759–765

Wertz PW, Downing DT (1984) Cholesteryl sulfate: the major polar lipid of hoof. J Lipid Res 25:1320–1323

Wertz PW, Cho ES, Downing DT (1983) Effect of essential fatty acid deficiency on the epidermal sphingolipids of the rat. Biochim Biophys Acta 753:350–355

Wertz PW, Downing DT (1986) Covalent attachment of ω-hydroxyacid derivatives to epidermal macromolecules: a preliminary characterization. Biochem Biophys Res Commun 137:992–997

Wertz PW, Downing DT, Freinkel RK, Traczyk TN (1984) Sphingolipids of the stratum corneum and lamellar granules of fetal rat epidermis. J Invest Dermatol 83:193–195

Wertz PW, Miethke MC, Long SA, Strauss JS, Downing DT (1985) The composition of the ceramides from human stratum corneum and from comedones. J Invest Dermatol 84:410–412

Wertz PW, Swartzendruber DC, Abraham W, Madison KC, Downing DT (1987) Essential fatty acids and epidermal integrity. Arch Dermatol 123:1381–1384

Williams ML (1983) The ichthyoses-pathogenesis and prenatal diagnosis: a review of recent advances. Pediatr Dermatol 1:1–24

Williams ML, Elias PM (1981) Increased cholesterol sulfate content of stratum corneum in recessive X-linked ichthyosis. J Clin Invest 68:1404–1410

Williams ML, Elias PM (1982) **n**-Alkanes in normal and pathological human scale. Biochem Biophys Res Commun 107:322–328

Williams ML, Elias PM (1984) Elevated **n**-alkanes in congenital ichthyosiform erythroderma. Phenotypic differentiation of two types of autosomal recessive ichthyosis. J Clin Invest 74:296–300

Williams ML, Elias PM (1985) Heterogeneity in autosomal ichthyosis. Clinical and biochemical differentiation of lamellar ichthyosis and nonbullous congenital ichthyosiform erythroderma. Arch Dermatol 121:477–488

Williams ML, Elias PM (1986) The ichthyoses. In: Thiers BH, Dobson RL (eds) Pathogenesis of skin disease. Churchill Livingstone, New York, pp 519–551

Williams ML, Grayson S, Bonifas JN, Epstein Jr. EH, Elias PM (1983) Epidermal cholesterol sulfate and steroid sulfatase activity and recessive X-linked ichthyosis. In: Marks R, Plewig G (eds) Stratum corneum. Springer, Berlin Heidelberg New York, pp 79–84

Williams ML, Hughes-Fulford M, Elias PM (1985) Inhibition of 3-hydroxy-methylglutaryl coenzyme A reductase activity and sterol synthesis by cholesterol sulfate in cultured fibroblasts. Biochim Biophys Acta 845:349–357

Williams ML, Feingold KR, Grubauer G, Elias PM (1987 a) Ichthyosis induced by cholesterol-lowering drugs. Implications for epidermal cholesterol homeostasis. Arch Dermatol 123:1535–1538

Williams ML, Rutherford SL, Feingold KR (1987 b) Effects of cholesterol sulfate on lipid metabolism in cutured human keratinocytes and fibroblasts. J Lipid Res 28:955–967

Winkelmann RK, Perry HO, Achor RWP, Kirby TJ (1963) Cutaneous syndromes produced as side effects of triparanol therapy. Arch Dermatol 87:140–145

Wolff-Schreiner E (1977) Ultrastructural cytochemistry of the epidermis. Int J Dermatol 16:77–102

Yardley HJ (1983) Epidermal lipids. In: Goldsmith LA (ed) Biochemistry and physiology of the skin, vol 1. Oxford University Press, New York, pp 363–381

Yardley HJ, Summerly R (1981) Lipid composition and metabolism in normal and diseased epidermis. Pharmacol Ther 13:357–383

Yoshiike T, Matsui T, Kimura T, Yamada H, Ogawa H (1985) The effect of steroid sulfatase on stratum corneum shedding in patients with X-linked ichthyosis. Br J Dermatol 113:641–643

2 Isolated Vulgar Ichthyoses

2.1 Autosomal Dominant Ichthyosis Vulgaris

2.1.1 Historical Aspects

Alibert [1] is credited with the first description of autosomal dominant ichthyosis vulgaris (ADI) under the designation "ichthyose nacrée." Peukert [14] noted the frequent familial occurrence of the disease and concluded that it was inherited as a dominant trait. A number of reports in the older literature mention that ADI seems frequently to skip a generation [13]. The skipping of a generation is typical for X-linked recessive inheritance, and in a number of families in which skipping of ichthyosis vulgaris is mentioned in the literature the disease may in fact have been X-linked recessive ichthyosis (XRI). The clinical and genetic features of ADI could be fully appreciated only after XRI had been delineated by Wells and Kerr [20, 21].

2.1.2 Incidence and Clinical Features

In most cases, ADI is a mild scaling disorder. Many patients are not aware that they are suffering from a skin disease, but rather describe their skin as being "a bit dry." Wells and Kerr studied 6061 pupils and found among them 24 children with ADI, which would correspond to a frequency of 1:250 in the general population [20]. Because of the mild manifestation of the gene defect in most cases, data obtained from dermatology departments are bound to be biased. Concomitant atopic dermatitis is a frequent motive for a patient with ichthyosis vulgaris to consult a dermatologist. ADI is about five times as frequent as XRI among patients who come to a dermatology department for treatment of keratinization disorders [17].

In contrast to congenital ichthyosis and to XRI, ADI is not present at birth. It usually develops during the first months of life. Wells and Kerr [20] found demonstrable hyperkeratosis in 40% of their patients at the age of 3 months. In many patients, however, ichthyosis does not become apparent until the first year of life. In my experience the onset of ichthyosis vulgaris in the first 6 months of life is typical of XRI, and onset after that time is usually associated with ADI. As a rule, fine hyperkeratoses are seen with light gray scales, covering mainly the extensor surfaces of the extremities and the trunk (Fig. 8). In general, the scales are much smaller than in XRI; the groin and the big flexures are always spared (Table 10). Follicular keratosis projecting above the skin surface is a further characteristic sign of the disease that is present especially in children and young

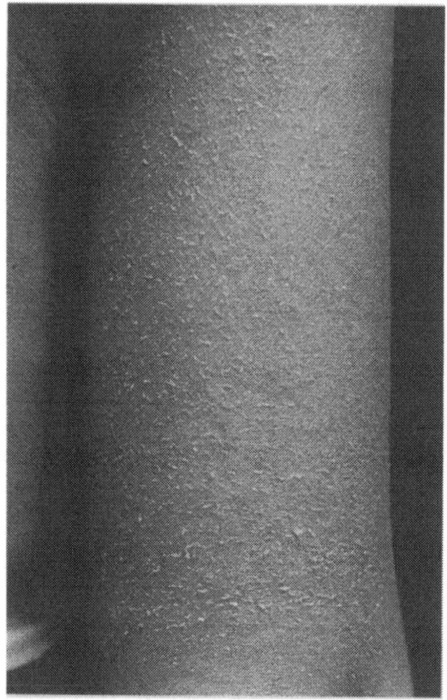

Fig. 8. Autosomal dominant ichthyosis vulgaris. Fine translucent scaling on the back of an arm

Table 10. Clinical findings in 65 patients with ADI, and other control patients (own results)

Characteristics/findings	Number of patients	Percent
Male	45[a]	69
Female	20	31
Sparing of the flexural folds	65	100
Accentuated palmoplantar creases	60	92
Light gray color of the scales	60	92
Atopic dermatitis	24	37
Cryptorchidism among 34 male dermatology patients	5	15
Cryptorchidism among 11 andrology patients	3	27
ADI among 35 patients with atopic dermatitis (control group)	13	37

[a] The male sex is overrepresented in this patient group because we were interested in the frequency of cryptorchidism in ADI.

patients (Fig. 9). According to Mevorah et al. [10], it occurs in 75% of all ADI patients, compared with 42% of the general population. In contrast, Voß and Voß [18] found keratosis follicularis in only 12.7% of the general population and noted a marked difference between patients with ADI alone (43%) and patients with ADI and associated atopic dermatitis (90%).

Accentuated palmoplantar markings are another characteristic feature of ADI found in 80%–90% of these patients. If the accentuation is marked it may be of

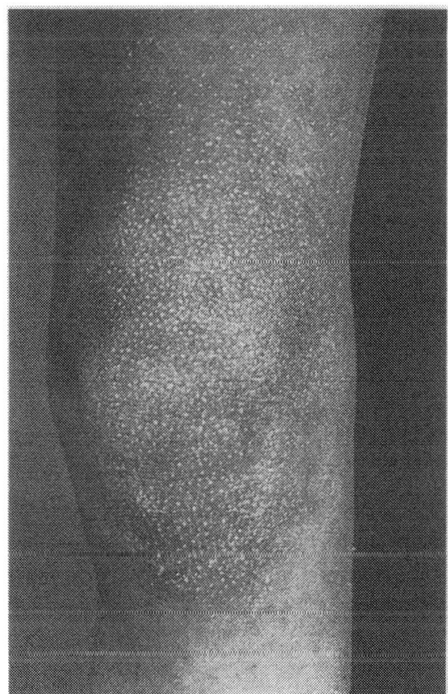

Fig. 9. Autosomal dominant ichthyosis vulgaris. Prominent follicular keratosis

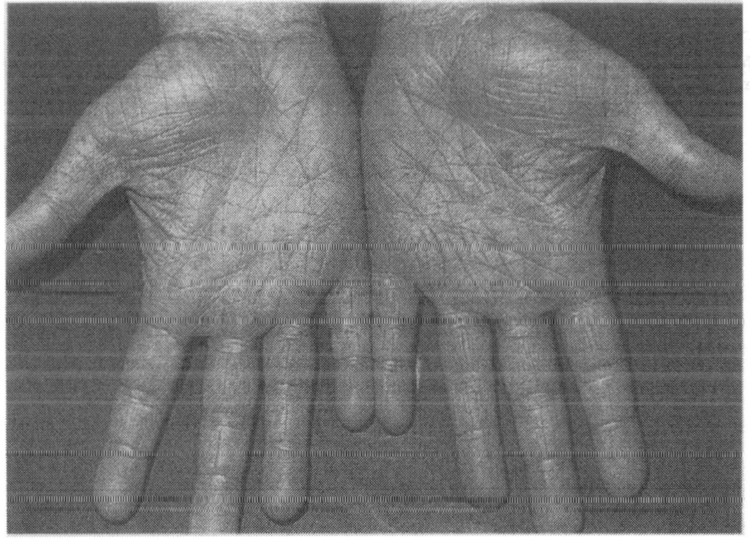

Fig. 10. Autosomal dominant ichthyosis vulgaris. Accentuated palmar creases. (From Traupe and Happle [17])

considerable diagnostic help (Fig. 10), but evaluation of accentuated palmoplantar creases proves rather difficult if this symptom is only mildly expressed. Using a subjective score ranging from 0 to 3+, Mevorah et al. [10] observed increased palmoplantar creases in 33% of patients with atopic dermatitis and also in 22% of a control group of dermatology patients (Table 11). If they accepted only marked accentuation (2+ and 3+), this was found in 48% of ADI patients, 8% of patients with atopic dermatitis, and 13% of the control group. From this it is evident that increased palmoplantar markings are strongly associated with ADI and may be considered pathognomonic. It is not a sign specific to ADI, however, since in our experience similar accentuated markings can be seen in patients with Refsum's disease and nonerythrodermic lamellar ichthyosis.

Voß and co-workers [19] found that scaling of the auricles is a typical sign of various types of ichthyosis. Though not specific for ADI, this symptom is usually found in ichthyosis vulgaris and may help to establish diagnosis of ADI in mildly affected cases. I was made aware of this finding by Dr. Voß on a recent visit to the German Democratic Republic; I had not paid much attention to auricular involvement in the past.

It is well known that ADI is associated with atopic dermatitis [9, 18]. Among 65 patients attending our department for treatment of ADI, I found concomitant atopic dermatitis in 37%; likewise, ADI was observed in 13 of 35 patients (also 37%) who came for treatment of atopic dermatitis (Table 10). The high prevalence of ADI in atopic dermatitis has been questioned very recently [6]. Based on clinical and histologic features (hyperlinear palms, reduced or lacking granular layer) Fartasch and co-workers [6] found that six of 32 patients with atopic dermatitis suffered from concomitant ADI, but electron microscopy confirmed this diagnosis in only one of these six patients. The authors accepted only the ultrastructurally confirmed case as true ADI and concluded that hyperlinear palms are a sign of atopic dermatitis. This latter conclusion would imply that up to 80% of all ADI patients displayed a phenotypic marker of atopic dermatitis. However, it might be argued that accentuated palmoplantar markings may be a more sensitive disease marker than the ultrastructural defect of keratohyalin granules in very mildly affected ADI patients. Sybert et al. [16] observed that the relative amounts of keratohyalin and profilaggrin present correlated with the severity of the disease.

Table 11. Prevalence of follicular keratosis and accentuated palmoplantar markings (From Mevorah et al. [10])

	Number of patients	Follicular keratosis		Accentuated palmoplantar markings	
		(*n*)	(%)	(*n*)	(%)
ADI	35	26	74	28	80
Atopic dermatitis	61	26	42	20	33
Control group	247	103	42	55	22

Another condition possibly linked with ADI is cryptorchidism, which was observed in five of 34 (15%) male patients in our dermatologic outpatient clinic and in three of 11 patients attending our andrology department. ADI is a frequent incidental finding in our andrology department (approximately one in 50 patients). The 15% occurrence of cryptorchidism in an unbiased patient group is more than the 1% to be expected in the German population as a whole [5]. To my knowledge, no other systematic studies on the simultaneous occurrence of cryptorchidism and ADI have been conducted. Therefore, it cannot be decided whether the two conditions are truly related. In contrast to views expressed in the older literature [15], ADI is not associated with mental retardation or other anomalies.

2.1.3 Histologic and Ultrastructural Features

A reduced granular layer, which may often even be completely lacking in parts of the biopsy, is the most outstanding histologic feature of ichthyosis vulgaris [7, 21] (Fig. 11a, b). The stratum corneum usually displays a mild but compact orthohyperkeratosis. It has been claimed that the epidermis is atrophic in ADI [7, 21]. Of ten patients I studied histologically, five had an epidermis of normal thickness; in three it was of increased thickness, and in only two patients was it of reduced thickness (Table 12). It is noteworthy that in the same biopsy it is possible to see parts showing atrophy of the epidermis and other parts where the epidermis is obviously acanthotic. A reduced rete-papillae pattern, occasional prominent follicular keratosis, and a significant reduction in the number of sebaceous glands are further features of ADI [7, 9]. Occasionally, slight perivascular infiltrates can be seen, but I find it difficult to decide whether these infiltrates are really more prominent than what would be expected in normal skin. The diminished granular layer is reflected at the ultrastructural level by reduced and abnormal keratohyalin granules [2, 3]. The keratohyalin granules display a crumbly or spongy appearance (Fig. 12). This defect of keratohyalin granules is a consistent ultrastructural finding. It permits a rapid distinction of ADI from XRI and other ichthyoses associated with a reduced granular layer (Refsum's disease, X-linked dominant ichthyosis) [2, 3].

2.1.4 Biochemical Aspects

The biochemical basis of ADI is unknown. Michaëlsson et al. [11] demonstrated a reduced binding of the epidermis for retinol-binding protein in 15 ADI patients, whereas the epidermis of patients suffering from congenital ichthyosis and from XRI showed a normal affinity for the retinol-binding protein. The authors discussed this finding as a secondary phenomenon which may be related to the defect in the keratohyalin granules.

Filaggrin is the major protein component of keratohyalin. It is especially rich in the basic amino acids. Filaggrin and its precursor profilaggrin are absent in severely affected ADI patients and reduced in intensity in less severely affected

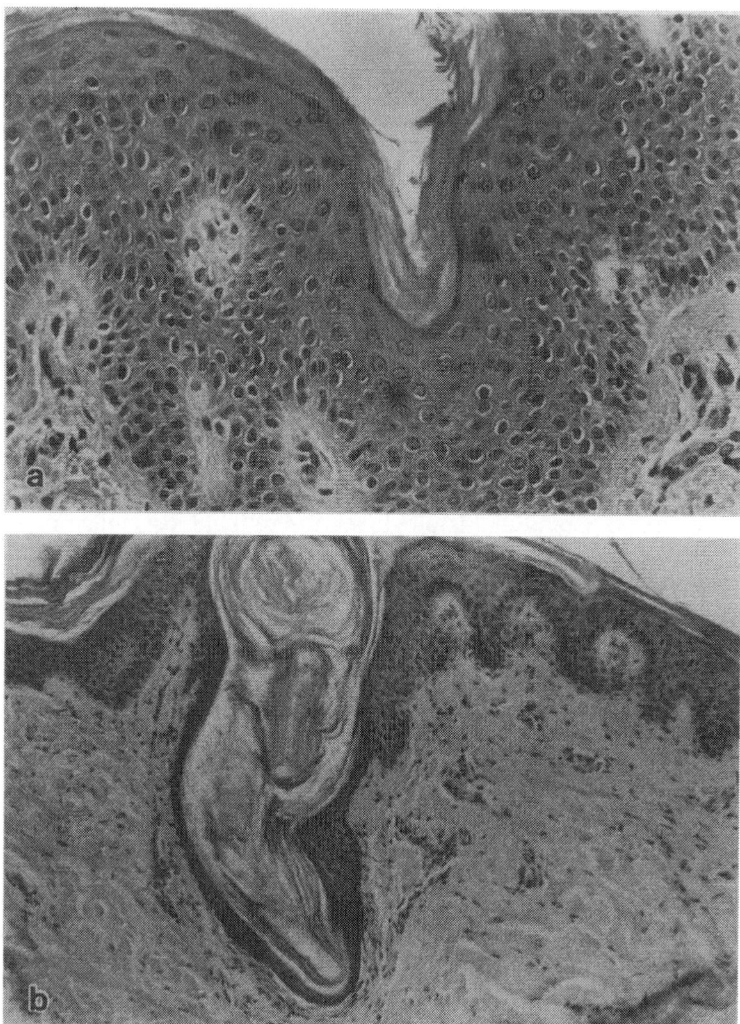

Fig. 11a, b. Autosomal dominant ichthyosis vulgaris. *a* Histology of ADI. The granular layer is reduced and lacking in part. Hematoxylin and eosin, × 100. (From Traupe and Happle [17]). *b* Follicular keratosis with prominent keratotic plugging. Note again the reduction of the granular layer. Hematoxylin and eosin, × 20

patients [16]. As ADI is a dominant disease in which affected individuals are heterozygous for a normal and an abnormal allele, one would expect both gene products, the normal and the abnormal protein, in the affected patients. Hence, the absence of profilaggrin and filaggrin and likewise the ultrastructural defect of keratohyalin cannot be the primary genetic defect of the disease, but rather are secondary to an abnormality in a factor which modulates profilaggrin/filag-

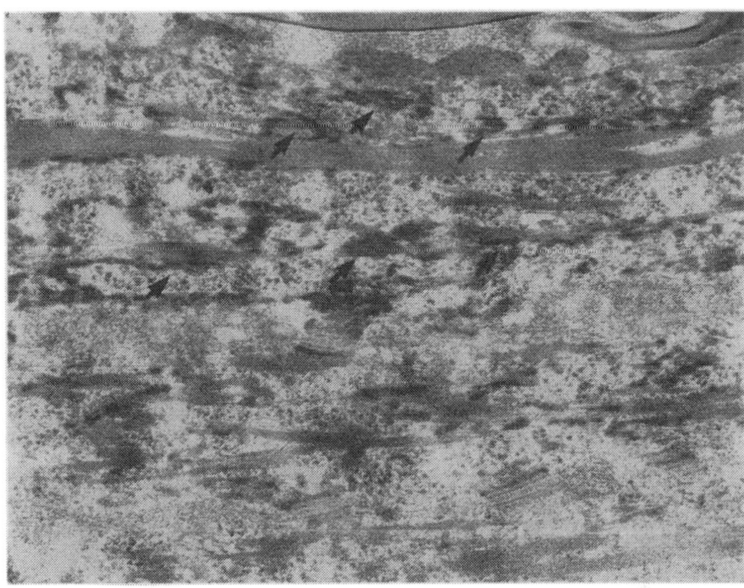

Fig. 12. ADI: electron microscopy of the upper granular layer. Note scarce and crumbly keratohyalin granules *(arrow)*. × 18200. (Courtesy of Dr. Kolde, Münster, Federal Republic of Germany)

Table 12. Histologic features in ten patients with ADI (own results)

Features		Number of patients
Stratum corneum	orthohyperkeratosis	10
	focal parakeratosis	1
	normal thickness	8
	increased thickness	2
Granular layer	reduced or lacking in part	10
Malpighian layer	normal thickness	5
	increased	3
	atrophic	2
Sebaceous glands	present	1
	lacking	9
Eccrine glands	present	10
Perivascular infiltrate	none	3
	slight	6
	moderate	1

grin synthesis [16]. Furthermore, the demonstration of an orderly keratin pattern casts doubt on the presumptive role of filaggrin in the aggregation and organization of keratin filaments to form bundles [4].

Cultured keratinocytes from patients with ADI exhibit the ultrastructural defect in keratohyalin and fail to react with a monoclonal antibody to filaggrin [8].

The structural and biochemical phenotypic characteristics of the disease appear to be maintained in epidermal cell cultures [8], and this should facilitate the eventual elucidation of the biochemical mechanisms involved. A recent study [12] showed that the cytokeratin pattern is normal in ADI.

2.1.5 Genetic Counseling

ADI is a monogenic autosomal dominant trait. Expression of the disease can vary from one generation to another. In parents of affected children I have often seen increased palmar markings and follicular keratosis, that is, a very mild disease manifestation only. The ultrastructural abnormality of the keratohyalin granules would most likely permit prenatal diagnosis, but it is generally agreed that prenatal diagnosis should not be offered for this rather mild condition. The frequent association with atopic dermatitis suggests that ADI may be one of the predisposing factors for atopic dermatitis [17]. In this case, the two conditions would share a common gene. Patients should be advised about the increased risk of developing atopic dermatitis, this usually being of greater concern than the ichthyosis.

References

1. Alibert L (1806) Description des maladies de la peau, observés à l'hópital Saint-Louis et exposition des meilleurs méthodes suivies pour leur traitement. Paris
2. Anton-Lamprecht (1973) Zur Ultrastruktur hereditärer Verhornungsstörungen. III. Autosomal-dominante Ichthyosis vulgaris. Arch Dermatol Forsch 248:149-172
3. Anton-Lamprecht I, Hofbauer U (1972) Ultrastructural distinction of autosomal dominant ichthyosis vulgaris and X-linked recessive ichthyosis. Hum Genet 15:261-264
4. Dale BA, Holbrook KA, Steinert PM (1978) Assembly of stratum corneum basic protein and keratin filaments in macrofibrils. Nature 276:729-731
5. Doepfmer R (1960) I. Hodendystopien (Kryptorchismus). In: Jadassohn J (ed) Handbuch der Haut- u. Geschlechtskrankheiten, vol 6/3. Springer, Berlin Göttingen Heidelberg, pp 517-531
6. Fartasch M, Haneke E, Anton-Lamprecht I (1987) Ultrastructural study of the occurrence of autosomal dominant ichthyosis vulgaris in atopic eczema. Arch Dermatol Res 279:270-272
7. Feinstein A, Ackerman AB, Ziprkowski L (1970) Histology of autosomal dominant ichthyosis vulgaris and X-linked ichthyosis. Arch Dermatol 101:524-527
8. Fleckman P, Holbrook KA, Dale BA, Sybert VP (1987) Keratinocytes cultured from subjects with ichthyosis vulgaris are phenotypically abnormal. J Invest Dermatol 88:640-645
9. Hofbauer M, Schnyder UW (1974) Zur Differentialdiagnose von autosomal dominanter Ichthyosis vulgaris and X-chromosomaler Ichthyose. Hautarzt 25:319-325
10. Mevorah B, Marazzi A, Frenk E (1985) The prevalence of accentuated palmoplantar markings and keratosis pilaris in atopic dermatitis, autosomal dominant ichthyosis and control dermatological patients. Br J Dermatol 112:679-685
11. Michaëlsson G, Forsum U, Malmnäs-Tjerlund U, Rask L, Vahlquist A (1979) Retinol-binding protein in serum and epidermis of patients with ichthyosis vulgaris. Clin Exp Dermatol 4:445-451
12. Moll I, Traupe H, Voigtländer V, Moll R (1988) Das Zytoskelett der hereditären Ichthyosen. Hautarzt 39:82-90

13. Orel H (1929) Die Vererbung der Ichthyosis congenita und der Ichthyosis vulgaris. Kleine Beiträge zur Vererbungswissenschaft. V. Mitteilung. Z Kinderheilkd 47:312-340
14. Peukert M (1899) Über Ichthyosis. Eine Übersicht. Dermatol Z:171-204
15. Salfeld K, Lindley J (1963) Zur Frage der Merkmalskombination bei Ichthyosis vulgaris mit Bambushaarbildung und ektodermaler Dysplasie. Dermatol Wochschr 147:118-128
16. Sybert VP, Dale BA, Holbrook KA (1985) Ichthyosis vulgaris: identification of a defect in synthesis of filaggrin correlated with an absence of keratohyalin granules. J Invest Dermatol 84:191-194
17. Traupe H, Happle R (1980) Klinik und Genetik der Ichthyosis vulgaris-Gruppe. Fortschr Med 98:1809-1815
18. Voß E, Voß M (1980) Genodermatosen in den Kreisen Heiligenstadt und Worbis. Dissertation A an der Medizinischen Akademie Erfurt
19. Voß M, Voß E, Schubert H (1982) Schuppung der Ohren. Ein Leitsymptom der Ichthyosisgruppe? Dermatol Monatsschr 168:394-397
20. Wells RS, Kerr CB (1966) Clinical features of autosomal dominant and sex-linked ichthyosis in an English population. Br Med J 1:947-950
21. Wells RS, Kerr CB (1966) The histology of ichthyosis. J Invest Dermatol 46:530-535

2.2 X-Linked Recessive Ichthyosis

2.2.1 Historical Aspects

X-linked recessive ichthyosis (XRI) is one of the most frequent genetic skin disorders. An apparently sex-linked type of ichthyosis vulgaris occurring only in males had been mentioned by Rayer [67] as early as 1835, but of course the genetic implications could not be understood at that time. X-linked recessive inheritance in ichthyosis vulgaris was clearly recognized by Lundborg [35] in 1927 (Fig. 13). Only 2 years later, Orel [61] collected a number of pedigrees showing the characteristics of X-linked recessive inheritance in ichthyosis vulgaris and concluded that this had to be a skin disease distinct from the more common ADI. In this early work on XRI, however, there was no attempt to correlate clinical and histologic features with pedigree analysis; therefore, the disease could not be recognized clinically and fell into oblivion until its rediscovery in the early 1960s. Wells and Kerr [93–97] actually "awoke" XRI from its status of a rare sleeping beauty to that of one of the most common genetic defects. In this context it may be of interest that their first publication concerned a genetic and not a clinical topic: the linkage of XRI to other X-linked markers.

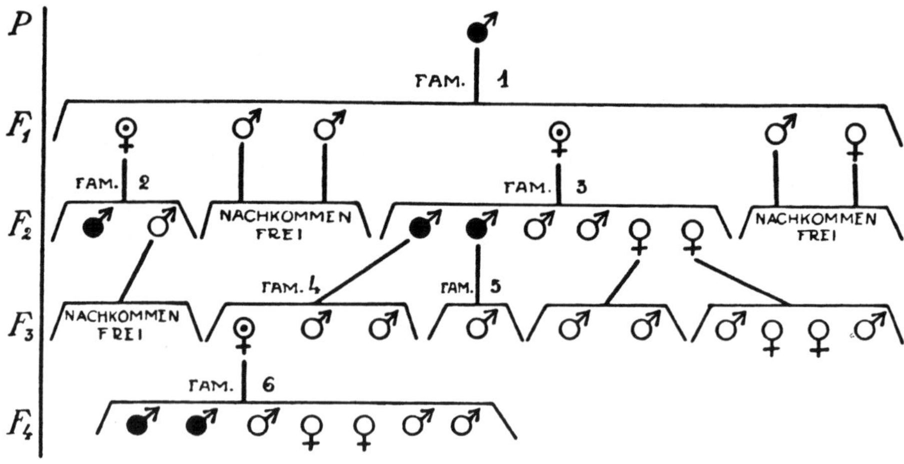

Fig. 13. X-linked recessive ichthyosis. Pedigree with characteristics of X-linked inheritance in ichthyosis vularis simplex, as drawn by Lundborg in 1927 [35]

Kerr and co-workers [32] were able to demonstrate a linkage between the newly discovered Xg blood group and XRI. This spectacular finding initiated a number of similar investigations, soon confirming the linkage [2, 98].

For quite some time dermatologists studied intensively the cutaneous features of XRI, and at the same time gynecologists established placental sulfatase deficiency as a distinct X-linked disorder [19], without realizing that they were dealing with the same entity. It was Mme. Marinkovic-Ilsen, working at the Department of Neonatology at the Wilhelmina Gasthuis in Amsterdam, who followed up the fate of the so-called risk births with placental sulfatase deficiency and noted in 1974 that such a child had developed ichthyosis 3 months after birth [45]. After a further two similar cases were observed, this group suggested that XRI and X-linked sulfatase deficiency were the same disease entity [30, 33]. This hypothesis was soon confirmed by an American group which - independently of the Dutch group - identified steroid sulfatase deficiency as the underlying biochemical defect of XRI [73].

2.2.2 Incidence

XRI is the second most common type of ichthyosis and, hence, one of the most frequent enzyme deficiencies. Population genetic studies disclosed a minimum prevalence in the male population of 1:6390 in South England [93], 1:9500 in Israel [106] and 1:4152 in the Spanish provence of Salamanca [86]. The actual incidence is probably even higher. Routine screening of pregancies for placental sulfatase deficiency by two groups from France and Denmark indicated that the incidence of XRI may be as high as 1:2000 in males [39].

2.2.3 Clinical Features

The clinical spectrum of steroid sulfatase deficiency includes XRI, birth complications, and cryptorchidism, a manifestation recognized only recently [81, 82]. Corneal opacities, not affecting visual acuity, seem to be a possible ophthalmologic manifestation of the underlying enzyme deficiency [72].

2.2.3.1 Cutaneous Findings at Birth

Prenatal diagnosis of placental sulfatase deficiency has made it possible to follow the course of the disease from birth in a Danish study. Of 21 boys prenatally diagnosed as suffering from placental sulfatase deficiency, 19 displayed a general peeling of the skin with rather large, light and loosely attached scales over the entire integument at the age of 1-3 weeks [28]. During the following weeks this fine scaling was replaced by the typical polygonal dark and firmly attached scales of XRI. In only two of the patients did visible hyperkeratoses occur at the age of 6-8 months. Careful inspection of prenatally diagnosed steroid sulfatase deficiency thus discloses cutaneous symptoms in 90% of all patients at birth. The fine scaling (Fig. 14) is not very striking, however, and usually escapes the attention of parents or nurses. Taking histories from parents, the disease is most often said to have started at the age of 2–6 months.

2.2.3.2 Cutaneous Findings During Later Life

Usually, large, thick, dark-brown to yellow-brown hyperkeratoses (Fig. 15) cover the trunk, the extremities, and the neck [93, 97]. The scalp is mildly involved, whereas the face is spared except for a preauricular scaling, and palms and soles are normal [39, 86]. Axillae, and antecubital and popliteal fossae may be involved in some patients. Wells and Kerr [93] emphasized that this involvement is more often seen in young children and becomes less frequent with increasing age. Dark hyperkeratoses giving the lateral aspects of the trunk and the back of the neck a "dirty" look is a further feature, which is typical of XRI and usually not found in ADI. The lack of hyperlinear palms and soles and of keratosis pilaris further helps to exclude ADI.

Early descriptions of the disease underlined that hyperkeratoses were usually very large and that the scales exhibited a dark-brown color. Therefore, XRI was considered to be identical with "ichthyosis nigricans" or "ichthyose noire" in the French literature [7, 64]. The presumptive identification of the purely descriptive term "ichthyosis nigricans" with XRI initially prompted the delineation of a "second" X-linked ichthyosis characterized by light-gray scales [7, 89]. This view seemed to be backed up by histologic features resembling those of ADI rather than of typical XRI. In the meantime, after careful clinical analysis of large,

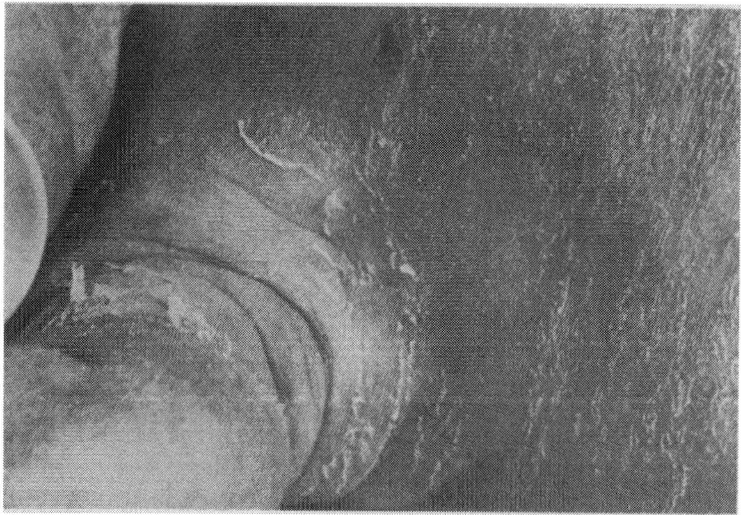

Fig. 14. X-linked recessive ichthyosis. Fine scaling, demonstrating skin peeling after birth in an 11-day-old boy. (Courtesy of Dr. Høyer, Rønne, Denmark with permission of Dr. H. S. Karger AG, Basel; from [28])

biochemically tested patient groups this possibility has been rejected, however. We have shown that up to 25% of all patients with XRI may exhibit light-gray

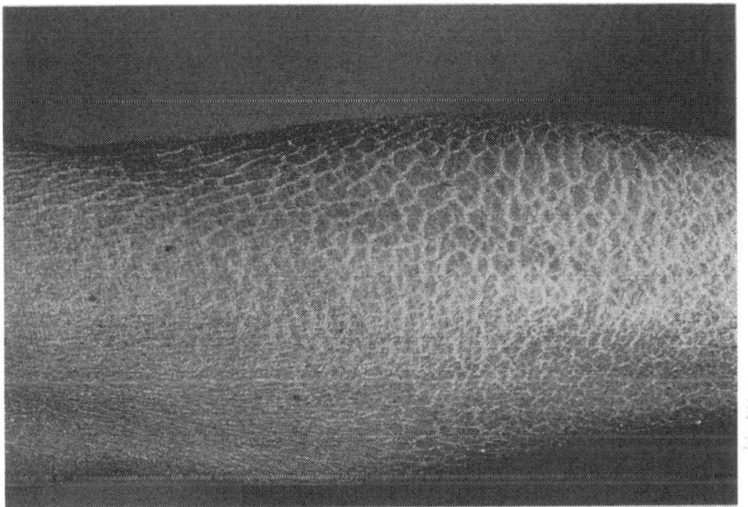

Fig. 15. X-linked recessive ichthyosis. Typical large, dark-brown hyperkeratoses with partial involvement of flexural fold of the arm. (From Traupe and Happle [81])

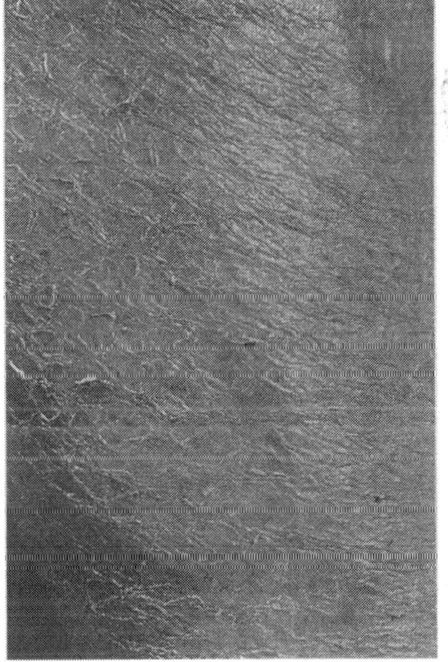

Fig. 16. X-linked recessive ichthyosis. Large, light-gray hyperkeratoses

hyperkeratoses (Fig. 16) which may be similar to those of severe ADI [81] (Table 13). Such patients are likely to be erroneously classified as having ADI, especially if the epidermis is also atrophic and the granular layer reduced. Recently, Voß [91] drew attention to a marked phenotypic variability of XRI even within the same family. Body sites showing marked scaling in one patient can be free in other affected family members.

2.2.3.3 Cutaneous Findings in Female Carriers

Female carriers are not affected by XRI unless they are homozygous for steroid-sulfatase deficiency, which is a very rare event and has so far been documented with certainty in only one family [48]. In many genetics textbooks, including McKusick's catalogue, reference is made to a paper by Csörsz [13] in 1928, in which he reported a second such family. A recent biochemical investigation verified the diagnosis of XRI in this family but failed to corroborate the homozygous status in one of the female members that had been claimed by Csörsz [71]. A clinical reexamination showed this woman now to be free of any skin symptoms. Arylsulfatase-C testing indicated that she was a heterozygous gene carrier. In 1928 Csörsz gave a very exact description of the woman's skin as follows: "On the whole trunk, on the upper as well as on the lower limbs, more expressed on the extensor surfaces of the extremities, the skin is rough and shows smudgy-brownish, lamellar scaling." This illustrates that female carriers of the gene can exhibit a forme fruste of XRI. Recently, Voß [91] emphasized that about 25% (eight of 29) obligate female carriers displayed a fine, silver-like scaling on the lower legs, especially the calves, and that four of them even suffered from dry skin with generalized involvement of the whole integument. It is now well known that the steroid-sulfatase locus does not fully escape X inactivation, and therefore enzyme acitivity in most female carriers is somewhat below that found in normal males [8, 38, 57]. Rather low enzyme activities in some of the female

Table 13. Cutaneous findings in 33 patients with biochemically confirmed XRI (own results)

Cutaneous findings	Number of patients	
	(*n*)	(%)
Onset during the first 6 months of life or occasionally at birth	33	100
Generalized involvement of the skin	31	94
Involvement of extremities only	2	6
Large dark-brown scales	24	73
Large gray scales	9	27
Clinical absence of follicular keratosis	33	100
Normal palmar creases	31	94
Possibly increased palmar creases	2	6
Atopic dermatitis	1	3

carriers may be just enough to account for this type of forme fruste involvement.

2.2.3.4 *Prenatal (Obstetric) Manifestations*

Insufficient cervical dilatation is often found in pregnant women with placental sulfatase deficiency and may cause weakness of labor and a prolonged delivery, necessitating cesarean section or forceps delivery. The duration of pregnancy may also be influenced by the metabolic defect [78]. The true incidence of these birth complications is much debated, however. Gynecology departments often perform routine screening for maternal estriol excretion in the urine to monitor placental function. If this is done, a prenatal diagnosis of placental sulfatase deficiency can be suspected, and apparently it is often decided to intervene and to perform elective cesarean sections with such pregnancies. Thus, of 84 patients reported in a literature review, 45 (= 53.6%) were delivered by cesarean section [79]. This approach has recently been questioned [21, 37]. In a study of boys diagnosed prenatally as having XRI, the course of pregancy and delivery did not seem to be adversely affected by the enzyme deficiency [37]. Among our own group of boys postnatally diagnosed as having XRI, there was a history of clinically manifest birth complications in ten of 33 patients (Table 14) [81]. Likewise, Unamuno et al. [87] reported a high rate of perinatal mortality (ten cases) and abortions (24 cases) in 17 XRI families from the province of Salamanca in Spain. With regard to the Danish data [37], however, it seems to be justified to follow a "wait-and-see" policy and to intervene only if obstetric complications actually occur.

2.2.3.5 *Gonadal Abnormalities*

Cryptorchidism is a recently recognized third manifestation of steroid-sulfatase deficiency [81]. We observed this association in eight of 33 patients (Table 15) and were surprised by the overlap between the patient group with a history of clinically apparent birth complications and that with cryptorchidism. Seven of the ten patients with a history of birth complications also exhibited cryptorchidism. Two recent systematic studies have confirmed the close association of XRI and cryptorchidism. Lykkesfeldt et al. [39] found nine instances of testicular maldescent among 76 XRI patients; in addition, they observed three patients with normally descended gonads who developed testicular cancer, which may be a

Table 14. Birth complications in 33 patients diagnosed postnatally with XRI (own results)

Birth complication	Number of patients
Infusion with oxytocin because of weakness of labor	6
Forceps delivery	3
Cesarean section	1

Table 15. Frequency of cryptorchidism (testicular maldescent) in 33 patients with XRI (own results)

	Dermatology clinic patients	Andrology clinic patients
Number of patients	29	4
Unilateral, inguinal cryptorchidism	4	0
Bilateral, inguinal-cryptorchidism	3	0
Bilateral, abdominal cryptorchidism	0	1
Total	7/29=24%	1/4

Testicular maldescent was found in seven of ten patients with a history of birth complications, but in only one of 23 patients without such a history

Table 16. Reports in the literature mentioning cryptorchidism or hypogenitalism in XRI

Case studies[a]	Cryptorchidism		Hypo-genitalism	Affected family members (*n*)
	unilateral	bilateral		
Lynch et al. [40]		+	+	3
York-Moore and Rundle [104]		+	+	2
Wells [95]			+	1
Wells [96]		+		1
Abe et al. [1]		+		2
Perrin et al. [63]		+	+	18
Tiepolo et al. [80]		+	+	1
Blanchet-Bardon et al. [9]	+		+	2
Metaxotou et al. [46]		+	+	2
Münke et al. [60]	+		+	1
Traupe et al. [85]		+	+	1
Andria et al. [3]		+	+	2
Steuhl et al. [76]		+		1

Systematic studies[b]	Country of study	Testicular maldescent (*n*/total)
Traupe and Happle [81]	Germany	7/25
Lykkesfeldt et al. [39]	Denmark	9/76
Unamuno et al. [87]	Spain	9/22

[a] Thirteen case studies of 37 patients
[b] In three systematic studies, 25 of 123 patients (=20%) suffered from testicular maldescent

further gonadal abnormality. Unamuno et al. [87] reported nine cases of testicular maldescent in a series of 22 patients. Taken together, these data indicate that about 20% of all patients with XRI suffer from associated testicular maldescent (Table 16). This figure is far above the prevalence of cryptorchidism to be expected in the male population after the first year of life, which is about 0.8%–1%.

How can the apparent association of cryptorchidism and XRI be explained? There are two conceivable mechanisms that could account for this association

[82]. The simplest answer is to consider testicular maldescent a further manifestation of steroid sulfatase deficiency. The considerable overlap between the subgroup of patients with manifest birth complications and the subgroup with cryptorchidism points to this. Even in the absence of cryptorchidism, patients with XRI exhibit an abnormal androgen and estrogen metabolism that is characterized by elevated levels of luteinizing hormone (LH) and estrone sulfate, lack of decline of dehydroepiandrosterone sulfate in older age, and low androstenedione and estradiol levels [39]. Surprisingly, basal testosterone remains normal, and the testosterone production reponse to human chorionic gonadotropin (HCG) is normal, too [70].

A second possible mechanism giving rise to cryptorchidism in XRI is tiny deletion mutations. If such deletions are rather large, they become visible at the cytogenetic level. In a considerable number of patients with XRI, such deletions due to X-Y translocations or due to the loss of the distal part of the short arm of the X chromosome (Xp-) have been observed (reviewed in Traupe et al. [85]). In these cases, steroid sulfatase deficiency occurs due to a deletion of the steroid sulfatase gene, and - depending on the size of the deletion - genes in the neighborhood of the steroid sulfatase locus may also be deleted or gene expression may be impaired. It should be borne in mind that the steroid sulfatase gene is located in the close vicinity of genes involved in sexual differentiation. Very recently it has been shown that the vast majority of XRI cases are actually due to deletion mutations, possibly as a result of impaired X-Y interchange during meiotic pairing [6, 11, 103]. Small deletions can segregate as mendelian traits. Due to a founder effect, the size and the percentage of deletions in XRI are most likely not distributed evenly in larger populations, which could account for the observed differences in the percentage of patients affected with cryptorchidism in the various regions of Europe (Table 16).

2.2.3.6 *Ophthalmologic Manifestation*

Deep stromal corneal opacities seem to be a frequent finding in XRI males [22, 25, 72]. Patients with this ocular manifestation exhibit tiny opacities of the deep ventral stroma, whereas the superficial parts of the cornea are less severely affected. In a recent study it was found that about 50% of all XRI patients had these mild opacities, which did not affect visual acuity and were not related to age [39], whereas in other studies, also comprising large patient groups, no opacities could be detected at all [86, 92]. It has been claimed that the possible ocular manifestation of steroid-sulfatase deficiency may even be useful in carrier identification [22]. Given the inconsistency of this mild corneal dystrophy and the special skills required for its detection (slit-lamp examination with retroillumination), this feature should not be relied upon for definite carrier identification. Recently, Steuhl et al. [76] reported bilateral corneal erosions in a patient suffering from XRI and epidermolysis bullosa simplex of the Köbner type. I have seen similar corneal erosions in one patient affected with XRI only. Corneal erosions caused by lid hyperkeratoses may therefore be a possible sequel of the gene defect which has not yet been fully appreciated.

2.2.4 Histologic and Ultrastructural Features

As early as 1904, Gassmann suggested that a distinction between two types of ichthyosis vulgaris be made and concluded that in one type the granular layer is absent, whereas in the other type it is rather prominent (see Sect. 1.2). It was not until the study by Wells and Kerr [94] in 1966, however, that these differences could be appreciated and were correlated with clinical findings and the results of pedigree analysis. Based on the examination of specimens from 12 patients, Wells and Kerr emphasized the following histologic features of XRI:

1. A marked orthohyperkeratosis with only occasional slight parakeratosis
2. A broad granular layer
3. An increased Malpighian layer

Furthermore, they noted marked perivascular infiltrates and the absence of follicular hyperkeratosis. According to Wells and Kerr, the thickness of the granular layer was the most outstanding feature, permitting a distinction between XRI, in which it was pronounced, and ADI, in which they found it reduced or even absent. Later studies largely confirmed their work [18, 27, 86]. It also became evident, however, that a clear-cut distinction between ADI and XRI is some-

Table 17. Histologic features in ten patients with biochemically confirmed XRI (own results)

Features		Number of patients
Stratum corneum	orthohyperkeratosis	10
	focal parakeratosis	1
	normal thickness	3
	increased thickness	7
Granular layer	reduced	1
	in part reduced, in part normal	3
	normal	3
	increased	3
Malpighian layer	normal thickness	3
	in part atrophic, in part normal	2
	atrophic	1
	increased	4
Sebaceous glands	present	10
	lacking	0
Eccrine glands	present	10
	lacking	0
Perivascular infiltrate	none	4
	slight	4
	moderate	1

Special findings: Three patients exhibited marked follicular plugging and three were found to have an increased stratum corneum associated with a reduced granular layer and an atrophic epidermis

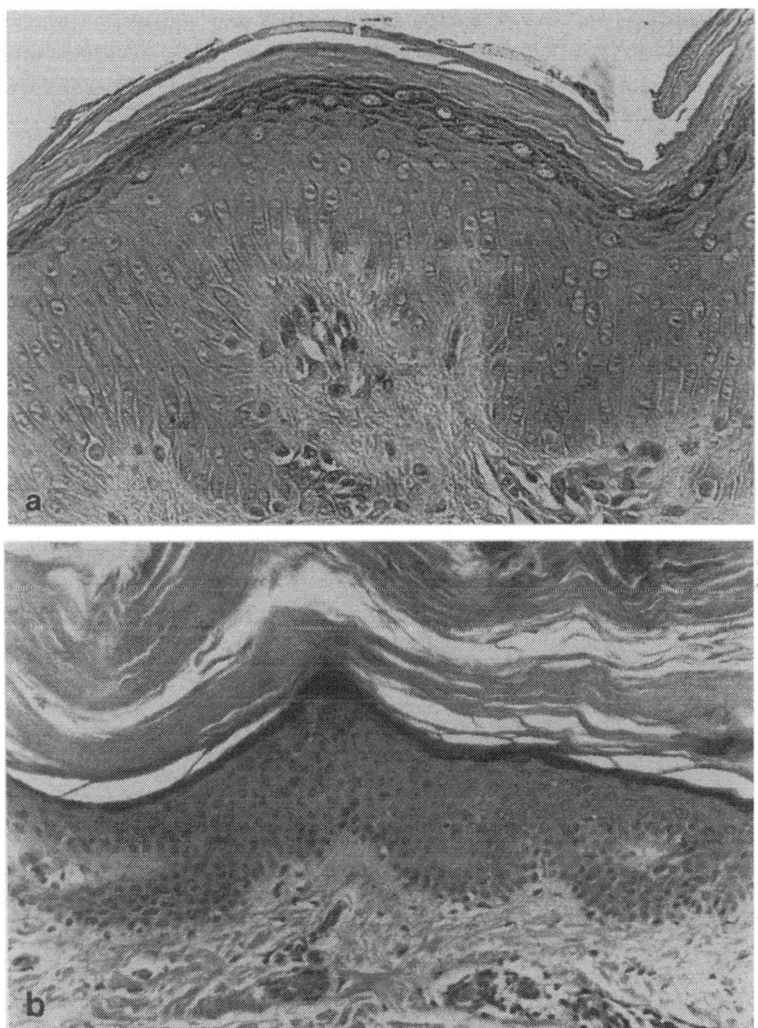

Fig. 17a, b. X-linked recessive ichthyosis. *a* Broadened granular layer and acanthosis. HE, ×100. *b* Reduced granular layer and almost atrophic epidermis, accompanied by marked broadening of stratum corneum. HE, ×50. (*a* From Traupe et al. [83])

times not possible on histologic grounds alone. In ADI the thickness of the granular layer is variable and dependent on the clinical severity of the disease; i.e., the granular layer may still be present in cases with only slight ADI and is absent in cases more severely affected [77]. Therefore, sites with maximal scaling (e.g., the upper leg) should be chosen for biopsy [18].

In contrast to Wells and Kerr, I observed that in XRI as well, the thickness of the granular layer can vary considerably from one patient to another and even within the same biopsy. I studied ten patients in whom diagnosis of XRI had been established by clinical and genetic means and confirmed biochemically

(Table 17). In all ten a preserved but sometimes reduced granular layer was observed (Fig. 17a). In one patient with a broadened stratum corneum, the granular layer was particulary reduced and the underlying epidermis almost atrophic (Fig. 17b). In three further patients large biopsies revealed a normal granular layer and a normal thickness of the epidermis in those parts where the stratum corneum was only moderately increased, but a decreased granular layer and an atrophic epidermis in those parts where the stratum corneum was markedly enlarged. Thus, if a small biopsy (i.e., punch biopsy) had been taken and if histologic examination alone had been relied upon, the same patient could have been classified as suffering from either ADI or XRI. The claim that the granular layer is always normal or even increased in XRI can no longer be upheld. In contrast to Wells and Kerr, I also observed follicular plugging in three of ten patients studied, as did Feinstein et al. [18] and Unamuno and co-workers [86]. Moreover, perivascular infiltrates need not be present in XRI or can be rather mild (Table 17) [18]. It can be concluded that XRI does not have distinctive histologic features, but is usually associated with rather nonspecific changes such as a broadened stratum corneum and a prominent granular layer. Similar changes can also be found in several types of congenital ichthyosis. In typical cases, the histologic features will help to distinguish between ADI and XRI. However, a clear-cut separation is not always possible. In these doubtful cases diagnosis should be confirmed biochemically.

As might be expected in a recessive disease, ultrastructural examinations disclosed no specific defect in XRI [5]. There are, however, a number of quantitative changes in XRI, such as an abnormal persistence of desmosomal disks, an increased number of transition cells, and an increased synthesis of keratohyalin [4]. Perrot and Ortonne [64] addressed the question of why the scales are usually dark brown. They suggested that this may be the result of a mixed epidermal and dermal hypermelanosis. According to their data, epidermal hyperpigmentation is due to hyperactivity of the melanocytes and increased melanosome transfer. The dermal component can be explained by a certain degree of pigment incontinence.

2.2.5 Biochemistry

2.2.5.1 Basic Aspects

Steroid sulfatase is the common name for a sulfohydrolase which cleaves the sulfate group of various sulfated steroids. The "correct" name for this enzyme is sterol sulfate sulfohydrolase, and it has been given the international Enzyme Commission (EC) number 3.1.6.2. Dehydroepiandrosterone (DHEA) sulfate and cholesterol sulfate are among the natural metabolic substances on which the enzyme acts. Arylsulfatase C is officially referred to as "arylsulfate sulfohydrolase C" and has been assigned the EC number 3.1.6.1. All substrates by which arylsulfatase C activity can be measured are artifical, such as *para*-nitrocatecholsulfate, *para*-nitrophenyl-sulfate, 4-methylumbelliferylsulfate, or 6-bromo-2-naphthylsulfate. Like steroid sulfatase, arylsulfatase C is a microsomal enzyme.

Most likely, steroid sulfatase is identical with one of the two isoenzymes of arylsulfatase C [88]. After electrophoretic separation on a polyacrylamide gel, Meyer and Schnyder [49] showed that steroid sulfatase and arylsulfatase C have only one activity band with the same electrophoretic mobility. Furthermore, all patients with XRI in whom both enzymes were measured showed the deficiency in both enzymes [49]. Moreover, both enzymes behave in the same way as far as the pattern of X inactivation is concerned [52]. Findings by van der Loos et al. [88] suggest that there may be two isoenzymes of arylsulfatase C, one of which is identical with steroid sulfatase. They performed polyacrylamide gel electrophoresis on extracts of cultivated skin fibroblasts. Then they compared arylsulfatase C activity, measured with the histochemical substrate 6-bromo-2-naphthylsulfate, with the activity determined with the biochemical substrate DHEA sulfate. They concluded that the histochemical substrate was hydrolyzed at two different bands (R_f – 0.49 and R_f = 0.58), whereas the biochemical substrate was hydrolyzed only at one band (R_f = 0.49). Recent biochemical investigations have allowed better characterization of the two arylsulfatase C isoenzymes, which have also been designated as "slow type" and as "fast type" [75]. The two types differed in their Km and – though not very much – in their pH optimum (slow type, pH 8.00; fast type; pH 7.67). Polyclonal antibodies raised against the slow type did not cross-react with the fast type [75]. Therefore, it is reasonable to assume that there are two different types of microsomal arylsulfatases, only one of which is identical with steroid sulfatase.

Some basic aspects of steroid-sulfatase deficiency are still unclear. Thus, MacNaught and France [44] postulated that steroid-sulfatase deficiency might not be due to the primary deficiency of the coding gene, but rather to a secondary defect of the membrane-bound enzyme. In microsomal placental fractions of affected patients low steroid sulfatase activities could be extracted by use of a detergent, and this remaining activity could be further enhanced by phosphatidylcholine.

Phosphatidylcholine is a phospholipid; it was found markedly reduced in microsomal membranes of placenta with steroid-sulfatase deficiency [43]. According to this concept, the gene defect would alter the normal structure of microsomal membrane and thus produce a deficient activation of steroid sulfatase. More recent studies seem to invalidate this concept, however. Patients with XRI not only lack steroid sulfatase activity; there is also no immunologically detectable steroid sulfatase protein [16] or synthesis of polypeptides related to steroid sulfatase [12]. Moreover, in most cases the gene defect seems to be due to deletions rather than to point mutations [6, 11, 103]. The proenzyme itself is synthesized as a membrane-bound 63 500-dalton polypeptide with asparagine-linked oligosaccharide chains and within 2 days is processed into the mature 61 000-dalton form [12].

2.2.5.2 Endocrine Functions of Sulfated Steroids

Steroid sulfatase cleaves sulfated steroid hormones such as DHEA sulfate. This reaction is of particular importance in pregnancy, since a defect blocks placental estrogen synthesis. In a normal pregnancy there is a steep rise of various estrogens after the 30th week of pregnancy. The maternal urinary excretion of estradiol and estrone increases 100-fold during pregnancy and that of estriol even increases by a factor of 10^3 [20]. This tremendous physiological increase in estrogens is used to monitor the normal function of the fetoplacental unit. In pregnancies where there is steroid-sulfatase deficiency the conversion of DHEA sulfate into DHEA and its cleavage products is disturbed and, as a consequence of this enzyme block, the sharp increase of estrogens is lacking. Even in pregnancies where there is steroid-sulfatase deficiency, estrogen excretion in maternal urine is still 20 times higher than estrogen excretion during the late follicle phase [78, 79]. Therefore, biosynthesis of estrogens during pregnancy can probably also use – to a certain extent – the classical delta-4 pathway. The excretion of sulfated steroids in the maternal urine allows prenatal diagnosis of placental sulfatase deficiency from specific steroid profiles [24, 78].

It is conceivable that sulfated steroids also play a role in testicular testosterone synthesis. The data addressing this question are sparse, however. Vihko and Ruokonen [90] studied the amounts of 24 neutral steroids in the testes after orchiectomy and found a high concentration of intermediate sulfated products of testosterone biosynthesis. Thus, DHEA sulfate was present at a concentration of 41 μg/100 g testicular tissue, whereas free DHEA was found only at a concentration of 1.3 μg/100 g. As far as the final product testosterone was concerned, the situation was inverted: testosterone sulfate was present at a concentration of 6.8 μg/100 g, while free testosterone predominated at 55 μg/100 g. It has been shown that the testicular steroid sulfatase can be inhibited by nonsulfated androgens [62]. Patients with steroid-sulfatase deficiency have an abnormal profile of sex hormones [39]. However, following HCG injections normal levels of testosterone are found, indicating that in these patients the classical delta-4 pathway can be used for testicular biosynthesis of testosterone as well.

2.2.5.3 Sulfated Steroids and Cell Membranes: Clues to the Pathophysiology of XRI

Cholesterol sulfate plays an important role in the stabilization of cell membranes. As a model for this function Bleau and co-workers [10] used erythrocytes which had been preincubated with cholesterol sulfate and were then exposed to different hypotonic salt solutions. Compared with the untreated erythrocytes, there was a broad range where the cholesterol sulfate-incubated erythrocytes resisted hemolysis. Cholesterol is a lipophilic molecule. Through sulfation it also takes on a hydrophilic function and thus becomes an amphoteric molecule especially well suited for membrane functions.

Williams and Elias [100] were able to demonstrate excessive amounts of cholesterol sulfate in the scales of patients with XRI. Under physiological conditions cholesterol sulfate represents only a small part of the stratum corneum lipids, but due to its amphoteric character it may play an important role in the maintenance of intercellular lipid lamellae [100]. Accumulation of cholesterol sulfate results in an enhanced stickiness of the corneocytes and in retention hyperkeratosis.

Further support for a direct role of cholesterol sulfate in the pathophysiology of scaling in XRI comes from an intriguing experiment performed by Maloney and co-workers [42]. They showed that topical application of cholesterol sulfate induced scaling in hairless mice. Furthermore, it has been shown that scaling of XRI patients can be improved if they are treated with a cream containing cholesterol [36]. The application of steroid sulfatase to the skin of XRI patients significantly increases the shedding of the stratum corneum in these patients, whereas no increased detachment of the stratum corneum was observed in normal subjects or ADI patients [105]. These experiments and clinical observations suggest that the accumulation of excess quantities of cholesterol sulfate within the lipid lamellae of the stratum corneum may result directly in "overstabilization" of the lamellae and retard desquamation.

Another mechanism that may be involved in scaling in XRI may be the regulation of hydroxymethylglutaryl-coenzyme A reductase by cholesterol sulfate. Cholesterol sulfate can inhibit this key enzyme of epidermal steroid synthesis [101]. Because cholesterol sulfate is an amphoteric molecule that can easily traverse cell membranes [66], the excessive accumulation of cholesterol sulfate in XRI is likely to disturb the orderly biosynthesis of epidermal steroids [99]. It is well known that drugs inhibiting cholesterol biosynthesis, such as 20–25-diazacholesterol, can cause an ichthyosis-like skin condition [102].

2.2.5.4 *Detection of Steroid-Sulfatase Deficiency*

Deficiency of arylsulfatase C or steroid sulfatase can be detected in a number of tissues: placenta [33], fibroblasts [73], keratinocytes [34], lymphocytes [57], and granulocytes [49]. Steroid sulfatase activity is determined either by tritium-labeled cholesterol sulfate or labeled DHEA sulfate. A histochemical assay is not available for steroid sulfatase, but arylsulfatase C can be assayed. For the histochemical reaction the substrate 6-bromo-2-naphthylsulfate is most often used [15, 33]. While the histochemical staining for arylsulfatase C is very clear-cut in placental tissue, it gives ambiguous results when skin biopsies are used [15, 51]. Using histochemical methods, de Groot and co-workers [15] found that 11 of 13 patients with ADI lacked arylsulfatase C activity; likewise, Meyer et al. [51] observed an apparent lack of arylsulfatase C activity in one of four histochemically studied ADI patients. The biochemical assay for arylsulfatase C is mostly done using 4-methylumbelliferyl sulfate and may be superior to STS testing as far as recognition of heterozygous gene carriers is concerned [52].

In healthy control persons, arylsulfatase C activity was found to depend on the body site from which the biopsy was taken [51]. An influence of the body area on enzyme activity was also observed for steroid sulfatase. In the same patient fibroblasts from ovarian tissue exhibited much less steroid sulfatase activity than fibroblasts obtained from the skin [68]. Steroid sulfatase is tissue dependent and its activity is decreased in skin fibroblasts from genital sites. A technical problem of steroid sulfatase testing is that the enzyme cannot be measured at a saturated concentration of DHEA sulfate. Therefore, the mean values for its activity can vary considerably in consecutive test series [68]. This problem can hamper detection of heterozygotes, especially when tissue is used where there is an overlap between the value found in normal and heterozygous women.

2.2.5.5 *Indirect Detection of Steroid-Sulfatase Deficiency by Lipoprotein Electrophoresis*

Direct demonstration of steroid-sulfatase or arylsulfatase-C deficiency is still a tedious and time-consuming procedure. The test is performed only in a few specialized laboratories around the world. A rapid biochemical confirmation of steroid sulfatase deficiency is possible, however, by an indirect assay now commonly used: lipoprotein electrophoresis. This new application of a well-established technique was introduced by Epstein and co-workers [17]. They discovered that patients with XRI exhibited an increased electrophoretic mobility of β-lipoprotein particles. The diagnostic value of lipoprotein electrophoresis (Fig. 18) has since then been confirmed by a number of groups [26, 29, 84]. Lipoprotein electrophoresis can be performed on an agarose gel using commercially available kits (e.g., Corning, Palo Alto, USA) without difficulty. Using this technique, clear-cut detection of patients with steroid-sulfatase deficiency is usually possible, whereas in heterozygous gene carriers, healthy control persons, and patients affected with other types of ichthyosis such as ADI, lamellar ichthyosis, and Refsum's disease, lipoprotein electrophoresis gives normal results. Meyer and Gilardi [50] studied a large series of patients with XRI ($n = 18$) or lamellar

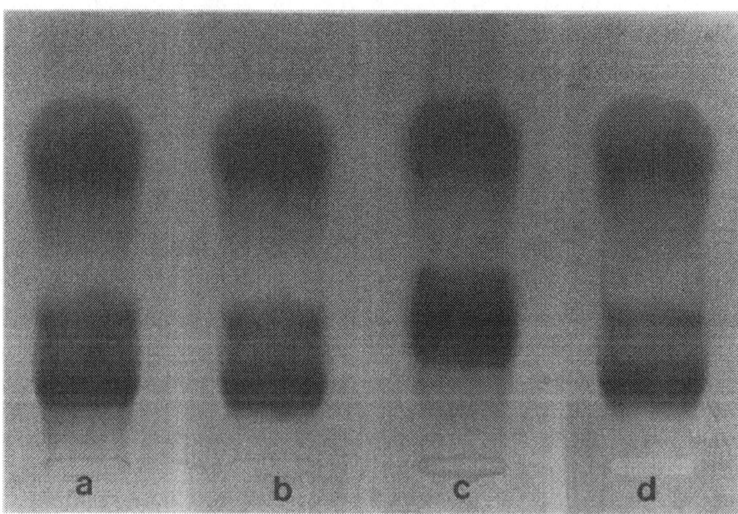

Fig. 18. Lipoprotein electrophoresis in steroid-sulfatase deficiency. Controls (**a** and **b**) and a heterozygous carrier (**d**) are normal. Note increased electromobility of β-lipoprotein in XRI (**c**). Anode at top. (From Traupe et al. [84])

ichthyosis ($n=7$) and healthy controls ($n=48$) using both arylsulfatase-C testing and lipoprotein electrophoresis. There were no false-positive results with lipoprotein electrophoresis, but in one of the 18 XRI patients the electrophoretic mobility remained normal despite arylsulfatase-C deficiency. It may be concluded that normal results do not rule out XRI with absolute certainty.

Increased electrophoretic mobility of β-lipoprotein as well as of pre-beta-lipoprotein can be attributed to an increased negative charge of the low-density lipoprotein particles. In patients with XRI, excessive amounts of cholesterol sulfate accumulate in the serum, thus altering the electric charge and the electrophoretic mobility of lipoprotein. Apart from the altered electrophoretic mobility of the lipoprotein, lipid metabolism is apparently not disturbed in XRI patients, and normal levels of triglycerides, cholesterol, and various lipoproteins are found [84] (Table 18).

Lipoprotein electrophoresis can be successfully carried out even when using serum of patients that has been stored at minus 20°C. Therefore, serum from patients with biochemically confirmed XRI can be stored in small aliquots and later used as an internal positive control together with serum from a normal healthy person. In many clinical settings all laboratory work is done in a department of clinical chemistry. In this case, the clinical chemist should be informed of the special interest in the electrophoretic mobility, for otherwise he will report normal results.

Table 18. Lipid analysis in eight cases of X-linked recessive ichthyosis (From Traupe et al. [84])

Case no.	Increased mobility		TG (mg/dl)	CH (mg/dl)	HDL-CH (mg(dl)	apoA$_1$ (mg/dl)	apoA$_2$ (mg/dl)	apoB (mg/dl)	Lp(a) (mg/dl)
	β-Lp	pre-β-Lp							
1	+	+	69	130	42	116	34	67	30
2	+	+	114	138	31	100	34	78	2
3	+	+	329	257	52	162	41	153	38
4	+	+	89	192	37	135	40	120	2
5	+	+	137	157	31	121	NT	107	2
6	+	+	56	137	38	121	37	77	3
7	+	+	62	108	35	120	38	92	8
8	+	+	124	136	34	130	38	85	5
Normal	0	0	< 200	< 260	27–65	102–176	30–50	60–130	< 10

TG, triglycerides; CH, cholesterol; HDL-CH, high density lipoprotein cholesterol; apoA$_1$, apolipoprotein A$_1$; apoA$_2$, apolipoprotein A$_2$; apoB, apolipoprotein B; Lp(a), lipoprotein(a); NT, not tested

2.2.6 Genetics

2.2.6.1 Detection of Heterozygous Carriers and X-Chromosome Inactivation

Identification of heterozygous female carriers seemed impossible at first. Shapiro et al. [73] studied eight obligate heterozygous gene carriers and found steroid sulfatase levels which were within the range of normal control patients. They did not, however, differentiate between female and male control patients. The inability to detect female gene carriers by simple testing of steroid sulfatase was not surprising; this was to be expected in X-linked diseases because of the Lyon hypothesis [41], according to which in each cell of a female individual only one X chromosome is active and can express its genes, while the other X chromosome is inactivated at an early stage of embryogenesis. By this mechanism the number of expressed X-linked genes in females parallels that in males. The inactivation occurs at random. Therefore, female carriers of an X-linked disorder exhibit a mosaic of defective and normal cells. In a skin biopsy both normal and defective cells are represented. Since the percentage of normal and defective cells can vary considerably in uncloned cultures, biochemical identification of the heterozygous state is usually possible only after subcloning of the cell cultures.

This strategy was followed by Shapiro et al. [74], who tested steroid sulfatase activity in subcloned skin fibroblasts in women who were obligate gene carriers for two X-linked traits: XRI and glucose-6-phosphate dehydrogenase (G6PD) deficiency. The expected mosaic was found for G6PD but not for steroid sulfatase, which showed normal values in all subcloned cultures. The Shapiro group concluded that the steroid-sulfatase locus escapes the common X-chromosome inactivation. At first glance, this finding seemed to exclude any test for heterozygous gene carriers once and for all, since even after subculturing, female carriers still had steroid sulfatase levels that could not be distinguished from those of healthy controls.

The Ropers group from Freiburg approached this problem from a different angle [57]. Their argument was as follows: If the gene for steroid sulfatase escapes X-chromosome inactivation in female carriers, then normal women should express the gene on both chromosomes. A linear gene-dosage relationship can be expected for this enzyme, since both X chromosomes are genetically active. Consequently, normal women should have twice the steroid sulfatase activity of normal men, and in female carriers the enzyme activity should be within the range found in normal men. An adequate evaluation of steroid sulfatase activity therefore required the splitting of the control groups into women and men.

This approach to the problem was confirmed by experimental data, and it was found that steroid sulfatase activity of fibroblasts in women was about 1.7 times higher than that in men [57]. In female carriers, steroid sulfatase activity was somewhat below that in normal men and could be clearly distinguished from the activity observed in normal women (Fig. 19). In lymphocytes, steroid sulfatase activity was about ten times lower than in fibroblasts. Sex differences of steroid sulfatase activity in lymphocytes were less pronounced, there being some over-

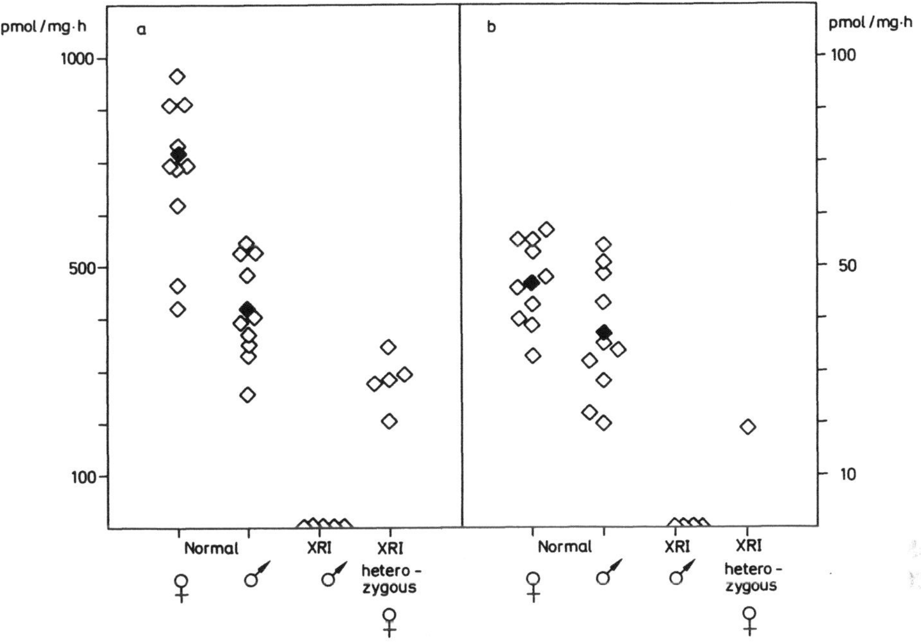

Fig. 19a, b. Recognition of heterozygous gene carriers by steroid sulfatase testing. In fibroblasts (*a*) steroid sulfatase activity of normal women is far above that of heterozygous women, whereas in lymphocytes (*b*) there can be some overlap. (Courtesy of Dr. C. Müller, Würzburg from [57])

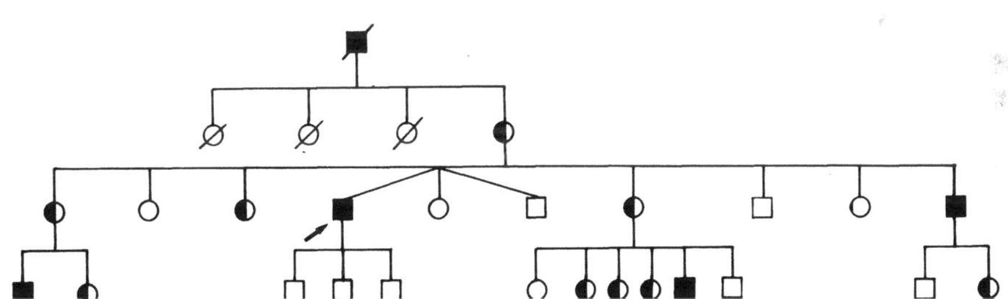

Fig. 20. Pedigree of family H. Several female gene carriers whose heterozygous steroid sulfatase status could not be deduced from the pedigree alone were recognized by steroid sulfatase testing. Testing was kindly done by Dr. C. R. Müller, now of Würzburg

lap between normal women and heterozygous carriers. Steroid sulfatase testing even allows recognition of those gene carriers whose status cannot be deduced from pedigree data because they have no affected offspring (Fig. 20).

In a later paper, Ropers et al. [68] studied steroid sulfatase activity in fibroblast cultures of patients with numerical and structural chromosome aberrations.

They demonstrated that steroid sulfatase activity correlates with the number of gene copies present. In recent years numerous studies have confirmed their main finding that STS activity is dependent on the number of gene copies present, and a ratio of 1.4:1 for steroid sulfatase activity in healthy women to that in healthy men was generally established [8, 37]. These studies suggest that the steroid sulfatase locus is not fully expressed, but participates to some extent in X-chromosome inactivation. In an elegant experiment, Migeon et al. [53] were able to corroborate this explanation. They studied two women who were heterozygous for both types of G6PD deficiency (A+B) and XRI. In subcloned fibroblast cultures steroid sulfatase activity was tested and the G6PD phenotype was determined by gel electrophoresis. Lower steroid sulfatase activity was found in those clones expressing the G6PD-B phenotype than in those clones expressing the G6PD-A phenotype. From this experiment it can be inferred that the steroid sulfatase gene is expressed differently on the two X chromosomes and does participate in part in X inactivation. In human beings, noninactivation of the steroid-sulfatase locus has also been verified by showing the expression of steroid sulfatase from isolated inactive X chromosomes in mouse-human hybrid cells [55].

The escape from X inactivation has aroused considerable interest in the steroid-sulfatase locus and may be an intrinsic feature of the gene. Normally, autosomal sequences attached to an X chromosome become inactivated, whereas steroid sulfatase even when flanked on either side by inactive X-chromosomal DNA, continues to be expressed [56]. The biochemical events leading to X inactivation are not yet known, but DNA methylation has been implicated in maintaining the inactivated state.

2.2.6.2 Regional Mapping of the Steroid Sulfatase Gene on the Human X Chromosome

Linkage studies done in the 1960s showed that the gene locus for XRI was in close vicinity to the locus for the blood group Xg [2, 32, 98]. A more precise localization of the steroid sulfatase gene became possible with the study of mouse-human cell hybrids. Using this tedious technique, in which a panel of defined structural X-chromosome aberrations is screened in human-mouse cell hybrids for steroid sulfatase activity, the steroid sulfatase gene could be assigned to the distal part of the X chromosome [54, 58]. An even more precise mapping became possible with the study of families in which an X-Y translocation resulted in loss of the steroid sulfatase gene and thus gave rise to the phenotype of XRI [59, 80]. Biochemical studies of such patients and of patients with a loss of Xp223-pter [14, 69] allowed assignment of the steroid sulfatase gene to the terminal part of the short arm of the X chromosome at Xp223.

Steroid-sulfatase deficiency can also occur in mice. At first, steroid-sulfatase deficiency in mice was believed to be inherited as a recessive trait, but Keitges et al. [31] recently demonstrated that the steroid sulfatase gene in mice is transmitted to XO offspring via the X chromosome and that the gene behaves as a pseudoautosomal trait due to the frequent crossovers between the X and the Y chromosomes. In human beings the steroid sulfatase gene is apparently located just below the pseudoautosomal region on the telomeric part of the X chromosome. This pseudoautosomal region is characterized by a frequent interchange between the X and the Y chromosomes.

2.2.6.3 Molecular aspects of the Steroid Sulfatase Gene

Very recently, several groups [6, 11, 103] were able to clone the steroid sulfatase gene and to prepare cDNA containing the entire coding sequence which could be isolated, sequenced, and expressed in autologous cells. This is a tremendous advance in our understanding of the molecular biology of steroid-sulfatase deficiency. Based on the work of Yen et al. [103], the following can be stated: The steroid-sulfatase locus appears to be large (greater than 80 kb). There are some nonfunctional steroid sulfatase-related sequences on the long arm of the Y chromosome. This is interpreted as very recent pericentric inversion with a relocation of steroid sulfatase sequences to the Y long arm. Most surprisingly, of ten patients with inherited steroid-sulfatase deficiency eight had complete gene deletions. The high incidence of deletions may explain why in several patients with steroid-sulfatase deficiency an immunologically cross-reacting protein could not be found [16]. With respect to the localization of the steroid sulfatase gene just below the pseudoautosomal region, it is likely that in many cases these deletions are caused by aberrant X-Y interchange. Aberrant X-Y interchange may occur more often than previously thought and has recently also been implicated in the pathogenesis of human XX males [65].

2.2.7 Genetic Counseling

The disease does not pose a threat to general health, but will be present throughout life and may result in some cosmetic disfigurement. Prenatal diagnosis of XRI is possible [23, 24, 78], but because the gene defect is rather mild, it should not be offered to patients with simple steroid-sulfatase deficiency. The situation is different in patients with associated symptoms who may suffer from a wide spectrum of clinical defects (hypogonadism, anosmia, mental retardation, short stature, chondrodysplasia, etc.). With the exception of cryptorchidism, all other associated diseases are rare. In our experience, cyptorchidism need not be present in all affected members of a given family; therefore, all families should be advised about this problem in order to ensure normal sexual development. From a practical point of view, even identification of heterozygous carriers by steroid sulfatase testing puts a psychological burden on these women, who now know in advance that they may have affected offspring. Therefore, carrier testing should be offered only if asked for. The occurence of both types of ichthyosis vulgaris (ADI and XRI) segregating in the same family has been reported twice [47, 83]. Given the high incidence of ADI in the general population, the concomitant presence of ADI and XRI is merely coincidental, but it may be a diagnostic problem.

References

1. Abe K, Matsuda I, Murayama T, Uzuki K, Endo M, Miyakoshi M, Okuno A (1976) X-linked ichthyosis, bilateral cryptochidism, hypogenitalism and mental retardation in two Siblings. Clin Genet 9:341–345
2. Adam A, Ziprkowski L, Feinstein A, Sanger R, Tippett P, Gavin J, Race RR (1969) Linkage relations of X-borne ichthyosis to the Xg blood groups. Ann Hum Genet 32:323–332
3. Andria G, Ballabio A, Parenti G, DiMaio S, Piccirillo A (1984) Steroid sulfatase deficiency and hypogonadism. Eur J Pediatr 142:304–305
4. Anton-Lamprecht I (1974) Zur Ultrastruktur hereditärer Verhornungsstörungen. IV. X-chromosomal-recessive Ichthyosis. Arch Dermatol Forsch 248:361–378
5. Anton-Lamprecht I, Hofbauer M (1972) Ultrastructural distinction of autosomal dominant ichthyosis vulgaris and X-linked recessive ichthyosis. Hum Genet 15:261–264
6. Ballabio A, Parenti G, Carrozzo R, Sebastio G, Andria G, Buckle V, Fraser N, Graig I, Rocchi M, Romeo G, Jobsis AC, Persico MG (1987) Isolation and characterization of a steroid sulfatase cDNA clone: genomic deletions in patients with X-chromosome-linked ichthyosis. Proc Natl Acad Sci USA 84:4519–4523
7. Bazex A, Bazex J, Gauthier Y, Surlève-Bazeille JE (1978) Ichthyose noire récessive liée au sexe. Étude clinique, examen en microscopie optique et microscopie électronique. Ann Dermatol Venereol 105:753–756
8. Bedin M, Weil D, Fournier T, Cedard L, Frezal J (1981) Biochemical evidence for the non-inactivation of the steroid sulfatase locus in human placenta and fibroblasts. Hum Genet 59:256–258
9. Blanchet-Bardon C, Bernheim A, Struz P, Passe P, Puissant A (1981) Syndrome olfacto-génital de Morsier avec ichthyose liée au sexe. Ann Dermatol Venerol (Paris) 108:605
10. Bleau G, Bodley FH, Longpré J, Chapdelaine A, Roberts KDC (1974) Cholesterol sulfate. I. Occurrence and possible biological function as an amphipatic lipid in the membrane of the human erythrocyte. Biochem Biophys Acta 352:1–9
11. Bonifas JM, Morley BJ, Oakey RE, Kan YW, Epstein EH Jr (1987) Cloning of a cDNA for steroid sulfatase: frequent occurrence of gene deletions in patients with recessive X-chromosome-linked ichthyosis. Proc Natl Acad Sci USA 84:9248–9251
12. Conary J, Nauerth A, Burns G, Hasilik A, von Figura K (1986) Steroid sulfatase. Biosynthesis and processing in normal and mutant fibroblasts. Eur J Biochem 158:71–76
13. Csörsz K (1928) Recessiv geschlechtsgebundene Vererbung bei Ichthyosis. Monatsschr Ungarischer Mediziner 2:180–187
14. Curry CJR, Magenis RE, Brown M, Lanman JT jr, Tsai J, O'Lague P, Goodfellow P. Mohandas T, Berner EA, Shapiro LJ (1984) Inherited chondrodysplasia punctata due to a deletion of the terminal short arm of an X chromosome. New Engl J Med 311:1010–1015
15. De Groot WP, Jobsis AC, Marinkovic-Ilsen A, Koppe JG, De Bruijn HWA (1980) Sex-linked ichthyosis and placental sulfatase-C deficiency. Br J Dermatol 103:73–79
16. Epstein EH Jr, Bonifas JM (1985) Recessive X-linked ichthyosis: lack of immunologically detectable steroid sulfatase enzyme protein. Hum Genet 71:201–205
17. Epstein EH, Krauss RM, Shackleton CHL (1981) X-linked ichthyosis: increased blood cholesterol sulfate and electrophoretic mobility of low-density lipoprotein. Science 214:659–660
18. Feinstein A, Ackermann AB, Ziprkowski L (1970) Histology of autosomal dominant ichthyosis vulgaris and X-linked ichthyosis. Arch Dermatol 101:524–527
19. France JT, Liggins GC (1969) Placental sulfatase deficiency. J Clin Endocrinol Metab 28:138–141
20. Geiger W (1976) Schwangerschaft. In: Deck KA (ed) Endokrinologie. Thieme, Stuttgart, pp 215–233
21. Giovangrandi Y, Magnin G, Sauvanet E, Soutoul JH, Cedard L, Bedin M, Moraine C, Nottin P. Hamard G (1984) Fault-il encore explorer les déficits en sulfatase placentaire? Réflexions a propos d'une observation. Rev Fr Gynecol Obstet 79:653–657
22. Grala PE (1985) Corneal changes in X-linked ichthyosis. J Am Optom Assoc 56:315–317
23. Grimm U, Herrmann FH, Machill G, Knoll W, Schütz M (1988) Zur pränatalen Diagnostik

bei X-chromosomal rezessiver Ichthyosis in unkultiviertem Choriongewebe. Dermatol Monatsschr 174:103-105
24. Hähnel R, Hähnel E, Wysocki SJ, Wilkinson SP, Hockey A (1982) Prenatal diagnosis of X-linked ichthyosis. Clin Chim Acta 120:143-152
25. Hammerstein W, Haensch R (1978) Die Differentialdiagnose der ophthalmologischen Befunde bei verschiedenen Formen der Ichthyosis. Fortschr Med 96:245-251
26. Hashimoto I, Tasaki M, Chiyoya S, Sato S, Nomura K, Onuma T, Kimura T (1982) Differentiation between X-linked ichthyosis and ichthyosis vulgaris with electrophoretic mobility rate of beta-lipoprotein. Med Genet Res (Jpn) 4:80-83
27. Hofbauer M, Schnyder UW (1974) Zur Differentialdiagnose von autosomal-dominanter Ichthyosis vulgaris und X-chromosomaler Ichthyose. Hautarzt 25:319-325
28. Høyer H, Lykkesfeldt G, Ibsen HH, Brandrup F (1986) Ichthyosis of steroid sulphatase deficiency. Clinical study of 76 cases. Dermatologica 172:184-190
29. Ibsen HH, Brandrup F, Blaabjerg O, Lykkesfeldt G (1986) Lipoprotein electrophoresis in recessive X-linked ichthyosis. Acta Dermatol Venereol 66:59-62
30. Jöbsis AC, van Duuren Chr Y, van de Vries GP, Koppe JG, Rijken Y, van Kempen GMJ, de Groot WP (1976) Throphoblast sulphatase deficiency associated with X-chromosomal ichthyosis. Ned Tijdschr Geneeskd 120:1980
31. Keitges E, Rivest M, Siniscalco M, Gartler SM (1985) X-linkage of steroid sulphatase in the mouse is evidence for a functional Y-linked allele. Nature 315:226-227
32. Kerr CB, Wells RS, Sanger R (1964) X-linked ichthyosis and the Xg groups. Lancet 2:1369-1370
33. Koppe JG, Marinkovic-Ilsen A, Rijken Y, De Groot WP, Jöbsis AC (1978) X-linked ichthyosis. A sulphatase deficiency. Arch Dis Child 53:803-806
34. Kubilus J, Tarascio AJ, Baden HP (1979) Steroid-sulfatase deficiency in sex-linked ichthyosis. Am J Hum Genet 31:50-53
35. Lundborg H (1927) Geschlechtsgebundene Vererbung von Ichthyosis simplex (vulgaris) in einer schwedischen Bauernsippe. Hereditas 8:45-48
36. Lykkesfeldt G, Høyer H (1983) Topical cholesterol treatment of recessive X-linked ichthyosis. Lancet 2:1337-1338
37. Lykkesfeldt G, Nielsen MD, Lykkesfeldt AE (1984) Placental steroid sulfatase deficiency: biochemical diagnosis and clinical review. Obstet Gynecol 64:49-54
38. Lykkesfeldt G, Lykkesfeldt AE, Skakkebaek NE (1984) Steroid sulphatase in man: a non-inactivated X-locus with partial gene dosage compensation. Hum Genet 65:355-357
39. Lykkesfeldt G, Høyer H, Ibsen HH, Brandrup F (1985) Steroid sulphatase deficiency disease. Clin Genet 28:231-237
40. Lynch HT, Ozer F, McNutt CW, Johnson JE, Jampolsky NA (1960) Secondary male hypogonadism and congenital ichthyosis: association of two rare genetic diseases. Am J Hum Genet 12:440-447
41. Lyon MF (1961) Gene action in the X-chromosome of the mouse (Mus musculus L). Nature 190:372-373
42. Maloney ME, Williams ML, Epstein EH Jr, Law MYL, Fritsch PO, Elisas PM (1984) Lipids in the pathogenesis of ichthyosis: topical cholesterol sulfate-induced scaling in hairless mice. J Invest Dermatol 83:252-256
43. McKee JWA, Abeysekera R, France JT (1981) Studies on the biochemical basis of steroid sulfatase deficiency. II. A finding of decreased phospholipid content in sulfatase-deficient placental microsomes. J Steroid Biochem 14:195-198
44. McNaught RW, France JT (1980) Studies on the biochemical basis of steroid sulfatase deficiency: preliminary evidence suggesting a defect in membrane-enzyme structure. J Steroid Biochem 13:363-373
45. Marinkovic-Ilsen A (1983) Placental sulfatase deficiency and recessive X-linked ichthyosis. Dissertation University of Amsterdam (Krips regio meppel Amsterdam 1983)
46. Metaxotou C, Ikkos D, Panagiotopoulous P, Mavrou A, Tsenghi C, Matsaniotis N (1983) A familial X/Y translocation in a boy with ichthyosis, hypogonadism and mental retardation. Clin Genet 23:239
47. Mevorah B, Frenk E, Pescia G (1978) Ichthyosis vulgaris showing features of the autosomal dominant and X-linked recessive variants in the same family. Clin Genet 13:462-470

48. Mevorah B, Frenk E, Müller CR, Ropers HH (1981) X-linked recessive ichthyosis in three sisters: evidence for homozygosity. Br J Dermatol 105:711–717
49. Meyer JC, Schnyder UW (1982) Mikrosomaler Sulfatasemangel bei X-chromosomaler Ichthyose. Hautarzt 33:82–88
50. Meyer JC, Gilardi S (1986) Biochemische Diagnose der X-chromosomalen Ichthyose. Hautarzt 37:205–209
51. Meyer JC, Groh V, Giger H, Weiss H, Varbelow H, Schnyder UW (1982) Rapid laboratory diagnostic of X-linked ichthyosis. Dermatologica 164:249–257
52. Meyer JC, Gilardi S, Sigg C, Bruckner-Tudermann L (1986) Intermediate levels of arylsulfatase C in human leukocytes of female carriers for X-linked recessive ichthyosis. Arch Dermatol Res 278:491–493
53. Migeon BR, Shapiro LJ, Norum RA, Mohandas T, Axelman J, Dabora RL (1982) Differential expression of steroid sulphatase locus on active and inactive human X chromosome. Nature 299:838–840
54. Mohandas T, Shapiro LJ, Sparkes RS, Sparkes MC (1979) Regional assignment of the steroid sulfatase-X-linked ichthyosis locus: implications for a noninactivated region on the short arm of human X chromosome. Proc Natl Acad Sci USA 76:5779–5783
55. Mohandas T, Sparkes RS, Hellkuhl B, Grzeschik KH, Shapiro LJ (1980) Expression of an X-linked gene from an inactive human X chromosome in mouse-human hybrid cells: further evidence for the noninactivation of the steroid sulfatase locus in man. Proc Natl Acad Sci USA 77:6759–6763
56. Mohandas T, Geller RL, Yen PH, Rosendorff J, Bernstein R, Yoshida A, Shapiro LJ (1987) Cytogenetic and molecular studies on a recombinant human X chromosome: implications for the spreading of X-chromosome inactivation. Proc Natl Acad Sci USA 84:4954–4958
57. Müller CR, Migl B, Traupe H, Ropers HH (1980) X-linked steroid sulfatase: evidence for different gene-dosage in males and females. Hum Genet 54:197–199
58. Müller CR, Westerveld A, Migl B, Franke W, Ropers HH (1980) Regional assignment of the gene locus for steroid sulfatase. Hum Genet 54:201–204
59. Müller CR, Wahlström J, Ropers HH (1981) Further evidence for the assignment of the steroid sulfatase X-linked ichthyosis locus to the telomer of Xp. Hum Genet 58:446
60. Münke M, Kruse K, Goos M, Ropers HH, Tolksdorf M (1983) Genetic heterogeneity of the ichthyosis, hypogonadism, mental retardation, and epilepsy syndrome. Clinical and biochemical investigations on two patients with Rud syndrome and review of the literature. Eur J Pediatr 141:8–13
61. Orel H (1929) Die Vererbung der Ichthyosis congenita und der Ichthyosis vulgaris. Kleine Beiträge zur Vererbungswissenschaft. V. Mitteilung. Z Kinderheilkd 47:312–340
62. Payne AH, Jaffe RB, Abell MR (1971) Gonadal steroid sulfates and sulfatase. III. Correlation of human testicular sulfatase, 3β-hydroxysteroid dehydrogenase-isomerase, histologic structure and serum testosterone. J Clin Endocrinol 33:582–591
63. Perrin JCS, Idemoto TY, Sotos JF, Maurer WF, Steinberg AG (1976) X-linked syndrome of congenital, ichthyosis, hypogonadism, mental retardation and anosmia. Birth Defects XII (5):267–274
64. Perrot H, Ortonne JP (1979) Ichthyosis nigricans: ultrastructural study of the melanin pigmentary disturbances. Arch Dermatol Res 265:123–131
65. Petit C, De la Chapelle A, Levilliers J, Castillo S, Nöel B, Weissenbach J (1987) An abnormal terminal X-Y interchange accounts for most but not all cases of human XX maleness. Cell 49:595–602
66. Ponec M, Williams ML (1986) Cholesterol sulfate uptake and outflux in cultured human keratinocytes. Arch Dermatol Res 279:32–36
67. Rayer P (1835) Traité theorique et pratique des maladies de la peau, vol 3. Baillière, Paris
68. Ropers HH, Migl B, Zimmer J, Fraccaro M, Maraschio PP, Westerveld A (1981) Activity of steroid sulfatase in fibroblasts with numerical and structural X-chromosome aberrations. Hum Genet 57:354–356
69. Ross JB, Allderdice PW, Shapiro LJ, Aveling J, Eales BA, Simms D jr (1985) Familial X-linked ichthyosis, steroid sulfatase deficiency, mental retardation, and nullisomy for Xp223-pter. Arch Dermatol 121:1524–1528
70. Ruokonen A, Oikarinen A, Vihko R (1986) Regulation of serum testosterone in men with

steroid sulfatase deficiency: response to human chorionic gonadotropin. J Steroid Biochem 25:113–119
71. Schlammadinger J, Meyer JC, Vajda I, Szabó G (1987) X-linked recessive ichthyosis. Reinvestigation of a family first described in 1928. Dermatologica 175:217–223
72. Sever RJ, Frost P, Weinstein G (1968) Eye changes in ichthyosis. JAMA 206:2283–2286
73. Shapiro LJ, Weiss R, Webster D, France JT (1978) X-linked ichthyosis due to steroid-sulphatase deficiency. Lancet 1:70–72
74. Shapiro LJ, Mohandas T, Weiss R, Romeo G (1979) Noninactivation of an X-chromosome locus in man. Science 204:1224–1226
75. Simard JP, Ameen M, Chang PL (1985) Biochemical characterization of arylsulfatase-C isozymes in human fibroblasts. Biochem Biophys Res Commun 128:1388–1394
76. Steuhl KP, Anton-Lamprecht I, Arnold ML, Thiel HJ (1988) Recurrent bilateral corneal erosions due to an association of epidermolysis bullosa simplex Köbner and X-linked ichthyosis with steroid-sulfatase deficiency. Graefe's Arch Clin Exp Ophthalmol 226:216–233
77. Sybert VP, Dale BA, Holbrook KA (1985) Ichthyosis vulgaris: identification of a defect in synthesis of filaggrin correlated with an absence of keratohyalin granules. J Invest Dermatol 84:191–194
78. Taylor NF, Shackleton HL (1979) Gas-chromatographic steroid analysis for diagnosis of placental sulfatase deficiency: a study of nine patients. J Clin Endocrinol Metab 49:78–86
79. Taylor NF (1982) Review: placental sulphatase deficiency. J Inherited Metab Dis 5:164–176
80. Tiepolo L, Zuffardi O, Fraccaro M, di Natale D, Gargantini L, Müller CR, Ropers HH (1980) Assignment by deletion mapping of the steroid sulfatase X-linked ichthyosis locus to Xp223. Hum Genet 54:205–206
81. Traupe H, Happle R (1983) Clinical spectrum of steroid sulfatase deficiency: X-linked recessive ichthyosis, birth complications and cryptorchidism. Eur J Pediatr 140:19–21
82. Traupe H, Happle R (1986) Mechanisms in the association of cryptorchidism and X-linked recessive ichthyosis. Dermatologica 172:327–328
83. Traupe H, Happle R, Ropers HH, Müller CR (1981) X-linked recessive ichthyosis and autosomal dominant ichthyosis segregating in the same family. Arch Dermatol Res 271:149–156
84. Traupe H, Kövary PM, Schriewer H (1983) X-linked recessive ichthyosis vulgaris: rapid identification by lipoprotein electrophoresis. Arch Dermatol Res 275:63–65
85. Traupe H, Müller-Migl CR, Kolde G, Happle R, Kövary PM, Hameister H, Ropers HH (1984) Ichthyosis vulgaris with hypogenitalism and hypogonadism: evidence for different genotypes by lipoprotein electrophoresis and steroid-sulfatase testing. Clin Genet 25:42–51
86. Unamuno P De, Martin-Pascual A, Garcia-Perez A (1977) X-linked ichthyosis. Br J Dermatol 97:53–58
87. Unamuno P, Martin C, Fernandez E (1986) X-linked ichthyosis and cryptorchidism. Dermatologica 172:326–327
88. van der Loos CM, van Breda AJ, Meijer AEFH, Jöbsis AC (1981) Biochemical investigation to the reliability of the histochemical demonstration of microsomal arylsulfatase activity in cryostat sections. Histochem 73:161–164
89. Vibrans U, Altwein JE (1970) An X-linked recessive variety of ichthyosis vulgaris different from the X-linked ichthyosis of Wells and Kerr. Clin Genet 1:304–309
90. Vihko R, Ruokonen A (1975) Steroid sulphates in human adult testicular steroid synthesis. J Steroid Biochem 6:353–356
91. Voß M (1985) Das klinische Bild der X-chromosomal-rezessiven Ichthyose. Dermatol Monatsschr 171:25–37
92. Voß M, Jünemann R (1986) Ophthalmologische Befunde bei X-chromosomal-rezessiver Ichthyose. Dermatol Monatsschr 172:209–211
93. Wells RS, Kerr CB (1966) Clinical features of autosomal dominant and sex-linked ichthyosis in an English population. Br Med J 1:947–950
94. Wells RS, Kerr CB (1966) The histology of ichthyosis. J Invest Dermatol 46:530–535

95. Wells RS (1966) Sex-linked ichthyosis, oligophrenia and hypogonadism. Br J Dermatol 78:308
96. Wells RS (1966) Sex-linked ichthyosis and oligophrenia. Br J Dermatol 78:309
97. Wells RS, Jennings MC (1967) X-linked ichthyosis and ichthyosis vulgaris. Clinical and genetic distinctions in a second series of families. JAMA 202:485–488
98. Went LN, de Groot WP, Sanger R, Tipett P, Gavin J (1969) X-linked ichthyosis: linkage relationship with the Xg blood groups and other studies in a large Dutch kindred. Ann Hum Genet 32:333–345
99. Williams ML (1986) A new look at the ichthyoses: disorders of lipid metabolism. Pediatr Dermatol 3:476–497
100. Williams ML, Elisas PM (1981) Stratum corneum lipids in disorders of cornification. Increased cholesterol sulfate content of stratum corneum in recessive X-linked ichthyosis. J Clin Invest 68:1404–1410
101. Williams ML, Hughes-Fulford M, Elias PM (1985) Inhibition of 3-hydroxy-3-methylglutaryl coenzyme A reducatase activity and sterol synthesis by cholesterol sulfate in cultured fibroblasts. Biochim Biophys Acta 845:349–357
102. Williams ML, Feingold KR, Grubauer G, Elias PM (1987) Ichthyosis induced by cholesterol-lowering drugs. Implications for epidermal cholesterol homeostasis. Arch Dermatol 123:1535–1538
103. Yen PH, Allen E, Marsh B, Mohandas T, Wang N, Taggart RT, Shapiro LJ (1987) Cloning and expression of steroid sulfatase cDNA and frequent occurrence of deletions in STS deficiency: implications for X-Y interchange. Cell 49:443–454
104. York-Moore ME, Rundle AT (1962) Rud's syndrome. J Ment Defic Res 6:108–117
105. Yoshiike T, Matsui T, Kimura T, Yamada H, Ogawa H (1985) The effect of steroid sulphatase on stratum corneum shedding in patients with X-linked ichthyosis. Br J Dermatol 113:641–643
106. Ziprkowski L, Feinstein A (1972) A survey of ichthyosis vulgaris in Israel. Br J Dermatol 86:1–8

3 Associated Ichthyoses of the Vulgaris Type

3.1 Refsum's Syndrome (Heredopathia Atactica Polyneuritiformis)

3.1.1 Historical Aspects

Refsum's syndrome is an autosomal recessive disorder that was first described under the name heredopathia atactica polyneuritiformis (HAP) by the Norwegian neurologist Sigvald Refsum in the years 1944–1946 [12]. Phytanic acid accumulation was identified in Refsum's disease by Klenk and Kahlke [8] more than 20 years ago and has since then been used as a diagnostic criterion. Prior to their publication, phytanic acid had been identified neither in plant nor in animal tissue. Recently, an infantile type was separated from the classical adult-onset type. This infantile type is characterized by a deficiency of catalase-containing particles (peroxisomes) [10, 14]. Infantile Refsum's syndrome does not seem to be associated with skin symptoms [10] and therefore will not be discussed in detail. Interestingly, it is a link to other peroxisomal diseases such as the cerebro-hepato-renal (Zellweger) syndrome, the rhizomelic type of chondrodysplasia puntata, and neonatal adrenoleukodystrophy. In all these conditions storage of phytanic acid can be detected [10, 14] and they share the defective alpha-oxidation capacity of phytanic acid.

3.1.2 General Clinical Features

In a few patients the condition begins in the first years of life. In most cases, however, there is a slow but continual evolution of the disease, with the onset well after puberty. HAP is characterized by numerous ophthalmologic, neurologic, otorhinological, and cardiological findings (Table 19) [13]. Its cutaneous manifestations are rather mild – at least in the beginning – and therefore the dermatologist usually is not the first physician consulted. Failing night vision and unsteadiness of gait [13] are often the first complaints. In late, prefinal stages, generalized wasting, severe paralysis, and severe skin symptoms can be seen [3]. At least nine cases with a fatal outcome have been recorded [3, 13]. The high mortality in late (usually undiagnosed and untreated) stages may be due to cardiological complications, mainly arrhythmia resulting from a block of AV and HIS bundle-branch conduction.

The protean course the disease may take, with periods of spontaneous improvement and inevitable deterioration, is obviously one of the reasons why a correct diagnosis is missed in many patients for a long time. Moreover, physicians from various specialties are usually involved. They may be unaware of the other

Table 19. Clinical features of heredopathia atactica polyneuritiformis (Refsum's disease)

Eye	Ear and nose	Nerves	Heart	Skin
Failing night vision Retinitis pigmentosa Constriction of visual fields	Anosmia Neurosensory deafness	Peripheral neuropathy Diminished deep tendon reflexes Cerebellar ataxia Intention tremor High cerebrospinal fluid protein	Nonspecific EEC changes Impaired AV conduction Bundle-branch block	Scaly skin mimicking ADI Accentuated palmar creases Dermal nevus cell nevi, presenting as yellowish papules

problems their patient has or blinded by the narrow section of complaints they care for.

Case History

This situation is well illustrated by the fate of a 39-year-old woman. It was 20 years after her first symptoms that the correct diagnosis of HAP was established by H. Feldmann, of Münster. A detailed report emphasizing the hearing loss has been published elsewhere [6]. At the age of 18 years she slowly developed night blindness, and at 25 she was involved in a car accident because of this. A diagnosis of retinitis pigmentosa and of bilateral cataracts was established. Four years later she was operated on because of the cataracts, and contact lenses were prescribed. At the same time beginning ataxia was noted. A lumbar puncture revealed high protein levels in the cerebrospinal fluid without pleocytosis. A brain tumor was suspected and the patient underwent neurosurgery the same year. No tumor could be found.

When she was 29 years old her skin became scaly. The patient consulted a dermatologist, who took a biopsy and entertained the diagnosis of ichthyosis vulgaris. When she was 36 years old a bilateral hearing loss was diagnosed and a hearing aid prescribed. Three years later, the almost blind patient presented for the first time at the department of otorhinology, University of Münster, where the definite diagnosis was finally made and confirmed biochemically by marked elevation of phytanic acid [6].

3.1.3 Cutaneous Manifestations

Though more than 50% of all patients affected with classical HAP exhibit an ichthyosis, there are only a few detailed reports dealing with the skin [1–5, 11]. My personal experience is confined to the case of a young boy suffering from the infantile type and showing no cutaneous symptoms at all, and to the above-mentioned 39-year-old woman with classical Refsum's disease.

Usually, the cutaneous involvement does not seem to be very marked and the condition mimics ichthyosis vulgaris (ADI). Scales are fair and light (Fig. 21),

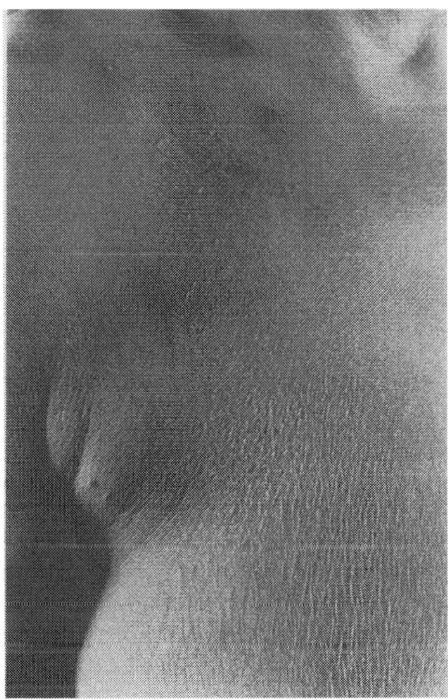

Fig. 21. Refsum's syndrome. Light and fair scaling with a wrinkled appearance of the skin

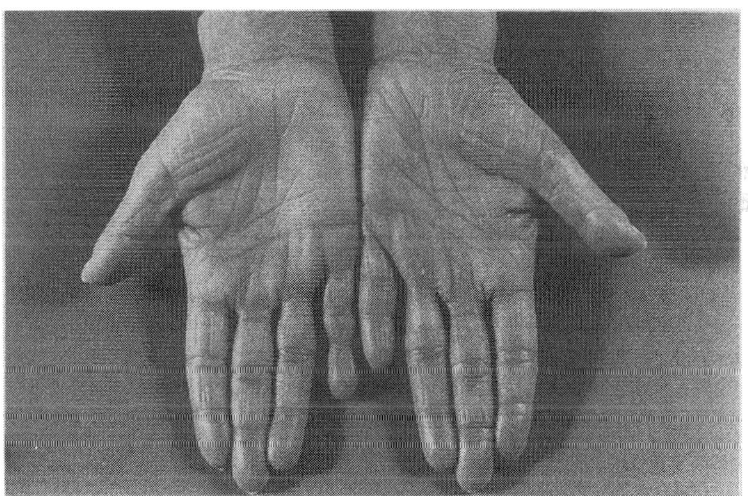

Fig. 22. Refsum's syndrome. Accentuated palmar creases. Note striking similarity to palmar involvement in ADI

sparing the big flexures, palms, and soles. The hyperkeratoses may give the skin a wrinkled appearance similar to exsiccation eczema. In my experience, even palmar creases can be accentuated (Fig. 22). Davies et al. [3] reported on a very severely affected patient with coarse, large hyperkeratoses for whom the diagnosis was established only a few weeks prior to death. Obviously, the severity of the cutaneous involvement can vary. It seems to correlate with the overall status of the disease, probably reflecting the extent of phytanic acid accumulation.

Puissant et al. [11] drew attention to the occurrence of peculiar disseminated dermal nevus cell nevi, which we observed in our patient, too. Clinically, these nevi have the appearance of yellowish papules and are rather inconspicuous. Histologic examination of these lesions may give an important clue for a correct diagnosis.

3.1.4 Histologic and Ultrastructural Findings

Routine hematoxylin-and-eosin-stained sections usually show a dimished granular layer, a normal epidermis, and slight orthohyperkertosis [1, 2]. In one case an increased granular layer has been reported [3]. If only routine histology is carried out, it may contribute to a misdiagnosis of ichthyosis vulgaris. Lipid stains such as Sudan red reveal vacuolated keratinocytes containing multiple lipid droplets in the basal and suprabasal cells of the epidermis (Fig. 23). Apparently, the dermal nevus cell nevi preferentially store phytanic acids, and vacuolated cells can also be found in such dermal nevi. Staining with Sudan red will disclose marked lipid droplets in these nevus cells, too.

The results of electron microscopy are ambiguous as far as the size of the

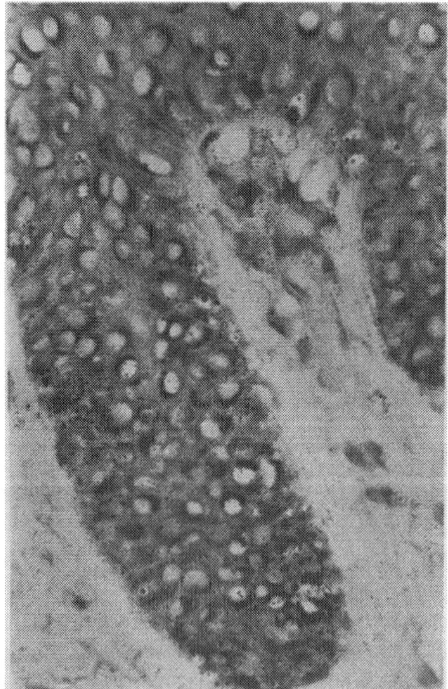

Fig. 23. Refsum's syndrome. The keratinocytes appear vacuolated and contain multiple lipid droplets. Sudan red, ×100

granular layer is concerned. Two studies indicate a reduction of the granular layer and a decreased amount of structurally normal keratohyalin [1, 2]. In contrast, the patient reported on by Davies et al. [3] had a markedly increased granular layer. On electron microscopy, lipid droplets can be seen in the cytoplasm of the keratinocytes and melanocytes. These lipid droplets often show a close proximity to the endoplasmic reticulum and to abnormal or giant degenerated mitochondria (Fig. 24). These giant degenerate mitochondria are a characteristic ultrastructural feature of HAP. They have a poorly developed internal membrane system and a matrix of poor contrast [1, 2]. Using all ultrastructural criteria available electron microscopy permits unequivocal distinction of HAP from ADI.

Labeling studies suprisingly showed an increased epidermal cell turnover [5] in one patient. According to these data, HAP would have to be regarded as a hyperproliferation hyperkeratosis. Electron-microscopic studies do not support this view, and it should be kept in mind that the histologic and ultrastructural features of this prefinal patient studied [3–5] were quite different from those seen in other cases.

3.1.5 Biochemical Aspects

Accumulation of phytanic acid in various tissues is the biochemical hallmark of HAP [8]. Phytanic acid cannot be synthesized by the human body and is entirely exogeneous. Therefore, a dietary therapy is possible. Though human beings do

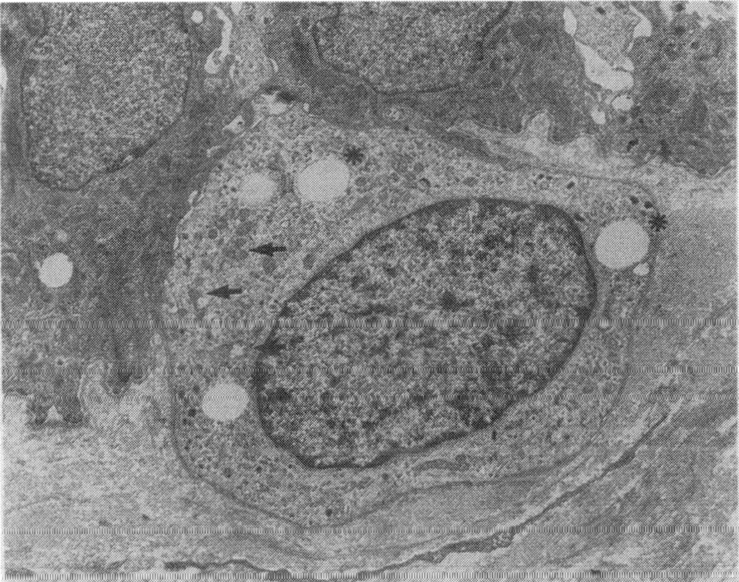

Fig. 24. Refsum's syndrome. Electron micrograph of a melanocyte with typical multiple cytoplasmic lipid inclusions *(asterisks)*. Note enlarged and degenerated mitochondria *(arrows)*. ×6100. (Courtesy of Dr. G. Kolde, Münster)

not produce phytanic acid on their own, they are usually able to degrade it by alpha-oxidation. Steinberg and co-workers showed that this alpha-oxidation is deficient in HAP and that conversion of phytanic acid to hydroxyphytanic acid is disturbed (phytanic acid oxidase deficiency, reviewed in Steinberg [13].

As far as a pathophysiologic explanation for the cutaneous manifestation is concerned, two different theories have been advanced. Blanchet-Bardon et al. [2] argue that considerable amounts of free cholesterol are esterified by phytanic acid and stored in the lipid droplets. The decrease of free epidermal cholesterol would result in a disturbed cholsterol/cholesterol-sulfate ratio, and thus the pathophysiologic pathway may be similar to that of XRI. Davies et al. [4] emphasize that phytanic acid substitutes for essential fatty acids in all lipid subfractions, especially in phospholipids. They assume that due to the incorporation of phytanic acid these altered epidermal lipids can no longer be degraded. Moreover, they found a striking reduction in linoleic acid content, from a mean of 30.6% in the controls to 5.4% in their patient. Therefore, they suggest that scaling in HAP may share a common pathogenesis with essential fatty-acid deficiency (see also Sect. 1.4).

3.1.6 Therapy

Prior to the elucidation of the basic biochemical defect, HAP was a life-threatening disease with an often fatal outcome. Therefore, low-phytol or phytol-free diet is a therapeutic breakthrough in the management of these patients. In this diet, dairy products and green vegetables have to be avoided since phytol is a side chain of the chlorophyl molecule and accumulates in dairy products. When such a diet is initiated, great care should be given to supply enough calories to keep the body weight unchanged. The patient we observed lost 5 kg within a few weeks after initiation of the therapy, and her general condition became worse. The reason for this seemingly paradoxical reaction is that the actual serum level of phytanic acid can rise when large amounts of phytanic acid are mobilized from the lipid tissue. Plasmapheresis is the therapy of choice in this situation [7].

3.1.7 Genetic Counseling

Heredopathia atactica polyneuritiformis is a monogenic autosomal recessive disorder. Onset of classical HAP is often late. Hence, questions like that of prenatal diagnosis may not become relevant, the parents of the affected patients no longer being in the reproductive age. Nevertheless, the enzyme is expressed in amnion cells and prenatal diagnosis is therefore possible [9]. Of course, a specialized center performing the actual enzyme test has to be found and consulted in advance. The same is true for heterozygote testing. As far as infantile HAP is concerned, an ultrastructural approach (looking for the absence or presence of peroxisomes) may be more feasible for prenatal diagnosis in many centers. Despite the new therapeutic modalities, HAP is still a severe handicap, warranting termination of a pregancy if it is desired by the parents.

References

1. Anton-Lamprecht I, Kahlke W (1974) Zur Ultrastruktur hereditärer Verhornungsstörungen. V. Ichthyosis beim Refsum-Syndrom (Heredopathia atactica polyneuritiformis). Arch Dermatol Forsch 250:185–206
2. Blanchet-Bardon C, Anton-Lamprecht I, Puissant A, Schnyder UW (1978) Ultrastructural features of ichthyotic skin in Refsum's syndrome. In: Marks H, Dykes PJ (eds) The ichthyoses. MTP Press, Lancaster, pp 65–69
3. Davies MG, Marks R, Dykes PJ, Reynolds D (1977) Epidermal abnormalities in Refsum's disease. Br J Dermatol 97:401–406
4. Davies MG, Reynolds DJ, Marks R, Dykes PJ (1978) The epidermis in Refsum's disease (heredopathia atactica polyneuritiformis). In: Marks H, Dykes PJ (eds) The ichthyoses. MTP Press, Lancaster, pp 51–64
5. Dykes PJ, Marks R, Davies MG, Reynolds DJ (1978) Epidermal metabolism in heredopathia atactica polyneuritiformis (Refsum's disease). J Invest Dermatol 70:126–129
6. Feldmann H (1981) Refsum-Syndrom. Heredopathia atactica polyneuritiformis in der Sicht des HNO-Arztes. Laryngol Rhinol Otol Ihre Grenzgeb (Stuttg) 60:235–240
7. Gibberd FB, Billimoria JD, Page NGR, Retsas S (1979) Heredopathia atactica polyneuritiformis (Refsum's disease) treated by diet and plasma exchange. Lancet 1:575–578
8. Klenk E, Kahlke W (1963) Über das Vorkommen der 3,7,11,15-Tetramethylhexadecansäure (Phytansäure) in den Cholesterinestern und anderen Lipoidfraktionen der Organe bei einem Krankheitsfall unbekannter Genese (Verdacht auf Heredopathia atactica polyneuritiformis (Refsum's syndrome). Hoppe Seyler Z Physiol Chem 333:133
9. Poll-The BT, Poulos A, Sharp P. Boue J, Ogier H, Odièvre M, Saudubray JM (1985) Atenatal diagnosis of infantile Refsum's disease. Clin Genet 27:524–526
10. Poll-The BT, Saudubray JM, Ogier HAM, Odièvre M, Scotto JM, Monnens L, Govaerts LCP, Roels F, Cornelis A, Schutgens RBH, Wanders RJA, Schram AW, Tager JM (1987) Infantile Refsum disease: an inherited peroxisomal disorder. Comparison with Zellweger syndrome and neonatal adrenoleukodystrophy. Eur J Pediatr 146:477–483
11. Puissant A, Dry J, Noury JY, Laudat P. Noury-Duperrat G (1972) Syndrome de Refsum-Thiebaut avec naevi xanthomateux disséminés. Bull Soc Franc Dermatol Syph 79:462–464
12. Refsum S (1946) Heredopathia atactica polyneuritiformis. Acta Psychiatr Scand [Suppl] 38:1–303
13. Steinberg D (1978) Phytanic acid storage disease: Refsum's syndrome. In: Stanbury J, Wyngaarden JB, Fredrickson DS (eds) The metabolic basis of inherited disease, 4th edn. McGraw-Hill, New York, pp 688–706
14. Wanders RJ, Schutgens RB, Schrakamp G, van der Bosch H, Tager JM, Schram AW, Hashimoto T, Poll-The BT, Saudubray JM (1986) Infantile Refsum disease: deficiency of catalase-containing particles (peroxisomes), alkyldihydroxyacetone phosphate synthase and peroxisomal beta-oxidation enzyme proteins. Eur J Pediatr 145:172–175

3.2 Associated Steroid-Sulfatase Deficiency

3.2.1 X/Y Translocations and Loss of Xp 223-pter

Occasionally, X-linked recessive ichthyosis is accompanied by other symptoms such as mental retardation, short stature, epilepsy, and severe hypogonadism. Until very recently, these cases were mostly classified under the diagnostic label of the so-called Rud syndrome [16] (see Sect. 3.3) In the past few years it has become apparent that many of these cases can be explained as X/Y-chromosome translocations [1, 15], reviewed in [16]. An X/Y translocation was first described in 1973 by Khudr [8], occurring in a woman who had undergone chromosome analysis on account of repeated miscarriages. Apart from being of short stature, she displayed a normal phenotype. X/Y-translocations are transmitted like mendelian traits. The translocation results in a deletion of genes located on the short arm of the X chromosome at p223. Males are more severely affected than females since they possess one X chromosome only and are unable to compensate for the loss of genes. In addition to short stature, males with an X/Y translocation therefore exhibit further features such as hypogonadism, mental retardation, and X-linked recessive ichthyosis, as discussed above.

X/Y translocations are due to an aberrant X-Y interchange. By the same mechanism the entire terminal short arm of the X chromosome may sometimes be deleted. Two families with total loss of the terminal part of the short arm of an X chromosome have been described, and their clinical features are very similar to those of X/Y translocation [5, 12]. Curry et al. [5] noted that the short stature was accompanied by epiphyseal stippling in infancy and that the condition should therefore be considered a mild form of chondrodysplasia punctata. Very recently, Langenbeck and Kollman [9] reported on a patient who, in addition to XRI and hypogonadism, displayed dyschondroosteosis but lacked signs of chondrodysplasia punctata.

3.2.2 XRI and Kallmann's Syndrome

A number of reports draw attention to the association of Kallmann's syndrome (hypogonadotropic hypogonadism with anosmia) with X-linked recessive ichthyosis [2, 10, 11]. Sunohara et al. [14] recently described a family containing three men affected with XRI, Kallmann's syndrome, and further features commonly found in some Kallmann patients such as nystagmus, mirror movements of the hands and feet, and ophthalmologic alterations. At a recent meeting of the

Dutch Dermatological Society a similar case featuring XRI, Kallmann's syndrome, neurologic alterations, and unilateral renal aplasia was reported [6]. Though an X/Y translocation was not detectable at the cytogenetic level, a deletion on the X chromosome could be demonstrated in this and other cases by the recently chracterized steroid sulfatase cDNA probe [3, 6, 17]. The complex syndromes in which X-linked recessive ichthyosis is an easy identifiable component help us to identify the genes located on the short arm of the X chromosome. From the foregoing it can be concluded that the Kallmann gene can be assigned to Xp223 [3, 16, 17].

3.2.3 XRI and Hypertrophic Pyloric Stenosis: Possible Implications for the Carter Effect

In two families the simultaneous occurrence of hypertrophic pyloric stenosis and X-linked recessive ichthyosis was observed [7, 13]. In the two families, altogether five patients showed this peculiar association. This raises the question of whether the concept of the Carter effect is still valid for hypertrophic pyloric stenosis. The effect is named after C.O. Carter [4] and is generally accepted among human geneticists as a way to prove polygenic inheritance. Carter [4] tried to explain why hypertrophic pyloric stenosis affects predominantly boys and why among the relatives of affected women the disease is much more common than among relatives of affected men. He suggested that the genetic disposition is the same in both genders, but that the threshold is lower in men than in women. A basic prerequisite of this assumption is that X-linked genes are not involved in the sex ratio observed. The simultaneous occurrence of pyloric stenosis and XRI indicates that this may not be true, but that at least one X-linked predisposition gene probably plays a role in hypertrophic pyloric stenosis.

3.2.4 Genetic Counseling

From the point of view of molecular biology, it can be argued that the distinction between isolated X-linked recessive ichthyosis and associated steroid-sulfatase deficiency is artificial. Both isolated and associated steroid-sulfatase deficiencies are caused by a gene deletion. For the clinician, however, the situation is quite different. Isolated XRI is a frequent disorder seen in one in 2000 male infants. In contrast, associated steroid-sulfatase deficiency is rather uncommon and probably affects not more than 1% of all XRI patients. Genetic counseling of affected families has to be different from that in cases of isolated steroid-sulfatase deficiency and should be guided by the clinical course of the disease in the individual family. It should be kept in mind that the deletions and the corresponding clinical pattern behave as X-linked traits. Prenatal diagnosis is possible via arylsulfatase C testing of chorion villi biopsies and, if deletions are present, also by recombinant DNA techniques (see Sect. 2.2).

References

1. Åkesson HO, Hagberg B, Wahlström J (1980) Y-to-X chromosome translocation observed in two generations. Hum Genet 55:39–42
2. Andria G, Ballabio A, Parenti G, DiMaio S, Piccirillo A (1984) Steroid sulfatase deficiency and hypogonadism. Eur J Pediatr 142:304–305
3. Ballabio A, Parenti G, Carrozzo R, Sebastio G, Andria G, Buckle V, Fraser N, Craig I, Rocchi M, Romeo G, Jöbsis AC, Persico MG (1987) Isolation and characterization of a steroid sulfatase cDNA clone: genomic deletions in patients with X-chromosome-linked ichthyosis. Proc Natl Acad Sci USA 84:4519–4523
4. Carter CO (1969) Genetics of common disorders. Br Med Bull 25:52–57
5. Curry CJR, Magenis RE, Brown M, Lanman JTJr, Tsai J, O'Lague P, Goodfellow P, Mohandas T, Bergner EA, Shapiro LJ (1984) Inherited chondrodysplasia punctata due to a deletion of the terminal short arm of an X chromosome. N Engl J Med 311:1010–1015
6. Fleuren E, van Oost B, Hamel B (1988) X-linked recessive ichthyosis in combination with the Kallmann syndrome as a manifestion of an X chromosome deletion (in Dutch.) Case demonstration at the 242 nd scientific meeting of the Dutch Society for Dermatology, Nijmegen, February 6
7. Garcia Perez A, Crespo M (1981) X-linked ichthyosis associated with hypertrophic pyloric stenosis in three brothers. Clin Exp Dermatol 6:159–161
8. Khudr G, Benirschke K, Judd HL, Strauss J (1973) Y-to-X translocation in a woman with reproductive failure. JAMA 226:544–549
9. Langenbeck U, Kollmann F (1987) Die Genetik der Dyschondroosteose. 6. Symposium klinische Genetik in der Pädiatrie, Bad Homburg, July 3–5
10. Lynch HT, Ozer F, McNutt CW, Johnson JE, Jampolsky NA (1960) Secondary male hypogonadism and congenital ichthyosis: association of two rare genetic diseases. Am J Hum Genet 12:440–447
11. Perrin JCS, Idemoto JY, Sotos JF, Maurer WF, Steinberg AG (1976) X-linked syndrome of congenital ichthyosis, hypogonadism, mental retardation and anosmia. Birth Defects XII (5):267–274
12. Ross JB, Allerdice PW, Shapiro LJ, Aveling J, Eales BA, Simms D Jr (1985) Familial X-linked ichthyosis, steroid sulfatase deficiency, mental retardation, and nullisomy for Xp233-pter. Arch Dermatol 121:1524–1528
13. Stoll C, Grosshans E, Binder P, Roth M (1983) Hypertrophic pyloric stenosis associated with X-linked ichthyosis in two brothers. Clin Exp Dermatol 8:61–64
14. Sunohara N, Sakuragawa N, Satoyoshi E, Tanae A, Shapiro LJ (1986) A new syndrome of anosmia, ichthyosis, hypogonadism and various neurological manifestation with deficiency of steroid sulfatase and arylsulfatase C. Ann Neurol 19:174–181
15. Tiepolo L, Zuffardi O, Fraccaro M, DiNatale D, Gargantini L, Müller CR, Ropers HH (1980) Assignment by deletion mapping of the steroid sulfatase X-linked ichthyosis locus to Xp223. Hum Genet 54:205–206
16. Traupe H, Müller-Migl CR, Kolde G, Happle R, Kövary PM, Hameister H, Ropers HH (1984) Ichthyosis vulgaris with hypogenitalism and hypogonadism: evidence for different genotypes by lipoprotein electrophoresis and steroid sulfatase testing. Clin Genet 25:42–51
17. Yen P, Allen E, Marsh E, Mohandas T, Wang N, Taggart RT, Shapiro LJ (1987) Cloning and expression of steroid sulfatase cDNA and the frequent occurrence of deletions in steroid sulfatase deficiency: implications for X-Y interchange. Cell 49:443–453

3.3 Ichthyosis and Hypogonadism: Reflections on the so-called Rud's Syndrome

3.3.1 General Remarks

In many textbooks of dermatology the designation "Rud's syndrome" is still used to describe the association of an ill-defined type of ichthyosis with hypogonadism (essential syndrome) and other features that are not obligatory, such as mental retardation and a variable type of neurologic involvement. As discussed in the foregoing section on associated steroid-sulfatase deficiency, we can now explain most of these cases in terms of molecular biology as deletion mutations affecting the X chromosome. Of course, some patients remain who are not deficient in steroid sulfatase, indicating genetic heterogeneity. Time has disproven the concept of Rud's syndrome as a distinct entity. The main reason for this is that the diagnostic label of "Rud's syndrome" was applied loosely to a varied clinical picture from the very beginning [20]. As the concept of Rud's syndrome is so deeply rooted in the medical literature, a brief review of the history of this textbook chimera is warranted. I want to thank Prof. Happle, now of Nijmegen, who translated the two original reports by Rud, written in Danish.

3.3.2 How a Syndrome was Made up

In 1927, the Danish physician Einar Rud [10] described a 22-year-old man who suffered from hypogenitalism, small stature, epilepsy, pernicious anemia, polyneuritis, and ichthyosis-like skin changes. Rud wrote that the patient had 15 brothers and sisters and that he was the only one so affected in this large family. The polyneuropathy began at the age of 18 years, growth retardation was said to have developed in childhood, and as far as the ichthyosis is concerned, no data regarding the onset of this symptom are given, Rud explicitly stated that the patient was mentally alert (*kvik* in Danish). Two years later, Rud [11] reported on a 29-year-old woman suffering from ichthyosis vulgaris, hypogonadism, eunuchoid body proportions, and diabetes mellitus. He explicitly mentioned that the mother, a brother, and a sister also suffered from ichthyosis vulgaris, but not from any of the other symptoms. This woman was not mentally retarded and did not show any neurologic involvement.

It is evident that the two cases have little in common and even less with what has later become known as the "Rud syndrome". In the first case, the ichthyosis was probably acquired and could be related to pernicious anemia. As both parents and all other children (15!) were unaffected, a genetic etiology is very unlikely. In the second case, there was obviously no relationship at all between the ichthyosis vulgaris segregating as an autosomal dominant trait in the family and the hypogonadism and diabetes mellitus observed only in the woman.

Six years later, Ludo van Bogaert [18] briefly described two patients presenting with ichthyosis and hypogenitalism. The first was a 16-year-old boy suffering from ichthyosis, hypogenitalism, and mental retardation, but not from neurologic abnormalities. The second was a 26-year-old man afflicted with ichthyosis vulgaris and epilepsy and lacking pubic hair. He was not said to be mentally retarded. Van Bogaert made reference to the above-mentioned two papers of Rud without stating whether his two cases should be considered to represent the same condition.

In 1939, Stewart [13] committed the cardinal sin of introducing the term "Rud's syndrome" for quite a different ensemble of clinical features. Actually, he observed a young man who exhibited congenital ichthyosis, hypogonadism, mental retardation, epilepsy, muscular hypotonia, dwarfism, contractures of the elbows, hips, and knee joints, arachnodactyly, and retinitis pigmentosa. Death occurred at the age of 21 years following an epileptic status.

In the following years, the term "Rud's syndrome" was used mostly to describe the association of ichthyosis with hypogonadism, mental retardation, and epilepsy. In a review that was excellent at its time (1962), York-Moore and Rundle [20] pointed out that Rud's syndrome probably comprised different clinical pictures. They suggested that ichthyosis and hypogonadism should be considered essential features of the syndrome and that mental retardation and epilepsy were commonly associated with it. Interestingly, the family reported by York-Moore and Rundle was later shown to suffer from X-linked recessive ichthyosis [19].

3.3.3 Current Concepts: Evidence for Genetic Heterogeneity

Both the neurologic involvement and the ichthyosis remain ill defined in the so-called Rud's syndrome. In many cases the neurologic involvement has been described as epilepsy [6–8, 18, 20] while in other cases polyneuropathy and retinitis pigmentosa have been found [4, 13]. Likewise, the ichthyosis is most often XRI [7, 9, 14, 17], while in some cases lamellar ichthyosis [5, 12, 13] and even atypical ichthyosis vulgaris [17, case 2] have been observed. Moreover, at least the Tay syndrome [3, 15] would also meet the criteria set out for diagnosis of "Rud's syndrome". It can be concluded that the so-called Rud's syndrome is a heterogeneous condition (Table 20). I therefore suggest that the designation "Rud's syndrome" be abandoned, as the term is misleading and the syndrome was not even described by Rud.

The clinical picture usually referred to as "Rud's syndrome" is most often caused by associated steroid-sulfatase deficiency. Figure 25 depicts such a patient. When we first reported on this patient, he suffered from XRI, bilateral cryptorchidism, and hypogenitalism only [17, case 1]. In the meantime he is also afflicted with epilepsy. While hypogonadism is of the hypogonadotropic type in

Table 20. Genetic heterogeneity of the so-called Rud's syndrome

Diagnosis	Inheritance	Ichthyosis	Hypo-gonadism	Mental retardation	Neurologic involvement	Reference
Isolated X-linked recessive ichthyosis	X-linked recessive	+	+ (possible)	–	–	Traupe and Happle [16] Andria et al. [2]
Associated steroid-sulfatase deficiency	X-linked (deletion)					Åkesson et al. [1]
(a) X-Y translocation		+	+	+	+	Metaxotou et al. [7]
(b) associated Kallmann's syndrome	X-linked (deletion)	+	+	+	+	Perrin et al. [9] Sunohara et al. [14] Andria et al. [2]
Tay syndrome	Autosomal recessive	+	+	+	–	Tay 1971 [15] Jorizzo et al. [3]
Atypical congenital ichthyosis	Recessive(?)	+	+	+	+	Ruiz-Maldonado et al. [12] Münke et al. [8]
Atypical ichthyosis vulgaris	Recessive(?)	+	+	–	–	Traupe et al. [17] (case 2)

Differential diagnosis should also include the following "neuroichthyoses": multiple sulfatase deficiency, neutral lipid storage disease, Sjögren-Larsson syndrome, Netherton syndrome, and Refsum's disease. In most case reports of the "Rud literature" these neuroichthyoses are not properly considered nor ruled out

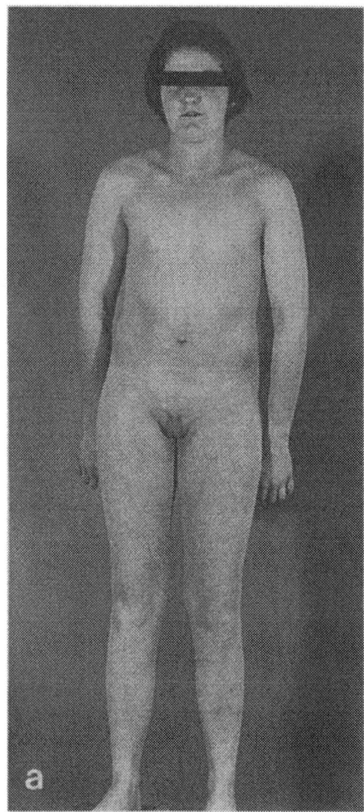
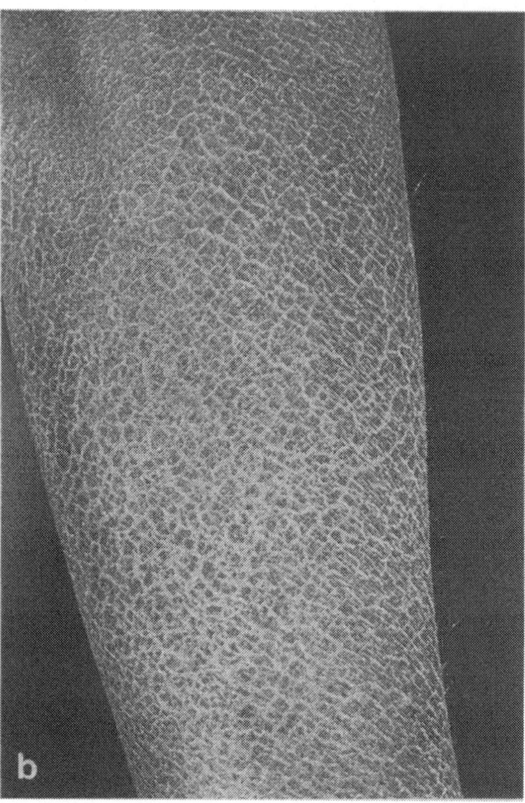

Fig. 25a, b. Associated steroid-sulfatase deficiency syndrome. *a* Hypogonadism with eunuchoid body proportions. *b* X-linked recessive ichthyosis. (From Traupe et al. [17])

most cases of associated steroid-sulfatase deficiency, hormone studies disclosed elevated levels of LH and FSH in this patient.

In several cases featuring ichthyosis and hypogonadism the exact type of ichthyosis cannot yet be classified. Thus, we observed a 26-year-old Pakistani exhibiting a peculiar type of ichthyosis vulgaris, somewhat resembling XRI (Fig. 26). In this patient, steroid sulfatase testing and lipoprotein electrophoresis ruled out steroid-sulfatase deficiency.

A well-preserved granular layer and ultrastructurally normal keratohyalin granules excluded ADI as well (Fig. 27). This latter observation underlines the concept of clinical and genetic heterogeneity in the association of ichthyosis and hypogonadism.

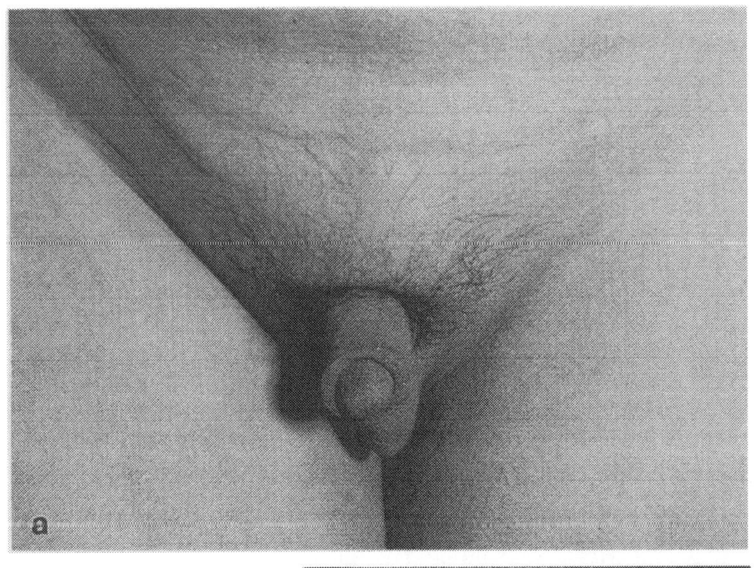

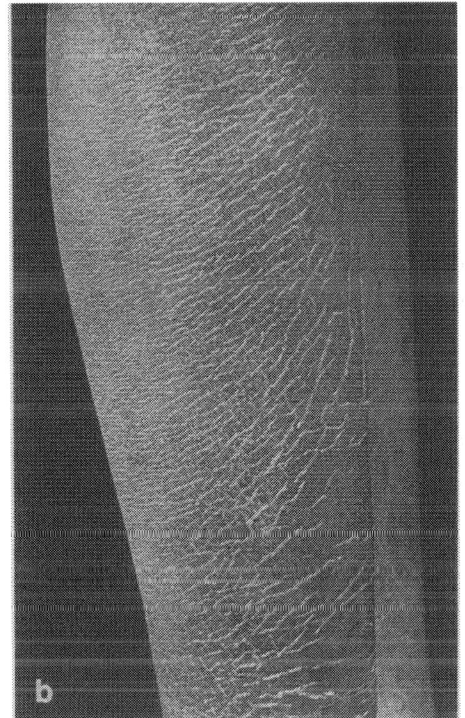

Fig. 26a, b. Atypical ichthyosis vulgaris with hypogonadism. *a* Genital involvement; *b* ichthyosis resembling XRI. (From Traupe et al. [17])

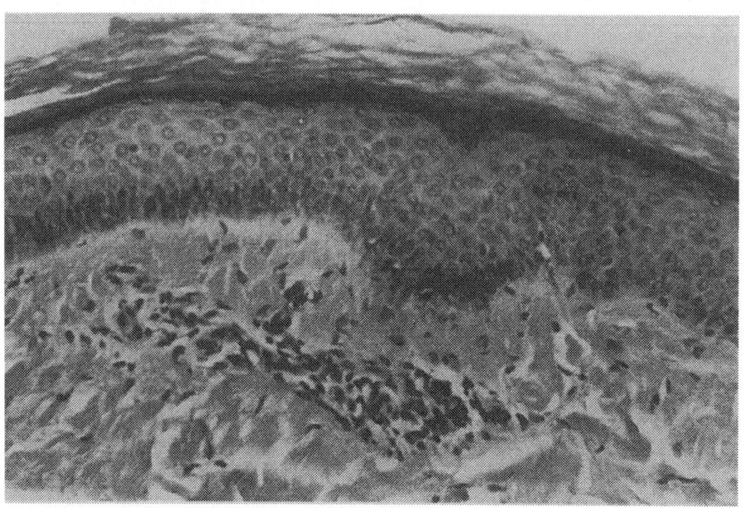

Fig. 27. Atypical ichthyosis vulgaris with hypogonadism. A prominent granular layer excludes ADI in this case. HE, ×50

References

1. Åkesson HO, Hagberg B, Wahlström J (1980) Y-to-X chromosome translocation observed in two generations. Hum Genet 55:39–42
2. Andria G, Ballabio A, Parenti G, DiMaio S, Piccirillo A (1984) Steroid sulfatase deficiency and hypogonadism. Eur J Pediatr 142:304–305
3. Jorizzo JL, Crounse RG, Wheeler CE Jr (1980) Lamellar ichthyosis, dwarfism, mental retardation, and hair shaft abnormalities. A link between the ichthosis-associated and BIDS syndromes. J Am Acad Dermatol 2:309–317
4. Larbrisseau A, Carpenter S (1982) Rud syndrome: congenital ichthyosis, hypogonadism, mental retardation, retinitis pigmentosa and hypertrophic polyneuropathy. Neuropediatrics 13:95–98
5. Marxmiller J, Trenkle I, Ashwal S (1985) Rud syndrome revisited: ichthyosis, mental retardation, epilepsy and hypogonadism. Dev Med Child Neurol 27:335–343
6. MacGillivray RC (1954) The syndrome of Rud. Am J Ment Defic 59:67–72
7. Metaxotou C, Ikkos D, Panagiotopoulou P, Alevizaki M, Mavrou A, Tsenghi C, Matsaniotis N (1983) A familial X/Y translocation in a boy with ichthyosis, hypogonadism and mental retardation. Clin Genet 24:380–383
8. Münke M, Kruse K, Goos M, Ropers HH, Tolksdorf M (1983) Genetic heterogeneity of the ichthyosis, hypogonadism, mental retardation, and epilepsy syndrome. Clinical and biochemical investigations on two patients with Rud syndrome and review of the literature. Eur J Pediatr 141:8–13
9. Perrin JCS, Idemoto JY, Sotos JF, Maurer WF, Steinberg AG (1976) X-linked syndrome of congenital ichthyosis, hypogonadism, mental retardation and anosmia. Birth Defects XII (5):267–274
10. Rud E (1927) The disease of infantilism with tetany, epilepsy, polyneuritis, ichthyosis, and anemia of the pernicious type. (in Danish: Et tilfaelde af infantilisme med tetani, epilepsi, polyneuritis, ichthyosis og anaemi af pernicios type.) Hospitalstidende (Copenhagen) 70:525–538
11. Rud E (1929) The disease of hypogenitalism (female eunuchoidism) with partial gigantism

and ichthyosis. (in Danish: Et tilfaelde af hypogenitalisme (eunuchoidismus femininus) med partiel gigantisme og ichthyosis.) Hospitalstidende (Copenhagen) 72:426–433
12. Ruiz-Maldonado R, Tamayo L, Carnevale A (1975) Neuroichthyosis with hypogonadism (Rud's syndrome). Int J Dermatol 14:347–352
13. Stewart RM (1939) Congenital ichthyosis, idiocy, infantilism and epilepsy - the syndrome of Rud. J Ment Sci 85:256–263
14. Sunohara N, Sakuragawa N, Satoyoshi E, Tanae A, Shapiro LJ (1986) A new syndrome of anosmia, ichthyosis, hypogonadism and various neurological manifestations with deficiency of steroid sulfatase and arylsulfatase C. Ann Neurol 19:174–181
15. Tay CH (1971) Ichthyosiform erythroderma, hair shaft abnormalities, and mental and growth retardation. A new recessive disorder. Arch Dermatol 104:4–13
16. Traupe H, Happle R (1983) Clinical spectrum of steroid sulfatase deficiency: X-linked recessive ichthyosis, birth complications and cryptorchidism. Eur J Pediatr 140:19–21
17. Traupe H, Müller-Migl CR, Kolde G, Happle R, Kövary PM, Hameister H, Ropers HH (1984) Ichthyosis vulgaris with hypogenitalism and hypogonadism: evidence for different genotypes by lipoprotein electrophoresis and steroid sulfatase testing. Clin Genet 25:42–51
18. van Bogaert L (1935) Les dysplasies neuroectodermiques congénitales. Rev Neurol (Paris) 63:353–398
19. Wells RS (1966) Sex-linked ichthyosis, oligophrenia and hypogonadism. Br J Dermatol 78:308
20. York-Moore ME, Rundle AT (1962) Rud's syndrome. J Ment Defic Res 6:108–117

3.4 Multiple Sulfatase Deficiency

3.4.1 Historical Aspects

Multiple sulfatase deficiency (MSD) is a very severe neuropediatric disorder, closely resembling the late-infantile-onset type of metachromatic leukodystrophy (MLS) [1, 6, 11]. The disease was separated from classical MLD on biochemical grounds. In 1965, Austin et al. [1] demonstrated that some of their patients exhibited not only the expected arylsulfatase-A deficiency. but also deficiencies of the arylsulfatases B and C. MSD is very uncommon, and the dermatologist is not likely to be confronted with these children, who are usually taken care of by pediatricians and neurologists since ichthyosis is only a minor complaint.

3.4.2 Clinical Features

The clinical spectrum of MSD was described in detail by Rampini and co-workers in 1970 [11]. The signs and symptoms of the disease resemble those of the late infantile form of MLD [6, 11]. Psychomotor retardation usually starts in the second year of life. The affected child, who may already have learned to walk, then becomes unsteady and requires support to stand or walk. A flabby weakness and hypotonia of all four limbs develops. During the third year the patient's condition rapidly deteriorates. An obvious mental regression, speech deterioration, and severe motor deficits are observed. In the final stage the children are blind, without speech, and must be fed, usually through a nasogastric tube [6]. Death usually occurs between 4 and 12 years of age. These neurologic findings correspond to the spectrum and course of disease found in the late-onset type of infantile MLD and can be related to arylsulfatase A deficiency. In addition, patients with MSD display some features typical of mucopolysaccharidosis, such as a coarse facial appearance, growth retardation, lumbar kyphosis, pectus excavatum, and hepatosplenomegaly. These symptoms can be attributed to arylsulfatase B deficiency. As a clinical correlate of steroid-sulfatase deficiency, the children usually present with mild ichthyosis.

Very recently, a neonatal variant of MSD was reported with onset of the disease at birth [3]. In these infants the presenting signs are more suggestive of a mucopolysaccharidosis [3]. These neonates exhibit a profound dysmorphic facies. Bone roentgenograms disclose severe hypoplasia of all vertebral bodies and multiple epiphyseal dysplasia. To my knowledge, a detailed study of the skin in MSD has so far not been carried out. The scaling seems to be much milder than in XRI. Very often the skin is simply said to be "dry". This mild cutaneous involvement reflects the considerable residual activity of steroid sulfatase (arylsulfatase C) in most cases.

3.4.3 Biochemical and Genetic Aspects

From a biochemical point of view, multiple sulfatase deficiency is a unique disorder in which all seven known sulfatases are deficient (Table 21). It is remarkable that the different enzymes are localized in different cellular compartments (lysosomes and microsomes) and that the genes for the various sulfatases are borne on different chromosomes. Arylsulfatase B maps to chromosome 5 [5, 8], whereas arylsulfatase A has been assigned to chromosome 22 [5] and steroid sulfatase is X-linked. To determine whether the same genes are involved in singular and multiple sulfatase deficiencies, complementation studies were done. In these investigations fibroblasts from patients with metachromatic leukodystrophy, Sanfilippo A syndrome, Hunter's syndrome, and X-linked recessive ichthyosis were fused with fibroblasts from individuals with multiple sulfatase deficiency. Surprisingly, in the fused heterokaryon cells activity of the various sulfatases could be partially restored, indicating that the genetic defect in MSD has to be different from that causing specific sulfatase deficiencies [2, 4, 9].

Biochemical evidence supports the notion that the singular sulfatase deficiencies and MSD are caused by different mechanisms (Table 22). In MSD, arylsulfatase-A deficiency depends on the pH of the medium in which the cells are grown [7]. In media maintained at low pH (<7) the cells express the enzymopathy, while in high-pH media (ph 7.4) the enzyme is produced. As the high- and low-enzyme states are reversible, it can be concluded that arylsulfatase-A deficiency in MSD is secondary and due to a different mutation. The initial synthesis of steroid sulfatase polypeptides is normal in MSD fibroblasts, but the half-life of the steroid sulfatase polypeptides is only 4–6 h, compared with a half-life of 6 days in normal cells [10]. This finding suggests that the basic defect in multiple sulfatase deficiency resides in an enhanced degradation of the various sulfatases [10].

Table 21. Biochemical and genetic aspects of multiple sulfatase deficiency

Deficient enzymes	Cellular localization	Chromosomal assignment	Corresponding phenotype of the singular deficiency
Arylsulfatase A	Lysosomes	22p	Metachromatic leukodystrophy
Arylsulfatase B	Lysosomes	5q	Maroteaux-Lamy syndrome
Arylsulfatase C (steroid sulfatase)	Microsomes	Xp223	X-linked recessive ichthyosis
Sulfoiduronate sulfatase	Lysosomes	X	Hunter's syndrome
Heparan sulfamidase	Lysosomes	?	Sanfilippo-A syndrome
Galactosamine-6 sulfatase	Lysosomes	?	Morquio-A syndrome
Glucosamine-6 sulfatase	Lysosomes	?	?

Table 22. Relationship of multiple to singular sulfatase deficiencies

Clinical level	Multiple sulfatase deficiency mimics the phenotype of the late-infantile-onset type of metachromatic leukodystrophy, of mucopolysaccharidosis and of X-linked recessive ichthyosis.
Genetic level	The genes for the various sulfatases involved are borne on different chromosomes. Complementation studies between cells from multiple and cells from singular sulfatase deficiencies show partial restoration of enzyme activity.
Biochemical level	In multiple sulfatase deficiency, but not in metachromatic leukodystrophy, arylsulfatase-A activity can be modulated by changes of pH. An enhanced degradation of regularly synthesized sulfatase molecules is probably responsible for the multienzyme deficiencies.

3.4.4 Genetic Counseling

Multiple sulfatase deficiency is a severe neurodegenerative disease, transmitted as an autosomal recessive trait. Diagnosis is confirmed by the absence of several singular sulfatases. A direct prenatal diagnosis by biochemical means should be possible, but to my knowledge this has not been done so far. Care will have to be given to the modulation of the enzyme deficiencies by the pH at which the amnion cells are cultured [7]. An indirect assay should also be feasible. As in X-linked recessive ichthyosis, low urinary estriol levels can be demonstrated in MSD pregnancies [12]. Given the severity of the disease and the absence of any treatment modalities, termination of the pregnancy would clearly be justified.

References

1. Austin J, Armstrong D, Shearer L (1965) Metachromatic form of diffuse cerebral sclerosis. V. Nature and significance of low sulfatase activity: a controlled study of brain, liver and kidney in four patients with metachromatic leukodystrophy (MLD). Arch Neurol 13:593-614
2. Ballabio A, Parenti G, Napolitano E, Di Natale P, Andria G (1985) Genetic complementation of steroid sulphatase after somatic cell hybridization of X-linked ichthyosis and multiple sulphatase deficiency. Hum Genet 70:315-317
3. Burch M, Fensom AH, Jackson M, Pitts-Tucker T, Congdon PJ (1986) Multiple sulphatase deficiency presenting at birth. Clin Genet 30:409-415
4. Chang P, Davidson RG (1980) Complementation of arylsylfatase A in somatic hybrids of metachromatic leukodystrophy and multiple sulfatase deficiency disorder fibroblasts. Proc Natl Acad Sci USA 77:6166-6170
5. DeLuca C, Brown JA, Shows TB (1979) Lysosomal arylsulfatase deficiencies in humans: chromosome assigments for arylsulfatase A and B. Proc Natl Acad Sci USA 76:1957-1961
6. Dulaney JT, Moser HW (1978) Sulfatide lipidosis: metachromatic leukodystrophy. In: Stanbury J, Wyngaarden B, Fredrickson DB (eds) The metabolic basis of inherited disease, 4th edn. McGraw-Hill, New York, pp 781-809
7. Fluharty AL, Stevens RL, De la Flor SD, Shapiro LJ, Kihara H (1979) Arylsulfatase A modulation with pH in multiple sulfatase deficiency disorder fibroblasts. Am J Hum Genet 30:249-255

8. Hellkuhl B, Grzeschik KH (1978) Assignment of a gene for arylsulfatase B to human chromosome 5 using human-mouse-somatic cell hybrids. Cytogenet Cell Genet 22:203–206
9. Horwitz AL (1979) Genetic complementation studies of multiple sulfatase deficiency. Proc Natl Acad Sci USA 76:6496–6499
10. Horwitz AL, Warshawsky L, King J, Burns G (1986) Rapid degradation of steroid sulfatase in multiple sulfatase deficiency. Biochem Biophys Res Commun 135:389–396
11. Rampini S, Isler W, Baerlocher K, Bischoff A, Ulrich J, Plüss HJ (1970) Die Kombination von metachromatischer Leukodystrophie und Mucopolysaccharidose als selbständiges Krankheitsbild (Mukosulfatidose). Helv Pediatr Acta 25:436–461
12. Steinmann B, Bieth D, Gitzelmann R (1981) A newly recognized cause of low urinary estriol in pregnancy: multiple sulfatase deficiency of the fetus. Gynecol Obstet Invest 12:107–109

4 Isolated Congenital Ichthyoses

4.1 Harlequin Fetus

4.1.1 Historical Aspects

Harlequin fetus is the most severe type of ichthyosis known. The American Rev. O. Hart is generally credited [9] with the first description of this devastating disease in the year 1750. The first medical report seems to be a dissertation by Richter in 1792 [11]. In 1900, Erhard Riecke [12] performed the first histologic study of a harlequin fetus which had been conserved in alcohol solution for more than 30 years at the University of Leipzig. In his classical paper entitled "Über Ichthyosis congenita" (On ichthyosis congenita) he reviewed the available literature from the nineteenth century and concluded that harlequin fetus (ichthyosis congenita type 1, according to Riecke) should be distinguished from what is today known as lamellar ichthyosis. Of the 54 case reports he reviewed, Riecke considered 25 cases to be harlequin fetus, whereas the remainder suffered from a less severe disease and were classified as ichthyosis congenita types 2 and 3. Riecke noted parental consanguinity in several instances, occurrence of the disease in siblings, and involvement of both sexes. In his detailed histologic description he emphasized the marked increase of the stratum corneum and prominent keratinization of hair follicles, contrasting with a normally developed Malpighian and granular layer.

4.1.2 Clinical Features

The clinical appearance of harlequin fetus is rather uniform. Directly after birth, the babies are covered by a hard, keratotic cast which cracks after some hours, resulting in deep, irregularly branched fissures (Fig. 28). The thick plates of stratum corneum covering the body surface impair normal food intake and breathing. Owing to the armor-like keratoses, the babies are immobile and the limbs are fixed in flexion. The affected babies are unable to move or suck effectively, but they can swallow. The face can have a frog-like appearance. The eyes often are covered with coagulated blood and turned out (severe ectropion), a flattened nose, and a wide-open mouth are further facial characteristics. It is of interest that most harlequin fetuses are born prematurely, usually at week 32–36. As these babies are preterm infants with a low birth weight and tremendous additional skin problems, most of them die in the neonatal period. The condition of those children who survive the first few weeks seems to evolve into lamellar ichthyosis [1, 3, 4, 9].

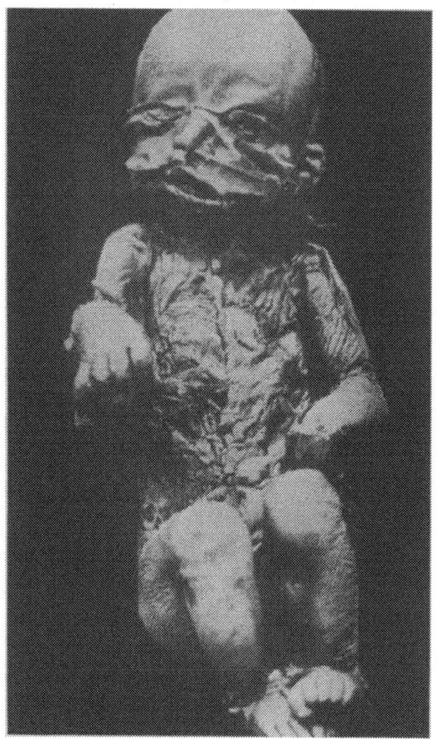

Fig. 28. Harlequin fetus. This case was first reported by Jahn in 1869. The corpse was conserved in alcohol solution at the Department of Pathology in Leipzig. The picture was taken 30 years later by Riecke and is reproduced from his publication [11]

4.1.2.1 Management of Harlequin Fetus

The usual fatal course of the disease may be overcome by treatment with etretinate directly from birth on and - perhaps even more important - by additional appropriate general measures [4, 9]. Careful attention should be given to fluid balance, calorie intake, and temperature control. Lawlor and Peiris [9] emphasize the need to place the infant in an incubator kept at 33 °C to which a humidifier is attached and to provide sufficient fluid and calories by nasogastric feeding. Etretinate seems to be very effective and slowly clears the skin. In a neonate treated with etretinate, Lawlor and Peiris [9] observed a dramatic reversal of the ectropion and a normal development of the nose and ears (Fig. 29a, b). They discontinued etretinate therapy after several months. In their case, no relapse of the armor-like keratoses was observed. The clinical picture seems to correspond to erythrodermic lamellar ichthyosis (Dr. F. Lawlor, 1988, personal communication). A similar experience was communicated by Cambazard et al. [4].

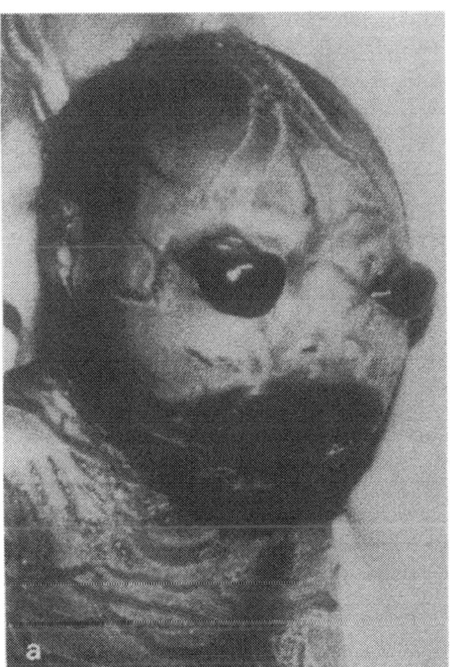

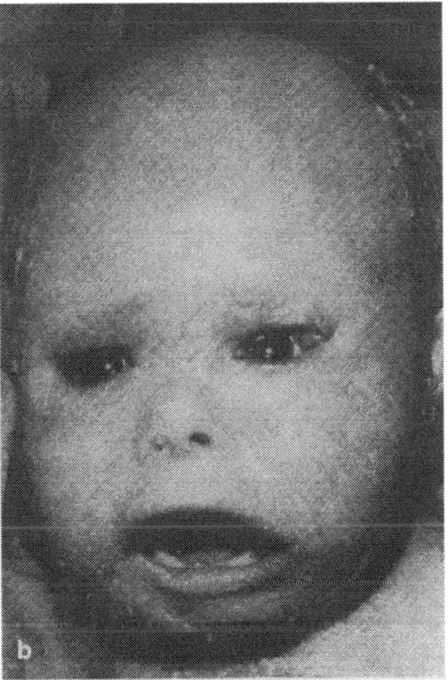

Fig. 29a. Harlequin fetus before etretinate therapy during first 24 h after birth. (Courtesy of Dr. Lawlor, London, from [8]). **b** The same patient at 16 weeks after etretinate therapy and additional general therapeutic measures. (Courtesy of Dr. Lawlor, London, from [8])

4.1.2.2 Differential Diagnosis

The striking clinical features of harlequin fetus are most impressive. Hence, a clear-cut diagnosis can usually be rendered on clinical grounds. Harlequin fetus can also be observed, however, in the recently delineated Neu-Laxova syndrome [6]. The cardinal features of the Neu-Laxova syndrome are: intrauterine growth retardation, generalized edema, microcephaly, abnormalities of the central nervous system, early death, and ichthyosis of varying degree. Curry [6] suggested splitting the Neu-Laxova syndrome into three different clinical subtypes. According to her, group 3 is associated with harlequin fetus and group 2 with lamellar ichthyosis, whereas in group 1 only a scaly skin is found. Detailed studies of the cutaneous involvement of Neu-Laxova syndrome cases are so far lacking. As harlequin fetuses are prematurely born and usually present with edema of the hands and feet, it is conceivable that type 3 of the Neu-Laxova syndrome could be identical with classical harlequin fetus.

Differential diagnosis of harlequin fetus should also include restrictive dermopathy. Outstanding features of this newly delineated disorder [8, 14] are a scaly skin, contracture of all joints, ectropion and eclabium, and premature delivery [8, 14]. In restrictive dermopathy microcephaly and polyhydramnion can be seen. The children usually die in the perinatal period, presumably because of restriction of respiratory movements. The skin in restrictive dermopathy has peculiar histologic and ultrastructural features [8] permitting differential diagnosis from harlequin fetus.

4.1.3 Histologic Features

The results of histologic studies are equivocal and seem to indicate the existence of two different types of harlequin fetus. In the vast majority of cases, the stratum corneum is grossly enlarged and orthokeratotic [1, 10]. The size of the granular layer is variable and is often diminished. There may be some acanthosis and papillomatosis. However, the overall appearance of the epidermis is normal and it is surprisingly small compared with the markedly broadened stratum corneum. Based on these histologic findings, it was suggested that harlequin fetus should be regarded as a retention hyperkeratosis [10].

In a few cases pronounced parakeratosis that cannot be explained by tangential sectioning is seen. In these cases the granular layer is also diminished or lacking and, again, the epidermis appears normal. Since parakeratosis is generally attributed to an enhanced cell turnover (hyperproliferation hyperkeratosis), it is possible that these cases represent a distinct type of harlequin fetus.

4.1.4 Biochemical Aspects

Until now, only a few cases of harlequin fetus have been studied biochemically. Therefore, a clear-cut picture has not yet emerged. The results obtained so far are contradictory and also indicate that harlequin fetus may be a heterogeneous condition [1]. In 1970, Craig and co-workers [5] reported that beta instead of normal alpha keratin was seen in the stratum corneum of a harlequin baby. X-ray diffraction analysis of three further harlequin fetuses failed to confirm this finding. In a later study, a poorly oriented alpha keratin pattern was found instead [1]. Studies of the molecular weight of the stratum corneum keratins gave conflicting results, too. In two of three cases an abnormal pattern of the keratin polypeptides and a lack of the 64-kD fraction was found, whereas the third patient showed a normal keratin polypeptide pattern. In this latter case, lipid biochemical studies disclosed elevated cholesterol and triglyceride levels in the scales [3].

4.1.5 Genetic Counseling

For a long time the mode of inheritance of the harlequin fetus was unclear. Today it has been established beyond doubt that the disease is transmitted as an autosomal recessive trait in most families (Fig. 30) [9, 13]. However, given the frequent sporadic occurrence of the trait a second dominant subtype cannot be ruled out with certainty. The sporadic cases could represent new mutations of a dominant gene. Because of the lethal character of the disease, transmission of

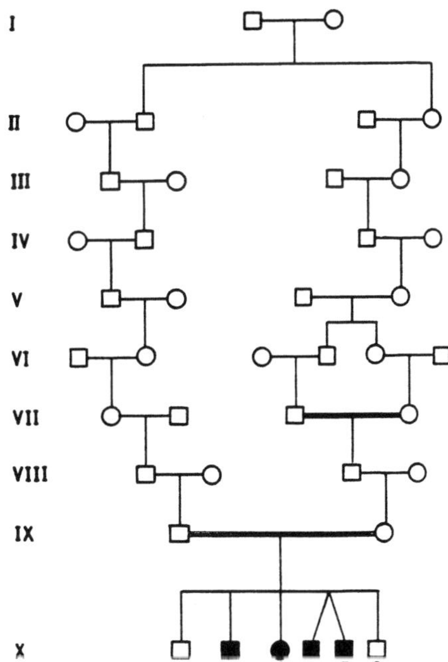

Fig. 30. Pedigree of a family affected with harlequin fetus. Note confinement of the disease to one generation and consanguinity indicating autosomal recessive inheritance. (Courtesy of Dr. Unamuno, Salamanca, Spain [12])

the trait from one generation to the other cannot be expected in a possible dominant subtype. In the future, this might pose a problem if sporadic patients successfully treated with etretinate ask for their genetic risk. Currently, it seems wise to counsel sporadic cases as being due to a recessive gene. As discussed above, histologic and biochemical studies point to the possibility that the condition could still be heterogeneous.

The birth of a harlequin fetus is a traumatic experience for the family. Prenatal diagnosis is possible and may be offered for further pregnancies [2, 7]. In this context the new therapeutic possibilities (e.g., etretinate) should also be discussed with the family, as this may influence their decision.

References

1. Baden HP, Kubilus J, Rosenbaum K, Fletcher A (1982) Keratinization in the harlequin fetus. Arch Dermatol 118:14–18
2. Blanchet-Bardon C, Fahrenbach WH, Diamond RL (1983) Prenatal diagnosis of harlequin fetus. Lancet 1:132
3. Buxman M, Goodkin Pe (1979) Harlequin ichthyosis with epidermal lipid abnormality. Arch Dermatol 115:189–193
4. Cambazard F, Haftek M, Hermier C, Lachaud A, Dutruge J, Gallet S, Armand J-P, Staquet MJ, Thirolet J (1988) Foetus arlequin traité par l'étrétine (Ro 10–1670) Ann Dermatol Venereol 115:1128–1130
5. Craig JM, Goldsmith LA, Baden HP (1970) An abnormality of keratin in the harlequin fetus. Pediatrics 46:437–440

6. Curry CJ (1982) Further comments on the Neu-Laxova syndrome. Am J Med Genet 13:441-444
7. Elias S, Mazur M, Sabragha R, Esterly NB, Simpson JL (1980) Prenatal diagnosis of harlequin ichthyosis. Clin Genet 17:275-280
8. Holbrook KA, Dale BA, Witt DA, Hayden MR, Toriella HV (1987) Arrested epidermal morphogenesis in three newborn infants with a fatal genetic disorder (restrictive dermopathy). J Invest Dermatol 88:330-339
9. Lawlor F, Peiris S (1985) Harlequin fetus successfully treated with etretinate. Br J Dermatol 112:585-590
10. Luderschmidt C, Dorn M, Bassermann R, Linderkamp O (1980) Kollodiumbaby und Harlekinfetus. Gegenüberstellung zweier Beobachtungen. Hautarzt 31:154-158
11. Richter CF (1792) Dissertatio medica de identificatio in artis obstetricae exercitio non sempers evatibili. Richter, Leipzig (Quoted according to Riecke [11])
12. Riecke E (1900) Über Ichthyosis congenita. Arch Dermatol Syph (Vienna and Leipzig) 54:289-340
13. Unamuno P, Pierola JM, Fernandez E, Roman C, Velasco JA (1987) Harlequin foetus in four siblings. Br J Dermatol 116:569-572
14. Witt DR, Hayden MR, Holbrook KA, Dale BA, Baldwin VJ, Taylor GP (1986) Restrictive dermopathy: a newly recognized autosomal recessive skin dysplasia. Am J Med Genet 24:637-648

4.2 The Lamellar Ichthyoses

4.2.1 Classification, History, and Remarks on Nomenclature

Today, the lamellar ichthyoses form a heterogeneous group of at least six, but possibly even more types of nonbullous congenital ichthyosis. In my definition, the term "lamellar ichthyosis" is used for all nonbullous (nonepidermolytic) and isolated types of congenital ichthyoses, except for harlequin fetus. The term "lamellar ichthyosis" does not apply to self-healing collodion baby [8, 21] which historically has also been called "lamellar ichthyosis of the newborn" [8, 21]. The relationship of self-healing collodion baby to lamellar ichthyosis is quite unclear. The fact that collodion baby is a transient feature of several types of lamellar ichthyosis as well as of several types of associated congenital ichthyoses [17] does not imply that self-healing collodion baby should be regarded as an ich-

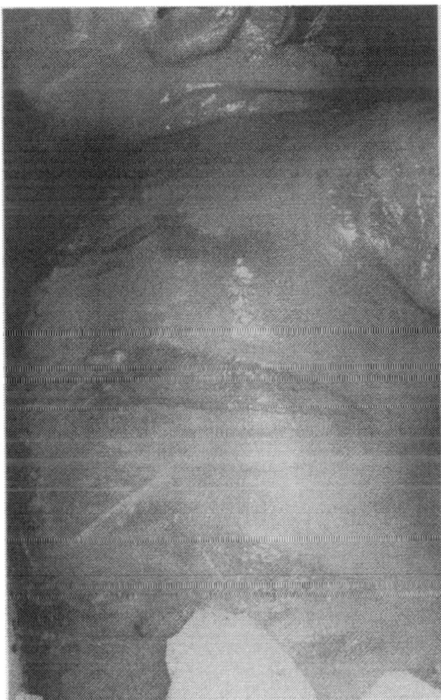

Fig. 31. Typical collodion baby at birth. This case later evolved into lamellar ichthyosis. (Courtesy of Dr. Happle, Nijmegen)

thyosis, too. Rather, it indicates that collodion baby (Fig. 31) is a transient and in itself heterogeneous condition of the neonate that can be caused by a variety of inborn errors of epidermal metabolism. Ultrastructural studies performed by Frenk allowed the distinction between self-healing collodion baby and those types evolving into lamellar ichthyosis [8]. It is noteworthy that even among the various types of lamellar ichthyosis, collodion baby is not a constant feature and does not necessarily precede the onset of ichthyosis [17].

Until very recently, lamellar ichthyosis was considered a single entity. In 1984, Traupe et al. [28] delineated a distinct autosomal dominant subtype of lamellar ichthyosis. Ultrastructural investigations by Kanerva and co-workers [15, 19] and the Anton-Lamprecht group [1–4], lipid biochemical studies by Williams and Elias [30, 31], and very recent enzymatic studies by the Happle group from Nijmegen [5] indicate further heterogeneity of autosomal recessive lamellar ichthyosis (Table 23). However, the process of identifying distinct subtypes of lamellar ichthyosis has not been completed yet. Thus, at the recent symposium, "Advances in Ichthyosis Research", held in Nijmegen, The Netherlands, Nov. 3, 1988, Dr. Gedde-Dahl (Tromsø, Norway) reported a further distinct type of lamellar ichthyosis (Table 23) [12]. As far as the skin is concerned, this type resembles the Sjögren-Larsson syndrome and displays marked keratotic lichenification (Fig. 32), but is not associated with spastic paresis, mental retardation, or glistening dots in the retina. In a preliminary communication concerning this type, Gedde-Dahl et al. [13] still discussed the possibility that they were dealing with a genetic compound between the gene for autosomal recessive lamellar ichthyosis and the gene for Sjögren-Larsson syndrome. In the meantime, Anton-Lamprecht [2] has observed a new type which may be identical to this Sjögren-Larsson syndrome-like type and has been able to identify specific ultrastructural characteristics. Her ultrastructural studies of this ichthyosis, which she preferes to call "ichthyosis congenita type IV" were presented at the 35th meeting of the German Dermatological Society in Munich, April 27 – May 1, 1988. Curved, often trilaminar lipid membranes in the granular layer and the stratum corneum are the outstanding ultrastructural feature of this new type of autosomal recessive lamellar ichthyosis [2].

Obviously, any classification of lamellar ichthyoses has to be provisional at the moment. Very likely, biochemistry and DNA studies will lead to recognition of further subtypes in the near future and may result in significant changes in the current classification. The situation may become similar to that of xeroderma pigmentosum, where many subtypes can be recognized biochemically. The comparison to xeroderma pigmentosum also seems appropriate, since even now it is rather difficult to correlate clinical phenotypes with underlying genotypes as recognized by ultrastructural and biochemical means.

Different nomenclatures introduced by various research groups in the past have contributed a great deal to a general confusion when it comes to the classification of lamellar ichthyosis. Therefore, a short treatise on the history and nomenclature of the lamellar ichthyoses is warranted.

As discussed in Sects. 1.2 and 4.1, lamellar ichthyosis was separated from harlequin fetus by Riecke in 1900 [22]. Two years later, Brocq [7] independently described lamellar ichthyosis as an ichthyosis-like condition and emphasized its

Table 23. Current classification of lamellar ichthyoses

Designation	Inheritance	Lipid biochemistry	Enzymology	Ultrastructure
Autosomal dominant lamellar ichthyosis	Autosomal dominant	Excessive free fatty acids, elevated n-alkanes	Normal butyrase and beta-glucosidase	Increased transition layer, lipid inclusions in the stratum corneum
Erythrodermic lamellar ichthyosis				
A	Autosomal recessive	Elevated n-alkanes	Beta-glucosidase deficiency, normal butyrase	Lipid vacuoles in the stratum corneum
B	Autosomal recessive	Not done	Not done	Massive cholesterol deposition in corneocytes
Nonerythrodermic lamellar ichthyosis				
A	Autosomal recessive	Not done	Low butyrase, normal beta-glucosidase	Laminated membrane structures, vesicular lamellar bodies
B[a]	Autosomal recessive	Not done	Not done	Laminated structures different from type NELI-A
C[b]	Autosomal recessive	Increased free sterols, normal n-alkanes	Not done	Not done

[a] Described by Dr. Gedde-Dahl at the Nijmegen Symposium on Ichthyosis, Nov. 3, 1988 [12a]

[b] Dr. Mary Williams refers to this type simply as "lamellar ichthyosis".

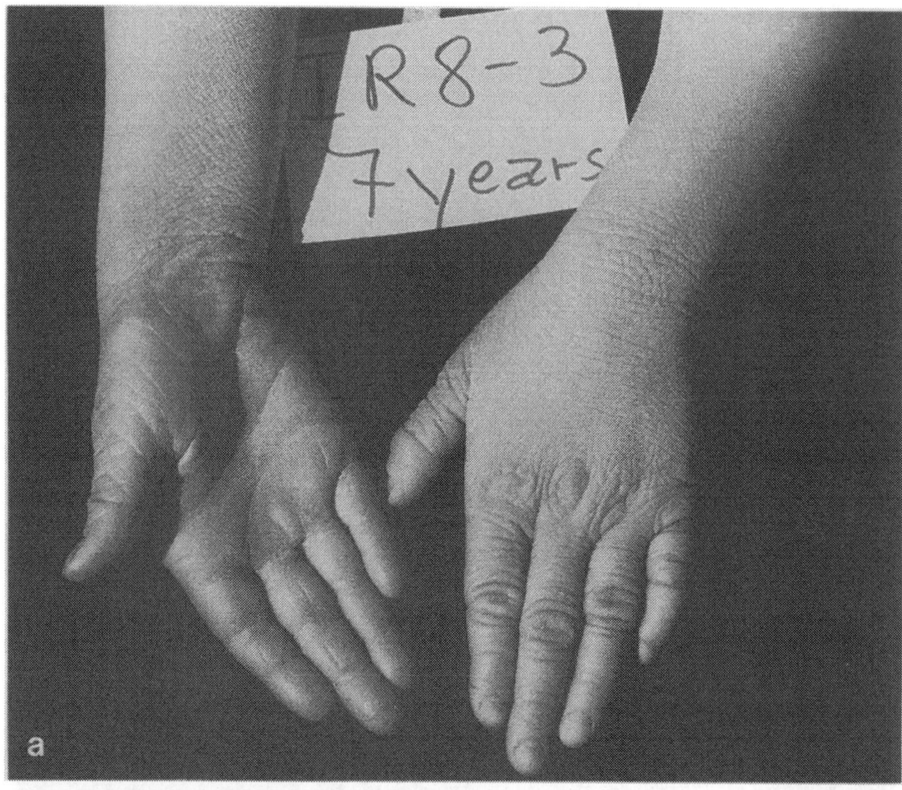

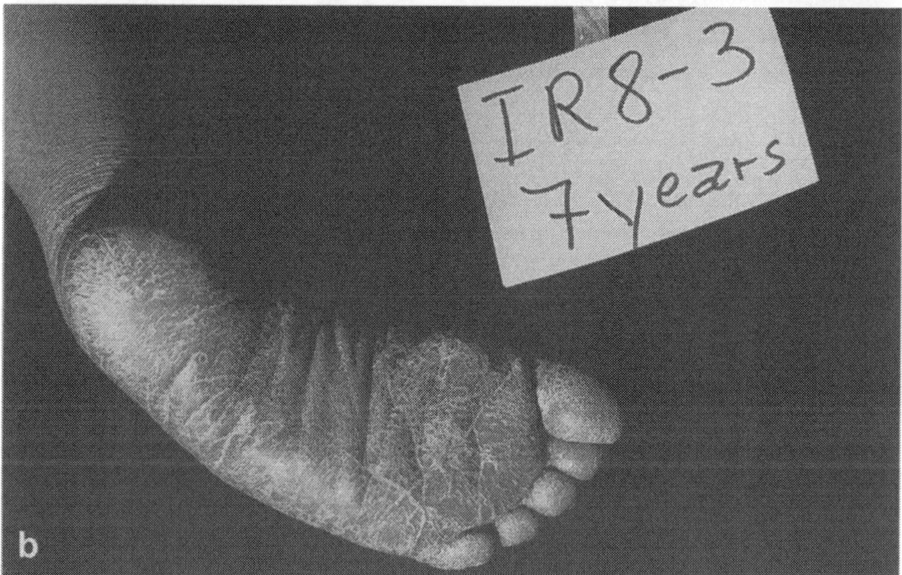

Fig. 32 a, b. Lamellar ichthyosis (NELI type B) resembling Sjögren-Larsson syndrome. **a** Note keratotic lichenification; **b** pronounced plantar keratosis. (Courtesy of Dr. Gedde-Dahl, Tromsø, from [13])

erythrodermic character introducing the term "erythrodermie congénitale ichthyosiforme". He already distinguished between a dry and a bullous type of this condition. Most likely, he used the attribute "ichthyosiform" (i.e., ichthyosis-like) since at his time the designation "ichthyosis congenita" was still identical with harlequin fetus and reserved for this far more severe disease. The definition of ichthyosis has changed considerably since the turn of the century and now encompasses all **genetic** disorders of cornification that affect the entire body (see Sect. 1.1). The appropriate adjective for ichthyosis is "ichthyotic" and not "ichthyosiform". Today terms like "congenital ichthyosiform erythroderma" should therefore better be avoided. Instead, I use "ichthyotic erythroderma", "erythrodermic ichthyosis", or "erythrodermic lamellar ichthyosis".

Riecke and Brocq stand at the beginning of two different nomenclatures that prevailed for many years. The descriptive designation "erythrodermie congénitale ichthyosiforme" (congenital ichthyosiform erythroderma) was used mostly in France and Great Britain, whereas in German-speaking and Scandinavian countries the Latin designation "ichthyosis congenita" was popularized by the work of Hermann Werner Siemens. Riecke called harlequin fetus "ichthyosis congenita type I" and referred to lamellar ichthyosis as "ichthyosis congenita type II". Moreover, he distinguished "ichthyosis congenita type III" with a delayed onset and called this type "ichthyosis congenita tarda". In contrast to Riecke, Siemens firmly believed in the importance of proper language since it influences the way we perceive diseases. He [24] therefore criticized the misleading term "ichthyosis congenita tarda" and argued that this was a "contradictio in adjecto." He accepted, however, the distinction between harlequin fetus and lamellar ichthyosis. Instead of using Roman numerals for the two types of congenital ichthyosis, he preferred the term "ichthyosis congenita gravis" for harlequin fetus and "ichthyosis congenita mitis" for lamellar ichthyosis [24]. In my opinion, the great advantage of "ichthyosis congenita mitis" was that this designation was noncommittal and did not evoke preconceived notions about the disease, a danger inherent to descriptive terms like "congenital ichthyotic erythroderma" or "lamellar ichthyosis".

The designation "lamellar ichthyosis" was originally used to describe what we now call "self-healing collodion baby" [8, 21]. In the late 1960s, Frost and van Scott [10, 11] studied the cell kinetics of epidermal turnover in various types of ichthyoses and distinguished between two different basic pathomechanisms causing ichthyosis: retention hyperkeratosis and proliferation hyperkeratosis. Their work was a significant milestone in our understanding of the pathophysiology of ichthyosis. Unfortunately, they advanced a new nomenclature, too. They introduced the term "lamellar ichthyosis" for ichthyosis congenita mitis (nonbullous congenital ichthyosis) and characterized this disease as a hyperproliferation hyperkeratosis. The first three patients they studied presented with thick, large, dark-brown scales and exhibited no appreciable erythroderma. Therefore, this type of involvement in nonbullous congenital ichthyosis is still sometimes called "classical lamellar ichthyosis". In later work, Frost [9] conceded that lamellar ichthyosis has a broad clinical spectrum and that many patients exhibit only fine translucent scales often accompanied by marked erythema.

Though much can be said in favor of the Latin designation "ichthyosis congenita mitis", the term "lamellar ichthyosis" has made the game and actually has replaced the older designations. Throughout this book I use "lamellar ichthyosis" as a synonym for all types of nonbullous congenital ichthyoses that do not form part of a syndrome. I do not restrict the term to refer to a certain clinical phenotype and use it much in the same way as "ichthyosis congenita mitis" was once used.

Hopefully, the basic biochemical defects underlying the various types of lamellar ichthyosis will be elucidated in the near future. The enzymatic defect may likewise be attached to lamellar ichthyosis, once unraveled. To me, this approach seems to be more didactic than simply numbering the various types of lamellar ichthyoses [4]. For the time being, numbering or attaching letters (A, B, C ...) to the various types is of course acceptable.

4.2.2 Autosomal Dominant Lamellar Ichthyosis

4.2.2.1 Introduction

For many years it was a dogma that lamellar ichthyosis is an autosomal recessive disorder. In 1984, Traupe and co-workers [28] reported on a family in which lamellar ichthyosis was transmitted through three generations, obviously following an autosomal dominant mode of inheritance (Fig. 33). This family observation provided first evidence for genetic heterogeneity of lamellar ichthyosis. In the meantime, the existence of autosomal dominant lamellar ichthyosis (ADLI) has been confirmed by groups from Spain [25], France [17], and Sweden [23]. Toribio et al. [25] reported on a family with ADLI in three generations. Rossmann-Ringdahl and co-workers [23] published a detailed study dealing with a mother and two children, all suffering from an erythrodermic type of lamellar

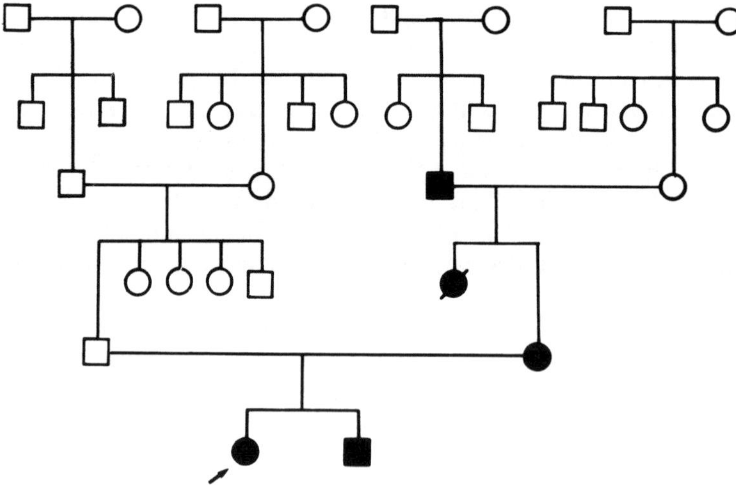

Fig. 33. Pedigree of a family showing an autosomal dominant mode of inheritance in lamellar ichthyosis. The disease is transmitted through three generations. (From [27])

ichthyosis. Finally, Larrègue et al. [17] briefly reported on five families in which collodion baby and lamellar ichthyosis occurred in two generations and on a similar family spanning four generations. In these latter families detailed histopathologic and ultrastructural studies have not yet been performed. It is noteworthy that there is some variation as far as the clinical features are concerned. Thus, the Swedish and French cases presented at birth as collodion babies and during later life showed an erythrodermic phenotype, while our own cases exhibited nonerythrodermic lamellar ichthyosis. Whether these differences are due to a variable clinical expression of ADLI or reflect possible further genetic heterogeneity of ADLI cannot be answered at the moment.

4.2.2.2 Clinical Features

Because of the above-mentioned phenotypic variation, I confine myself describing the clinical features found in our own family observation [28] and in that of Toribio [25]. In ADLI the ichthyosis is present at birth and hence truly congenital. Our cases and those of Toribio did not have a history of collodion baby, however. The entire body, including palms and soles, is covered by large, dark-gray scales (Fig. 34), though the flexural folds are less severely involved. Our own patients show no facial involvement, whereas in the Spanish family facial tautness and slight ectropion are seen. There is pronounced plantar keratosis (Fig. 35). The palms are less severely involved but exhibit accentuated creases. Prominent lichenification on the back of the hands, feet, wrists, knees, and ankles (Fig. 36) is a further conspicuous finding. In the absence of any other signs of atopic dermatitis this lichenification can be attributed to the cornification dis-

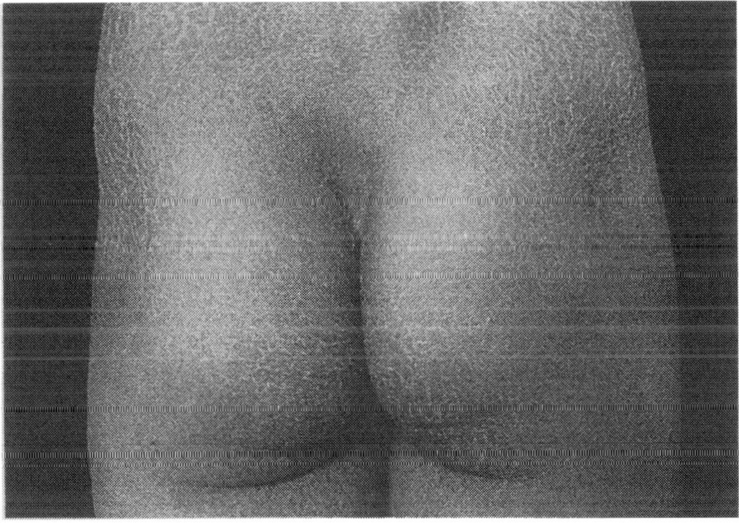

Fig. 34. Autosomal dominant lamellar ichthyosis. Note large, dark-gray scales. (From [28])

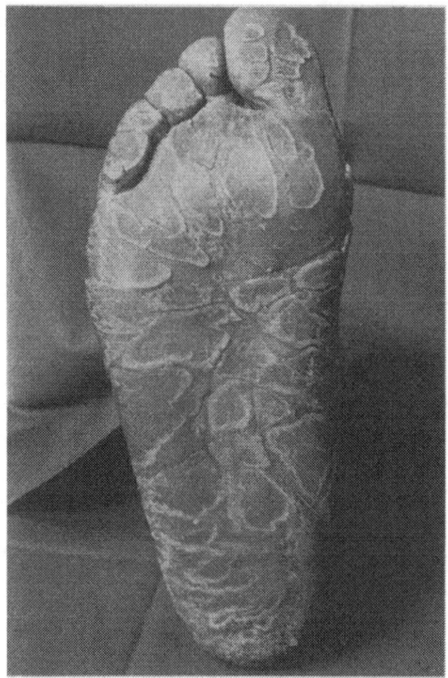

Fig. 35. Autosomal dominant lamellar ichthyosis. Pronounced plantar keratosis

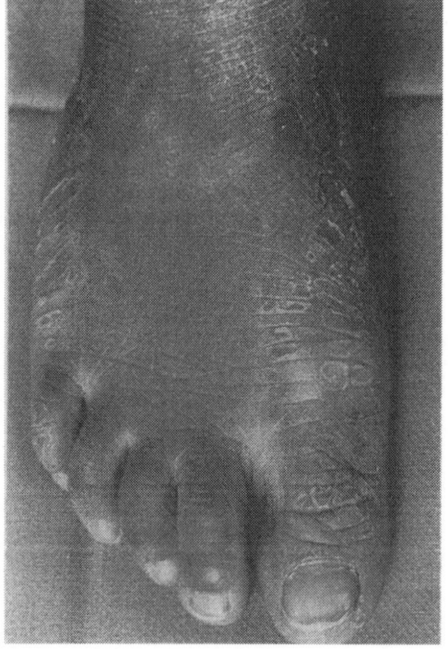

Fig. 36. Autosomal dominant lamellar ichthyosis. Prominent lichenification over the back of the feet. (From [28])

order. The patients do not suffer from blistering or bullous episodes. Severe caries with childhood onset may be an additional feature of the condition. The cases reported by Toribio and co-workers [25] exhibit very similar clinical findings, but they also present mild ichthyotic erythroderma, not encountered in our family. Considerable pruritus is a problem in their family and was also observed in one of our patients.

4.2.2.3 Histologic and Ultrastructural Features of ADLI

Histologically, ADLI is characterized by acanthosis and papillomatosis of the epidermis. Within the same biopsies, parts show orthohyperkeratosis with a normal and slightly increased granular layer, whereas other parts exhibit marked parakeratosis with a conspicuous broadening of the granular layer (Fig. 37). Parakeratosis is usually associated with a decreased or even lacking granular layer. The concomitant presence of orthohyperkeratosis and marked parakeratosis above a well-preserved granular layer is an unusual histologic finding. Unfortunately, it is not specific. I have seen this constellation in two patients suffering from very mild autosomal recessive lamellar ichthyosis (ELI type B?). Thus, histologic examinations do not allow a clear-cut distinction between ADLI and the more common recessive types of lamellar ichthyosis. This difficulty may be overcome by electron microscopy, as demonstrated by Kolde et al. [16]. The most prominent ultrastructural finding is an increased transforming zone of up to six cell layers. This transforming zone is situated between the granular and horny layers [16] (Fig. 38). In normal skin this transforming zone measures only one cell layer. The transition (transforming) layers reflect the structural and biochemical conversion of fully developed granular cells into horny cells at the stratum corneum/stratum granulosum interface. So far, the transformation layer has not

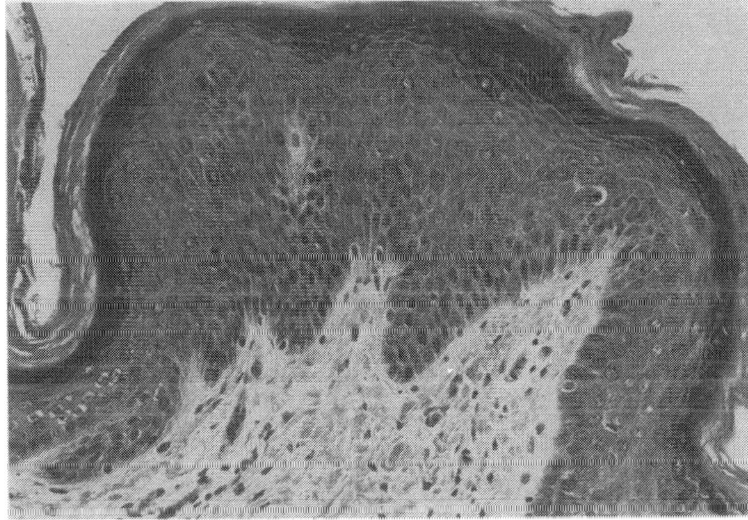

Fig. 37. Autosomal dominant lamellar ichthyosis. Some parts of the biopsy show marked parakeratosis associated with an increased granular layer, other parts show orthokeratosis. (From [27]) HE, ×50

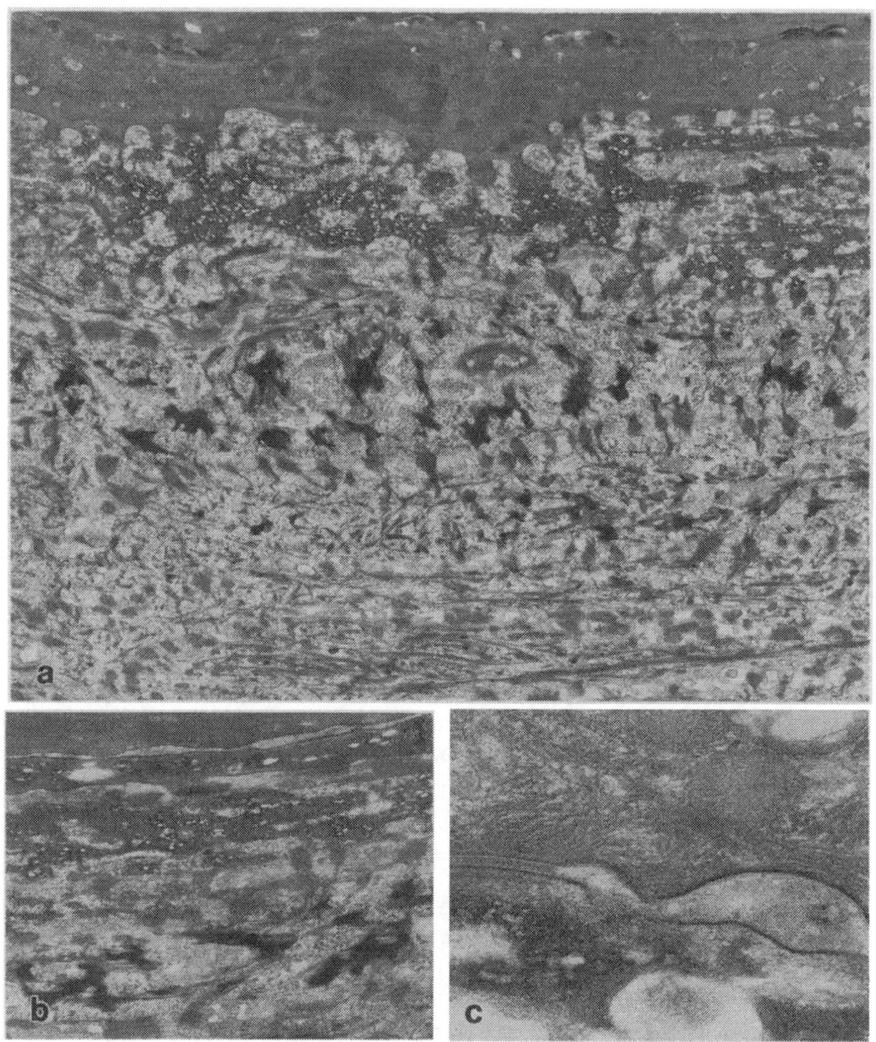

Fig. 38a–c. Autosomal dominant lamellar ichthyosis; electron micrographs. **a** Survey of the upper epidermal layers. Note the prominent transformation zone between the granular keratinocytes and corneocytes. ×7800. **b** Transformation zone with multiple vacuoles. ×10200. **c** Interface between the lower stratum corneum and the transformation zone. Note regular tonofilament structure of corneocytes. ×42000 (Courtesy of Dr. G. Kolde, Münster)

been reported to be markedly increased in any other types of ichthyosis. Tonofilaments and keratohyalin granules are regular in structure and number in ADLI [16]. As in the recessive types, keratinocytes show ultrastructural signs of increased cellular metabolism, such as a large number of mitochondria and numerous free ribosomes, indicating proliferation hyperkeratosis. A normal keratin pattern and lipid inclusions in the stratum corneum are further ultrastructural features [16, 25].

4.2.2.4 Biochemical Aspects

The basic biochemical defect of ADLI is still unknown. Melnik et al. [18] recently found that ADLI has a characteristic scale lipid pattern which distinguishes it from all other types of recessive lamellar ichthyosis (see also Sect. 1.4). The two patients studied showed pronounced elevations of free fatty acids, triglycerides, sterol ester, and elevated n-alkanes, whereas free sterol and total ceramides were decreased. The significantly increased levels of free fatty acids and triglycerides are an important finding so far not reported in other keratinization disorders. Probably, these alterations reflect the ultrastructurally recognized lipid inclusions in the stratum corneum.

Surprisingly, the n-alkane levels were about five times higher in the plantar materials studied than in normal controls. This shows that increased n-alkane levels are not always associated with ichthyotic erythroderma. The finding of elevated n-alkane levels is difficult to explain. It casts some doubt on the specificity of increased n-alkane values in erythrodermic lamellar ichthyosis (see Sect. 4.2.3). Enzymatic investigations have so far revealed no striking defect or characteristic pattern. Scale enzyme analysis for butyrase and beta-glucosidase were both normal (P. Mier 1988, personal communication).

4.2.3 Heterogeneity of Autosomal Recessive Lamellar Ichthyosis

4.2.3.1 Historical Aspects

For a long time it has been known that lamellar ichthyosis can have a very variable clinical picture. In 1928, Siemens [24] reported on three patients whose development he had followed from birth for several years. Siemens stressed the remarkable improvement observed in these three children, who had been born as collodion babies and had suffered from ichthyotic erythroderma, displaying severe ectropion in the neonatal period. In one child the lamellar ichthyosis cleared completely. Actually, this may have been a self-healing collodion baby. In the remaining two children erythroderma faded soon after birth. At the age of 5–7 years they presented only fine scaling reminiscent of ichthyosis vulgaris, but no longer displayed erythroderma or ectropion. In one case Siemens observed remarkable seasonal variation in the severity of scaling not related to therapy. In this case lamellar ichthyosis almost cleared in the summertime, underlining the importance of external factors such as weather and humidity. Three other patients Siemens studied as adults [24] were said not to have suffered from erythroderma at all and displayed moderate generalized scaling with small brown hyperkeratotic fields separated by erythematous stripes.

From these early observations and similar later studies it became quite clear that lamellar ichthyosis has a broad clinical spectrum. This spectrum is due in part to genetic heterogeneity. On the other hand, considerable variation of intrafamilial and intraindividual disease expression made it impossible to base a meaningful classification on the analysis of clinical phenotypes alone. Recognition of distinct entities had to await the advent of new ultrastructural and biochemical techniques.

4.2.3.2 Ultrastructural and Biochemical Evidence for Heterogeneity

In the early 1970s, electron microscopy performed on a limited number of patients with erythrodermic lamellar ichthyosis (ELI type A/ichthyosis congenita type I) failed to reveal specific ultrastructural defects [1, 29]. Instead, nonspecific changes reflecting enhanced cell turnover, such as an increased number of keratinosomes (lamellar bodies) or numerous and enlarged mitochondria, were found [1, 29]. The most prominent finding was lipid vacuoles in the stratum corneum.

In 1983, Kanerva and co-workers, from Helsinki [15], described in detail ultrastructural criteria delineating a distinct second type of ELI (ELI type B/ichthyosis congenita type II). So far, a clinical diagnosis of this type is not possible. Its clinical features have not been reported in detail. Massive cholesterol deposition within the stratum corneum in the form of large electron-lucent rods (30–60 nm thick, length up to several micrometers) and a lack of the marginal band of the corneocytes are the electron-microscopic markers of this entity (ELI type B) [15]. The work of Kanerva was soon confirmed by Arnold and Anton-Lamprecht [3], who noted that this type of lamellar ichthyosis mostly has an erythrodermic phenotype. In the huge patient series of 94 cases of lamellar ichthyosis studied ultrastructurally by the Heidelberg group, 18 of them belonged to the cholesterol deposition type [4]. Anton-Lamprecht [2] reported that some of her patients with this type presented with a nonerythrodermic phenotype. This indicates that clinical phenotypes do not correlate very well with genotypes.

Arnold et al. [4] recently delineated a third type of autosomal recessive lamellar ichthyosis (NELI type A/ichthyosis congenita type III). Clinically, this is nonerythrodermic lamellar ichthyosis (NELI type A). The main ultrastructural features are elongated membrane structures in the keratinocytes of the granular and spinous layer and abnormal vesicular keratinosomes (lamellar bodies) (Fig. 39). Figure 39 was kindly supplied by Dr. Anton-Lamprecht and Dr. Arnold, Heidelberg. In this figure the outstanding ultrastructural features of NELI type A (ichthyosis congenita type III) are compared with those of NELI type B (ichthyosis congenita type IV). In NELI type A the vacuoles in the granular layer can be seen by light microscopy, if semithin sections are used. The digitonin stain shows that these vacuoles contain cholesterol. Of the 94 patients studied in Heidelberg, 9 belong to this nonerythrodermic type (NELI type A), which the Heidelberg group prefers to call "ichthyosis congenita type III" [4]. The findings of Arnold et al. were recently confirmed by Niemi and Kanerva [19], who observed the same vacuolations of granular cells and keratinosome defects in a 75-year-old woman with lamellar ichthyosis.

Fig. 39a–e. Ultrastructural differentiation of ichthyosis congenita types III and IV. **a, b** Ichthyosis congenita type III. Ultrastructural characteristics: **a** Elongated membrane structures (*open arrows*) within the cytoplasm of the granular cells (*Sg*), residues of them in the horn cells

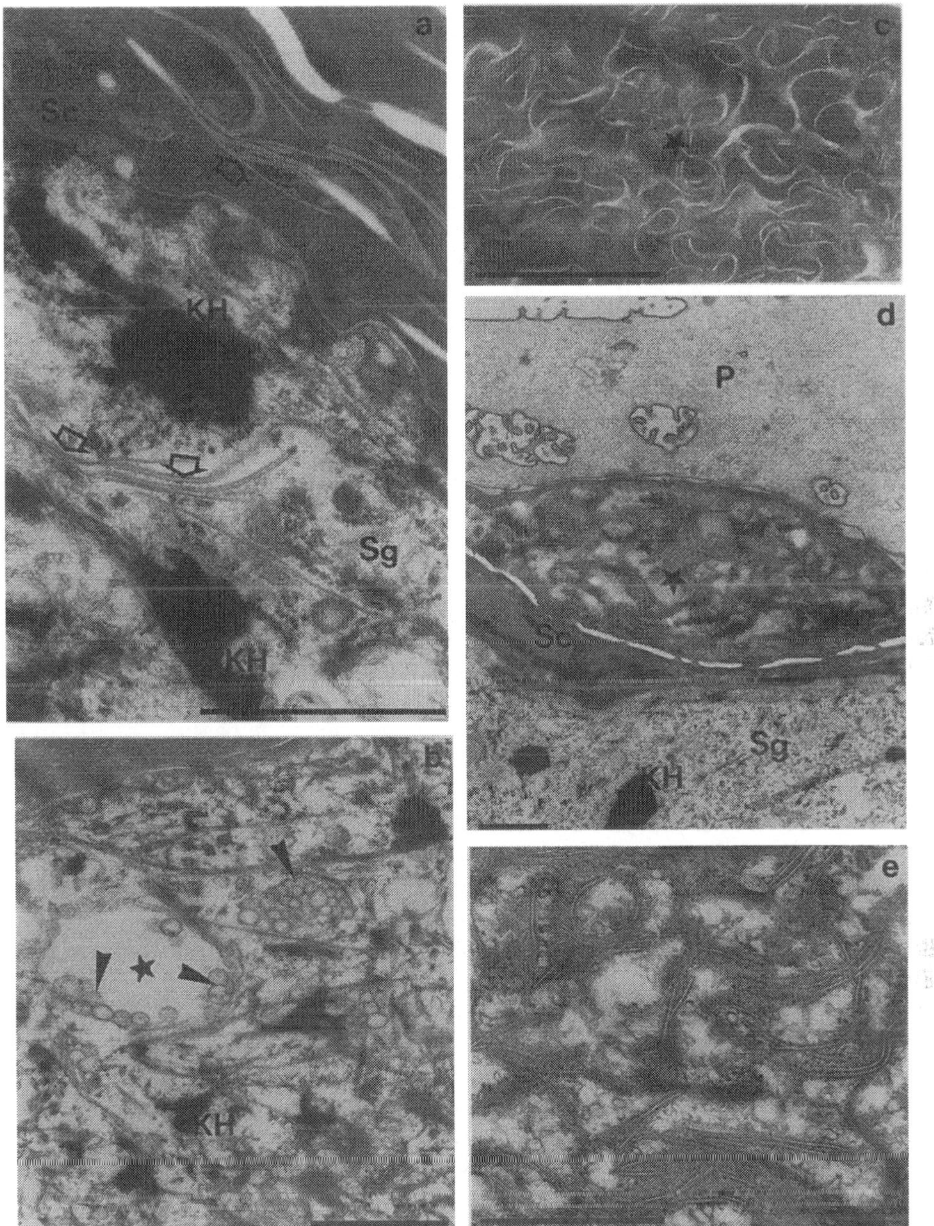

(*Sc*). ×33000. **b** Granular cell with a vesicular keratinosome complex (*single arrowhead*) and an ovoid vacuole (*) containing abnormal vesicular keratinosomes (*arrowheads*) on the inner leaflet of the limiting membrane. *KH*, Ultrastructurally normal keratohyalin. ×19000 (From [2]). **c–e** Ichthyosis congenita type IV. Groups of irregularly arranged curved lamellae (*) are concentrated in circumscribed blow-up regions of the horn cells (*Sc*) of a deceased newborn (**c**, re-embedded from paraffin material); the same pattern of synthesis and deposition of lipid lamellae is already manifest in an affected fetus of the same family (**d** and **e**) with the first onset of keratinization: trilaminar lamellae are present in blown-up regions (*) of keratinized fetal horn cells (*Sc*), while periderm cells (*P*) do not yet reveal the disturbance. *KH*, Ultrastructurally normal keratohyalin. (From [4], courtesy of Dr. I. Anton-Lamprecht and Dr. M.-L. Arnold, Heidelberg). c, ×25000; d, ×9000; e, ×25000

Independent of the ultrastructural work done in Europe, the Williams/Elias group from San Francisco approached the question of heterogeneity using newly elaborated lipid biochemical techniques. Based on their lipid biochemical findings, Williams and Elias [30, 31] suggested distinguishing between between an erythrodermic (ELI) and a nonerythrodermic (NELI) variant of lamellar ichthyosis. They found large quantities of n-alkanes (straight-chain, fully saturated hydrocarbons) in the scales of ELI patients. In ELI the n-alkanes made up 25% of the total scale lipids, whereas NELI patients had only slightly elevated n-alkane levels (7%) compared with a normal background of 5.5%. Moreover, in NELI significant elevations of free sterols were found, making up 24% of the total scale lipids and a significant increase of sphingolipids, whereas in ELI these values did not differ from the normal controls. Their findings suggested a clear-cut separation between ELI and NELI. This view seemed to be backed up by cell kinetic studies performed by Hazell and Marks [14]. They found an increased labeling index in patients with ELI, whereas in patients with NELI epidermal cell turnover was not significantly increased compared with normal controls.

Very recently, the Happle group [5] confirmed genetic heterogeneity of lamellar ichthyosis by enzyme studies. They found very low levels of beta-glucosidase in the scales of 10 ELI patients (ELI type A), whereas 13 patients with NELI (type A) had rather low values for soluble butyrase. The internal ratio of the two enzymes (butyrase: glucosidase ratio) yielded a clear-cut separation of ELI and NELI. A ratio below 11 was found in NELI, whereas a ratio above 40 was indicative of ELI. A decrease of butyrase may reflect a functional state of the epidermis, while a deficiency of soluble beta-glucosidase has so far not been found in a screening of the major and some of the rare types of ichthyosis (P. Mier 1988, personal communication). Very recent results indicate that beta-glucosidase is not missing in ELI type A, but that the enzyme firmly adheres to the lamellar body and is much less releasable than other lamellar body enzymes.

4.2.3.3 Clinical Phenotypes

As discussed above, dermatologists were – for good reasons – rather conservative about basing a nosologic classification of lamellar ichthyosis on phenotypic differences. However, the lipid biochemical findings of the Williams/Elias group [30–32] paved the way for a better clinical understanding of lamellar ichthyosis. It is possible to distinguish between two clinical phenotypes: erythrodermic (ELI) and nonerythrodermic (NELI) lamellar ichthyosis [26, 27, 31]. Unfortunately, the clinical phenotypes do not seem to correlate very well with genotypes as revealed by ultrastructural markers, according to very recent studies [2]. As already stated, the ELI phenotype still is genotypically heterogeneous and comprises the more common beta-glucosidase-deficient type and the less frequent cholesterol-deposition type. At the recent symposium "Advances in Ichthyosis Research", held at Nijmegen on Nov. 3, 1988, Dr. Gedde-Dahl showed that some of the cholesterol-deposition-type patients may also display the NELI phenotype [12]. Anton-Lamprecht came to the same conclusion [2]. The NELI phenotype certainly shows genetic heterogeneity, too. It includes a more common type characterized by moderate scaling, low butyrase activity in the scales, and vesicular keratinosomes (NELI type A/ichthyosis congenita type III), and at least a second type clinically reminiscent of the Sjögren-Larsson syndrome (NELI type B or ichthyosis congenita type IV). At the above-mentioned symposium, Dr. Mary Williams (San Francisco) presented her series of patients with the NELI phenotype. The majority of her NELI patients were much more severely affected than the average patients with the NELI phenotype observed in West Germany, The Netherlands, or Norway. The reason for this is unknown, but it can account for some differences between the European and American experience with lamellar ichthyosis. Probably, the extremely affected patients observed by Dr. Mary Williams represent a third subset of the NELI group (NELI type C). I regard ELI and NELI as clinical phenotypes but no longer as distinct genetic entities.

Bernhardt and Baden [6] recently questioned the value of such designations as ELI and NELI. They reported on a family with very mild nonerythematous lamellar ichthyosis which did not fit the descriptions given for NELI. Likewise, I have seen three patients with very mild nonerythematous lamellar ichthyosis who are difficult to assign to either the NELI or ELI groups. Moreover, I have observed a family consisting of two sisters and their brother who showed marked variation of the clinical phenotype (Fig. 40). The elder sister presented the typical NELI (type A) phenotype. The younger sister displayed large gray scales

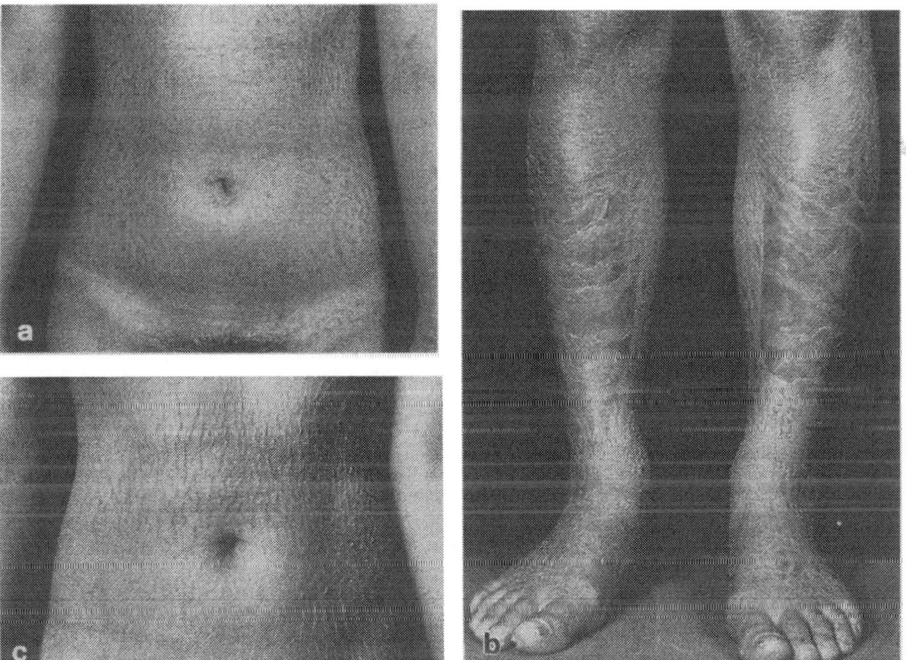

Fig. 40a–c. See explanation on the next page

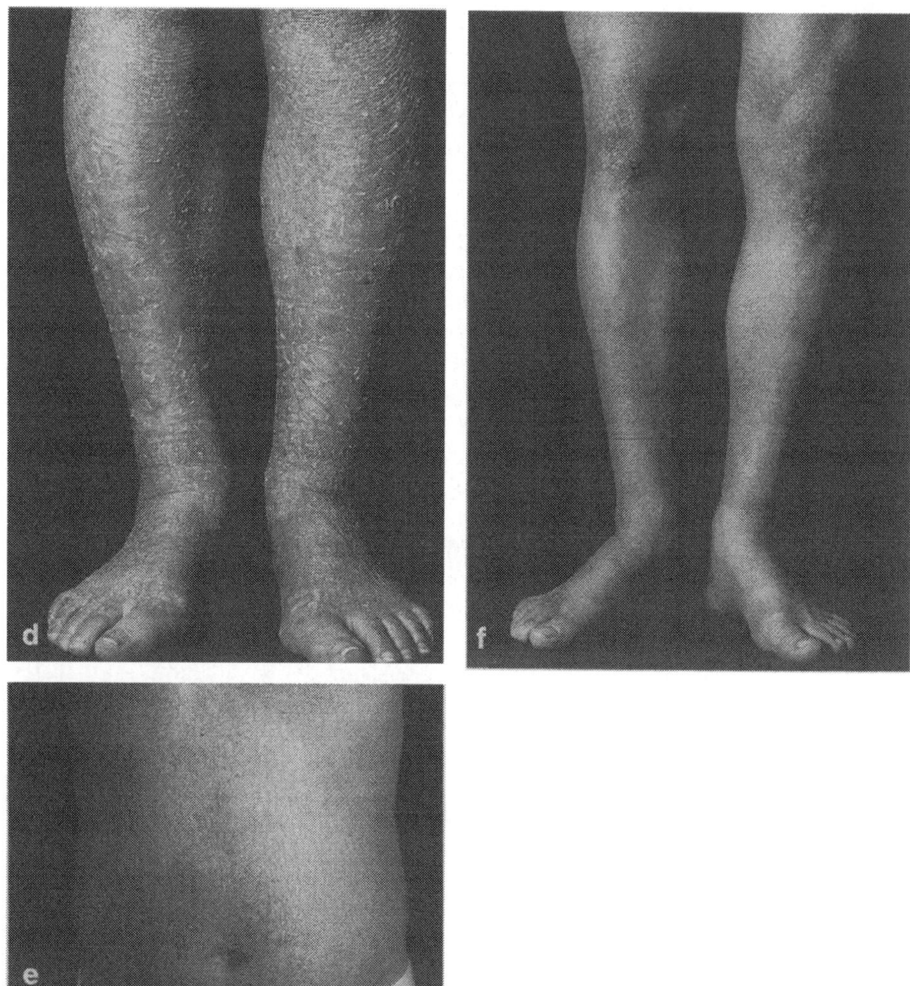

Fig. 40d–f. Marked variation of disease expression in a NELI family (type A). **a** and **b** The elder sister presents the typical NELI phenotype with large dark-brown scales (untreated, wintertime). **c** and **d** The younger sister shows only fine scaling with a reticulate pattern on the trunk and marked scaling accompanied with erythroderma over the legs (untreated, wintertime). **e** and **f** Mild scaling reminiscent of ichthyosis vulgaris in the brother (untreated, wintertime)

accompanied by considerable erythema over the extremities, but only fine scaling and slight erythematous stripes on the trunk. Her scaling had the reticulate pattern considered typical of ichthyosis congenita type III, according to Arnold et al. [4]. The brother, finally, suffered from very mild ichthyosis with no erythema at all. The low butyrase activity found in the scales of these three patients [5] suggests that they belong to the NELI group (type A). Despite my reservations concerning the true significance of terms like "ELI" and "NELI," I want to briefly discuss the "ideal" or "typical" features of these clinical phenotypes.

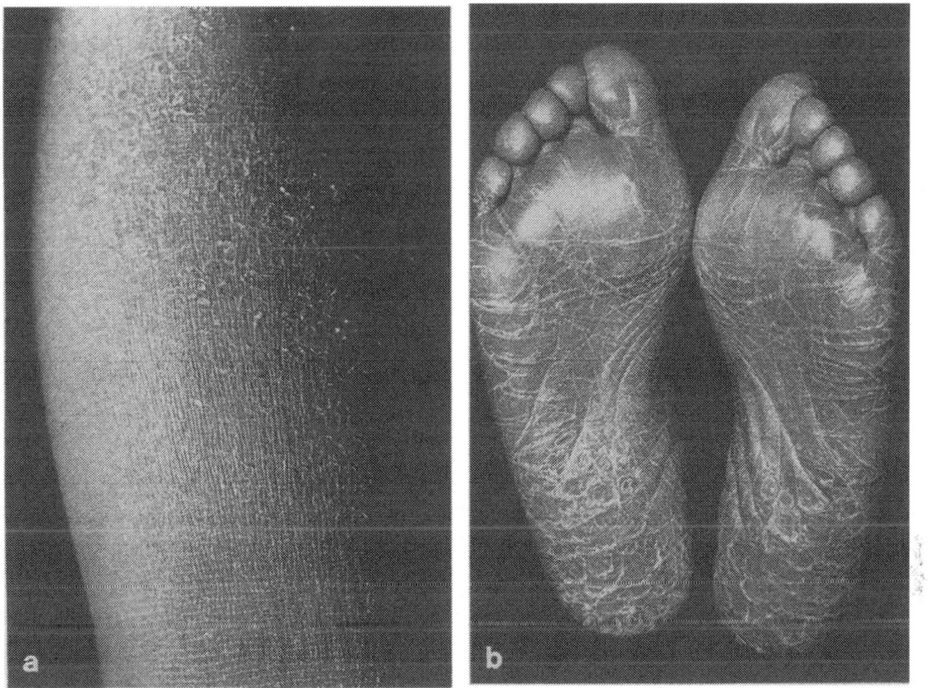

Fig. 41a, b. Erythrodermic lamellar ichthyosis (type A). **a** Fine translucent scaling, **b** marked plantar keratosis

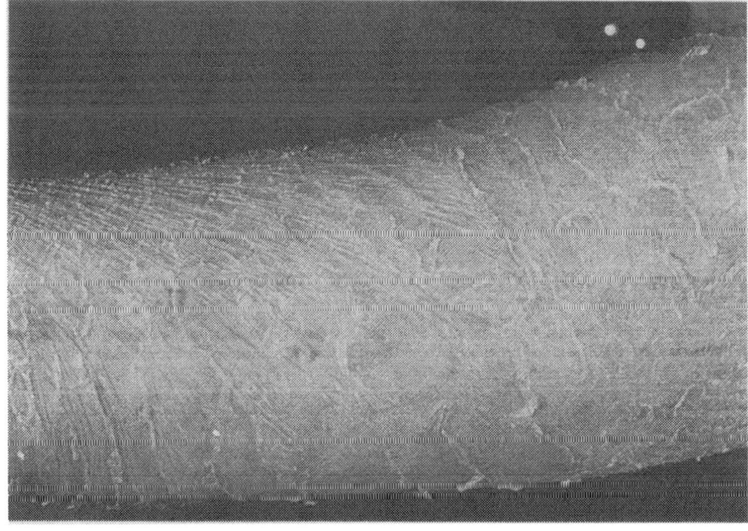

Fig. 42. Erythrodermic lamellar ichthyosis (type B?) Unusually large, coarse hyperkeratoses. (From [26])

Clinical Features of ELI

The most outstanding feature of ELI is erythroderma. At birth all ELI patients present ichthyotic erythroderma. Some, but not all of them, are also encased in a collodion-like membrane (collodion baby). In a few patients the erythroderma fades and is no longer present or hardly visible in later life, while in others it remains rather marked. It is not as severe, however, as in patients with Sézary syndrome, for example. Patients with very severe ichthyotic erythroderma usually suffer from the Comèl-Netherton syndrome and not from ELI. Most patients with ELI exhibit only fine scaling (Fig. 41), whereas in some, large, coarse hyperkeratoses can be noted (Fig. 42). The scaling usually involves the flexural folds, but may be less severe in this region. In most, but not all patients with ELI marked hyperkeratosis of the palms and soles can be seen, often in striking contrast to rather fine, translucent scales on the rest of the body. Ectropion is present in many ELI cases. It may be less marked than in NELI [31]. At the moment it is not possible to distinguish between the ELI type A and ELI type B by clinical analysis. The main reason for this is that a sufficient clinical description of the ELI type B (cholesterol-deposition type/ichthyosis congenita type II) is so far lacking.

Clinical Features of NELI

According to the descriptions given by Williams and Elias [31], NELI (type C) patients are very severely affected and display large, platelike dark-brown hyperkeratoses (Fig. 43). There is no erythroderma at birth, but they may also present as collodion babies. Appreciable erythroderma never develops, though between the cracks of the scales erythematous stripes can be seen. Palms and soles are usually dry and hyperkeratotic, but generally to a lesser extent than in ELI.

As stated above, I have observed one NELI family (type A) with remarkable phenotypic variations, ranging from moderate lamellar ichthyosis with dark-brown scales to a rather mild involvement resembling the phenotype of ichthyosis vulgaris. Likewise, Arnold et al. [4] stress that some of their NELI (type A) patients (ichthyosis congenita type III, according to their designation) presented with only a rather mild ichthyosis, while others were very severely involved. I take this as a clue that the background of other genes influences and modulates the clinical expression of lamellar ichthyosis in NELI type A (and in other types of lamellar ichthoyis). The clinical features of NELI type A have to be expanded to also include patients with rather mild, but nonerythematous lamellar ichthyosis (Fig. 44). Recent biochemical data support the notion that NELI type A has a broad clinical spectrum. Using the butyrase/beta-glucosidase ratio, several patients with mild nonerythematous lamellar ichthyosis were assigned to this group [5]. As stated above, NELI type B looks very similar to the Sjögren-Larsson syndrome as far as the cutaneous phenotype is concerned. It may be identical with ichthyosis congenita type IV.

4.2.3.4 Histologic Features

Routine histopathology fails to allow a definite recognition of the different subtypes of autosomal recessive lamellar ichthyosis. Using semithin sections cut

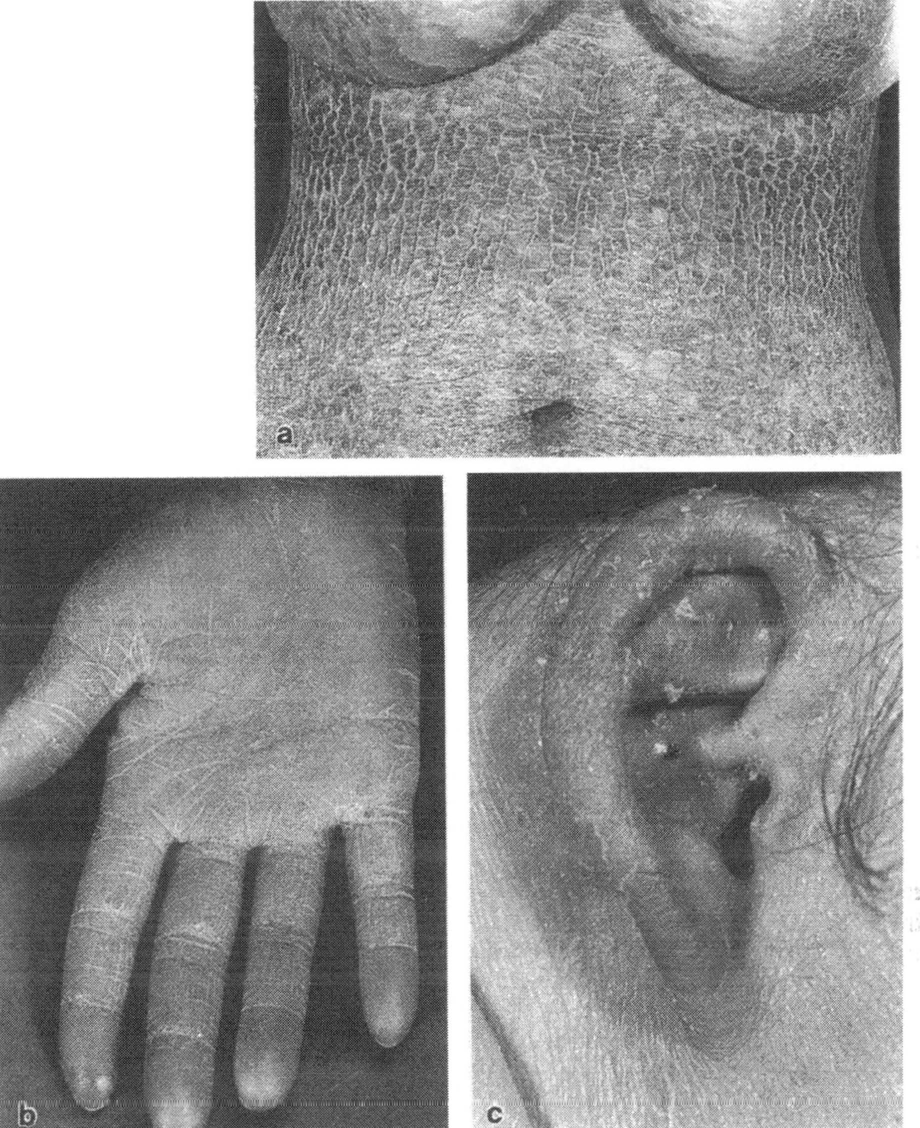

Fig. 43a–c. Nonerythrodermic lamellar ichthyosis (type C). **a** Note platelike dark-brown hyperkeratoses; **b** palmoplantar involvement is usually rather mild. This patient has a very severe form, similar to the cases of Dr. Williams; **c** deformed, small ears are typical of this severe type. (From [26])

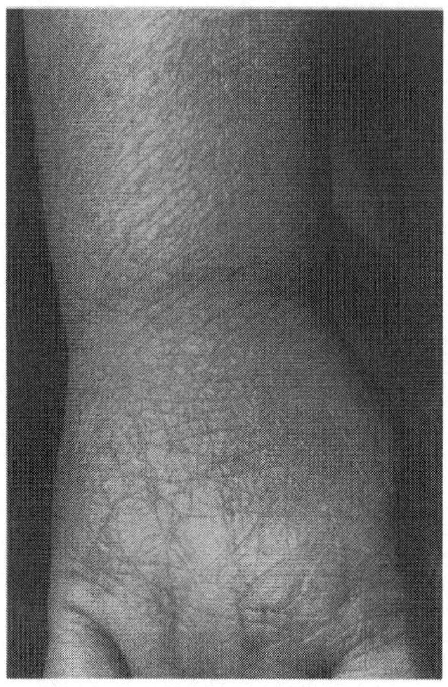

Fig. 44. Mild disease expression in lamellar ichthyosis. Low butyrase levels in the scales suggest that this patient with a clinically intermediate picture belongs to NELI type A

with an ultratome, it is possible to see vacuoles within the keratinocytes of the granular layer in NELI type A patients [4]. The characteristic rodlike electron-lucent vacuoles typical of the cholesterol-deposition type (ELI type B) cannot be seen on routine histology [15], though a special digitonin staining might visualize these structures in the stratum corneum. This question has not yet been studied. Finally, the more common beta-glucosidase-deficient type (ELI type A) lacks any specific histologic features. Quantitative differences in the thickness of the stratum corneum are also problematic since these differences reflect the extent of scaling, which at least in NELI type A is very variable.

In my opinion, the value of a histologic examination lies in the exclusion of epidermolytic hyperkeratosis (bullous types of ichthyosis) and in the possibility that some clues may be gained for a differential diagnosis of the Comèl-Netherton syndrome. This latter condition may masquerade as ELI [27]. In the Comèl-Netherton syndrome, marked parakeratosis can be found and the granular layer is decreased and often lacking. Prominent PAS-positive clumps appear within the stratum corneum. In contrast, in lamellar ichthyosis the stratum corneum predominantly shows orthohyperkeratosis, an increased or normal granular layer, and usually acanthosis (Fig. 45). A faint, but distinct PAS-positive staining of the stratum corneum may be seen in both ELI and NELI patients, in my experience, while according to Williams and Elias, this is more typical of ELI patients. In the dermis moderate perivascular infiltrates are usually observed, but the extent of this inflammation correlates poorly with the clinical phenotype. Very marked inflammatory changes, spongiosis, and exocytosis are usually a sign of the Comèl-Netherton syndrome and not of ELI.

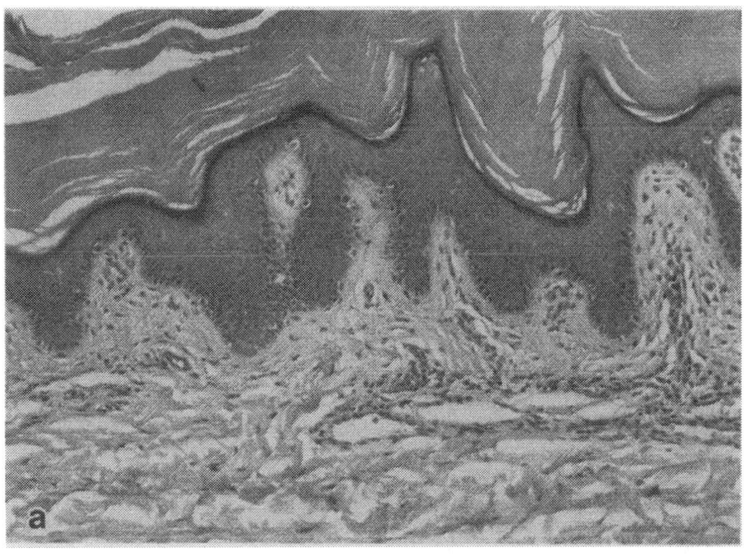

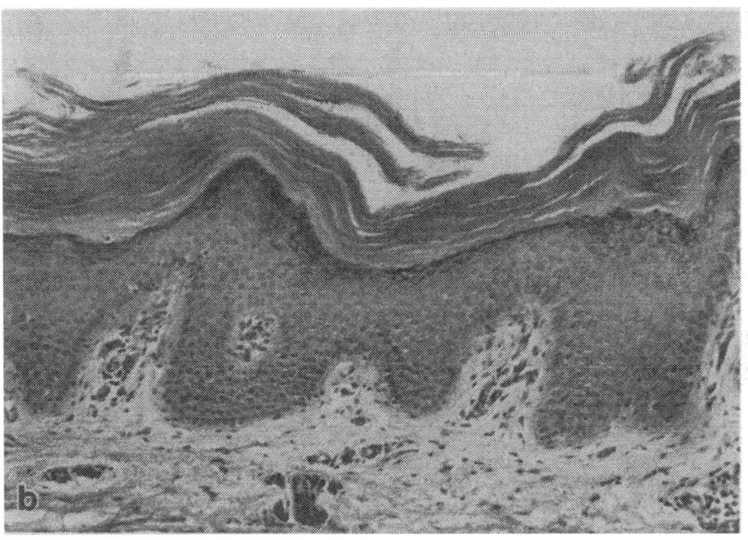

Fig. 45a, b. Histology of lamellar ichthyosis. **a** ELI. Nonspecific changes such as orthohyperkeratosis, an increased granular layer, acanthosis, and papillomatosis. Same patient as in Fig. 37. HE, ×50. **b** NELI. The upper portions of the stratum corneum are PAS positive, while the lowermost part of the stratum corneum is not. The rete/papillae pattern is flattened. The rete ridges are plump and confluent. Clinical features and enzymology assign this patient to NELI type A. PAS, ×100

4.2.4 Genetic Counseling in Lamellar Ichthyosis

Increasing genetic heterogeneity and intrafamilial variation of disease expression make genetic counseling a difficult task, especially when one is confronted with a sporadic case. In patients having a negative family history the question is: Is this case due to a recessive gene, or due to a new mutation of a dominant gene? Without access to the new diagnostic tools this question cannot be answered properly. Moreover, I want to caution that as far as ADLI is concerned, the new diagnostic advances (ultrastructural characteristics, typical scale lipid profile) are based on the study of one family only. It must still be established whether these findings are representative of all ADLI families.

It can be assumed that most sporadic cases will belong to one of the recessive types of lamellar ichthyosis. If it is not possible to make use of the newly described biologic disease markers I advise to assume the worst. Parents should be told that the risk for further children to be affected is at least 25% for each pregnancy. Even if diagnosis of a dominant type of congenital ichthyosis can be established in a sporadic case, this does not necessarily rule out any recurrence risk. Sporadic cases of a dominant disease cannot always be explained as de novo mutations, but may be due to an early somatic mutation affecting the germ line of a parent. Gonadal mosaicism in a parent is a problem that troubles genetic counselors.

Prenatal diagnosis of the lamellar ichthyoses would be desirable but is very problematic as far as a safe exclusion diagnosis is concerned [2, 3, 20]. The main reason is that onset of normal keratinization is after week 24 of gestational age and thus practically beyond the time when termination of a pregnancy can be advised without running into very serious ethical and legal problems. In contrast to harlequin fetus and Sjögren-Larsson syndrome, patients with lamellar ichthyosis do not always exhibit signs of precocious keratinization. Two cases of false-negative exlusion diagnosis have been reported [3, 20]. Using fetoscopy and electron microscopy, a safe exclusion may be impossible before 22 weeks of gestation [2, 3, 20]. According to Anton-Lamprecht [2], only two types (ELI type B/ichthyosis congenita type II, and NELI type B/ichthyosis congenita type IV) can be safely diagnosed antenatally.

In the future, polymorphic DNA markers may become a very powerful tool for prenatal diagnosis. At the moment these DNA techniques cannot be employed, as none of the various types of lamellar ichthyoses has been assigned to a specific chromosomal locus.

References

1. Anton-Lamprecht I (1972) Zur Ultrastruktur herreditärer Verhornungsstörungen. I. Ichthyosis congenita. Arch Dermatol Forsch 243:88–100
2. Anton-Lamprecht I (1989) Pränatale Diagnostik von Genodermatosen. Vortrag 35. Tagung der Deutschen Dermatologischen Gesellschaft, München, 27.4.–1.5.1988. Hautarzt Suppl. VIII:16–20
3. Arnold ML, Anton-Lamprecht I (1985) Problems in prenatal diagnosis of the ichthyosis congenita group. Hum Genet 71:301–311

4. Arnold ML, Anton-Lamprecht I, Melz-Rothfuss B, Hartschuh W (1988) Ichthyosis congenita type III. Clinical and ultrastructural characteristics and distinction within the heterogeneous ichthyosis congenita group. Arch Dermatol Res 280:268–278
5. Bergers M, Traupe H, Mier PD, Steijlen P, Happle R (1989) Enzymatic distinction between two subgroups of autosomal recessive lamellar ichthyosis. J Invest Dermatol (submitted)
6. Bernhardt M, Baden HP (1986) Report of a family with an unusual expression of recessive ichthyosis. Review of 42 cases. Arch Dermatol 122:428–433
7. Brocq L (1902) Erythrodermie congénitale ichthyosiforme avec hyperépidermotrophie. Ann Dermatol Syph (Paris) ser 4, 3:1–31
8. Frenk E (1981) Spontaneously healing collodion baby: a light and electron-microscopical study. Acta Derm Venereol (Stockh) 61:168–171
9. Frost P (1978) Less common scaling dermatoses. In: Marks R, Dykes PJ (eds) The ichthyoses. MTP, Lancaster, pp 107–126
10. Frost P, Van Scott EJ (1966) Ichthyosiform dermatoses. Classification based on anatomic and biometric observations. Arch Dermatol 94:113–126
11. Frost P, Weinstein G, Van Scott EJ (1966) The ichthyosiform dermatoses. II. Autoradiographic studies of epidermal proliferation. J Invest Dermatol 47:561–567
12. Gedde-Dahl T (1988) Genetic heterogeneity of congenital ichthyoses: evidence from clinical and epidemiological data. Lecture at the symposium "Advances in Ichthyosis Research", 3 Nov 1988, Nijmegen, The Netherlands
13. Gedde-Dahl T, Rajka G, Larsen TE, Jellum E (1984) Autosomal recessive ichthyosis in Norway. II. Sjögren-Larsson-like ichthyosis without CNS or eye involvement. Clin Genet 25:242–244
14. Hazell M, Marks R (1985) Clinical, histologic, and cell kinetic discriminants between lamellar ichthyosis and nonbullous congenital ichthyosiform erythroderma. Arch Dermatol 121:489–493
15. Kanerva L, Niemi K-M, Lauharanta J, Lassus A (1983) New observations on the fine structure of lamellar ichthyosis and the effect of treatment with etretinate. Am J Dermatopathol 5:555–567
16. Kolde G, Happle R, Traupe H (1985) Autosomal-dominant lamellar ichthyosis: ultrastructural characteristics of a new type of congenital ichthyosis. Arch Dermatol Res 278:1–5
17. Larrègue M, Ottavy N, Bressieux JM, Lorette J (1986) Bébé collodion. Trente-deux nouvelles observations. Ann Dermatol Venereol 113:773–785
18. Melnik B, Küster W, Hollmann J, Plewig G, Traupe H (1989) Autosomal dominant lamellar ichthyosis identified by an abnormal scale lipid pattern. Clin Genet 35:152–156
19. Niemi K-M, Kanerva L (1989) Ichthyosis with laminated membrane structures. Am J Dermatopathol 11 (2):149–156
20. Perry TB, Holbrook KA, Hoff MS, Hamilton EF, Senikas V, Fisher C (1987) Prenatal diagnosis of congenital nonbullous ichthyosiform erythroderma (lamellar ichthyosis). Prenat Diagn 7:145–155
21. Reed WB, Herwick RP, Harville D, Porter PS, Conant M (1972) Lamellar ichthyosis of the newborn. A distinct clinical entity: its comparison to the other ichthyosiform erythrodermas. Arch Dermatol 105:394–399
22. Riecke E (1900) Ueber Ichthyosis congenita. Arch Dermatol Syph (Wien) 54:289–340
23. Rossmann-Ringdahl I, Anton-Lamprecht I, Swanbeck G (1986) A mother and two children with nonbullous congenital ichthyosiform erythroderma. Arch Dermatol 122:559–564
24. Siemens HW (1928) Zur Differentialdiagnose und Prognose der überlebenden Fälle von Ichthyosis congenita. Arch Dermatol Syph 156:624–655
25. Toribio J, Redondo VF, Peteiro C, Zulaica A, Fabeiro JM (1986) Autosomal dominant lamellar ichthyosis. Clin Genet 30:122–126
26. Traupe H (1986) Die Ichthyosen: auf dem Weg vom Phän zum Gen. In: Macher E, Czarnetzki BM, Knop J (eds) Jahrbuch der Dermatologie 1986. Regensberg and Biermann, Münster, pp 35–48
27. Traupe H (1987) Clinical and genetic features of the lamellar ichthyoses: evidence for three different types. In: Happle R, Grosshans E (eds) Pediatric dermatology. Advances in diagnosis and treatment. Springer, Berlin Heidelberg New York, Tokyo, pp 30–40

28. Traupe H, Kolde G, Happle R (1984) Autosomal dominant lamellar ichthyosis: a new skin disorder. Clin Genet 26:457–461
29. Vandersteen PR, Muller SA (1972) Lamellar ichthyosis. An enzyme-histochemical, light- and electron-microscopic study. Arch Dermatol 106:694–701
30. Williams ML, Elias PM (1984) Elevated n-alkanes in congenital ichthyosiform erythroderma. Phenotypic differentiation of two types of autosomal recessive ichthyosis. J Clin Invest 74:296–300
31. Williams ML, Elias PM (1985) Heterogeneity in autosomal recessive ichthyosis. Clinical and biochemical differentiation of lamellar ichthyosis and nonbullous congenital ichthyosiform erythroderma. Arch Dermatol 121:477–488
32. Williams ML, Elias PM (1986) Ichthyosis: genetic heterogeneity, genodermatoses and genetic counseling. Arch Dermatol 122:529–531

4.3 Alopecia Ichthyotica: A Characteristic Feature of Many Types of Congenital Ichthyosis

Collodion skin and ectropion, involvement of palms and soles, and involvement of the big flexures are recognized features commonly found in many patients with congenital ichthyosis. In contrast, alopecia ichthyotica is a much neglected sign [4], though it may be of similar diagnostic value. Like the other symptoms mentioned, alopecia ichthyotica is not a specific marker of a single disease, but can be seen in various types of congenital ichthyosis (Table 24). We [10] observed this type of hair loss in adult patients suffering from both the erythrodermic (Fig. 46a) and nonerythrodermic (Fig. 46b) variants of lamellar ichthyosis. It can be found in patients with X-linked dominant ichthyosis, too [5]. Alopecia ichthyotica is also a feature of patients with neutral lipid storage disease [2] and of ichthyosis follicularis with photosensitivity [3, 7]. Recently, Jagell and coworkers reported on a Swedish family with nonerythrodermic lamellar ichthyosis, mental retardation, marked alopecia ichthyotica, ectropion, and eclabion. Apparently, they did not realize that alopecia ichthyotica, ectropion, and ecla-

Table 24. Alopecia ichthyotica in congenital ichthyoses

Diagnosis	Scalp biopsy	Reference
Erythrodermic lamellar ichthyosis (type A)	Inflammation around hair follicles, pseudopelade	Traupe and Happle 1983 [10], Williams and Elias 1985 [11]
Nonerythrodermic lamellar ichthyosis (type C)	Pseudopelade	Frost 1978 [4], Traupe and Happle 1983 [10], Williams and Elias 1985 [11], Jagell et al. 1987 [6]
Ichthyosis follicularis with alopecia and photosensitivity	Inflammation around hair follicles	MacLeod 1909 [7], Eramo et al. 1985 [3]
Neutral lipid storage disease	Not done	Dorfman et al. 1974 [2]
X-linked dominant ichthyosis	Not done	Happle 1979 [5], Manzke et al. 1980 [8]
Keratitis-ichthyosis-like hyperkeratosis-deafness syndrome[a]	Not done	Burns 1915 [1], Skinner et al. 1981 [9]

[a] The Burns syndrome (keratitis-ichthyosis-like hyperkeratosis-deafness syndrome) is often erroneously classified as congenital ichthyosis

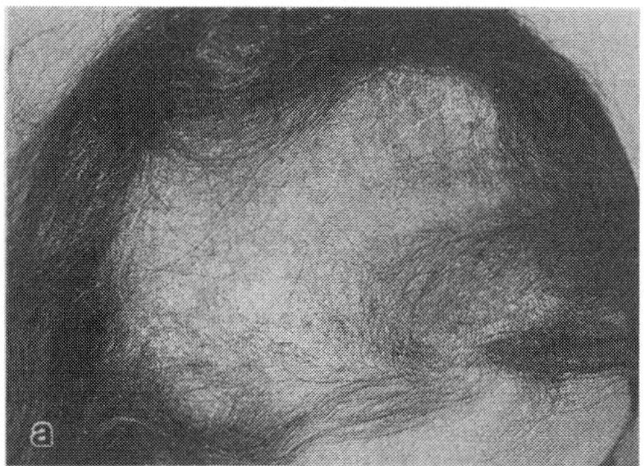

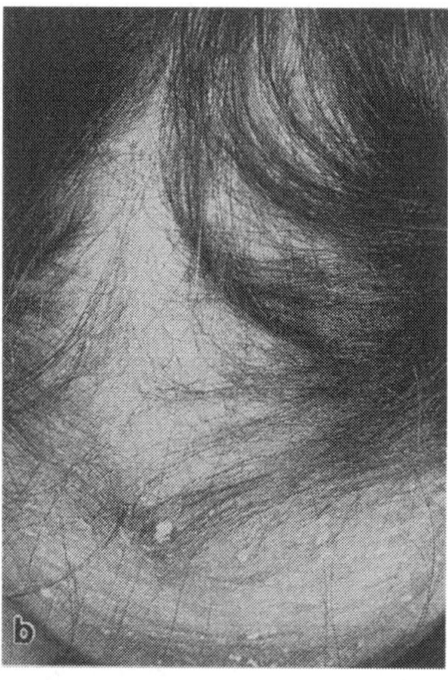

Fig. 46a, b. Alopecia ichthyotica **(a)** in a 24-year-old woman with ELI (type A), **(b)** in a 21-year-old woman with NELI (type C). (**a** From [10] with permission of Karger-Verlag, Basel)

bion are common features of various types of lamellar ichthyosis, and the presence of these nonspecific signs led them to assume a new genetic syndrome. The only unusual feature, however, was severe mental retardation, which could have been a chance association in this consanguineous family. According to Jagell et al. [6], alopecia ichthyotica is not a feature of the Sjögren-Larsson syndrome and I myself have never observed it in the epidermolytic ichthyoses.

In our series of 16 patients with autosomal recessive lamellar ichthyosis, four exhibited alopecia ichthyotica [10]. Alopecia ichthyotica usually starts during adolescence and can become very severe during adult life. Clinically, a circumscribed, scarring alopecia involving large parts of the scalp can be seen. In X-linked dominant ichthyosis usually only small patches are involved, probably reflecting X-chromosome mosaicism of the defective gene [5].

Light microscopy of hairs taken from the margin of the alopecic lesions reveals an uneven diameter and irregular torsions of the hair shaft along its axis and trichorrhexis nodosa. A biopsy taken from the margin of an active lesion in a patient with ELI showed pronounced inflammatory infiltrates around the hair follicles (Fig. 47), whereas biopsies obtained from the center of such a lesion displayed the typical features of pseudopelade [10]. Mostly, hair follicles are lacking completely in alopecia ichthyotica. They have been replaced by fibrous tracts reaching from the corium up to the epidermis. Moreover, the dermis is usually sclerotic and orphaned hair muscles can be seen.

Because of its scarring nature, alopecia ichthyotica is a permanent, irreversible hair loss that cannot improve with topical or retinoid therapy. The mechanisms causing this type of hair loss are not quite clear. It is resaonable to assume that

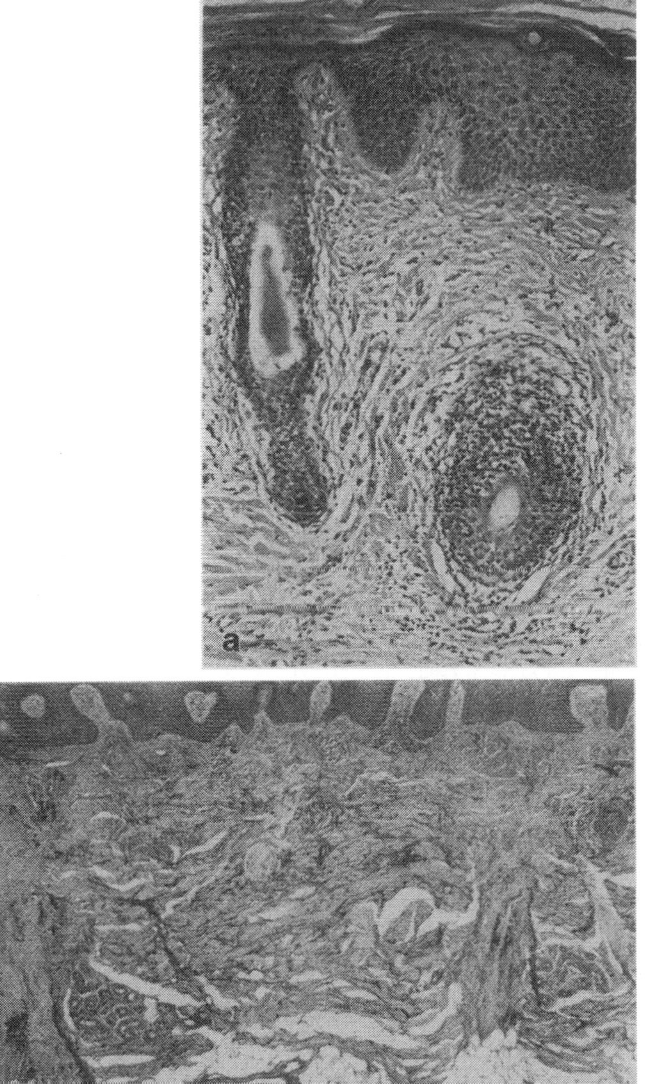

Fig. 47 a, b. Scalp biopsies in alopecia ichthyotica. **a** ELI (type A): Dense perifollicular round cell infiltrate contrasting with only slight infiltrate in the dermis. HE, ×40. **b** NELI (type C): Pseudopelade with sclerotic dermis. Orcein, ×12.5 (**a** From [10] with permission of Karger-Verlag, Basel)

the inflammatory changes accompanying the congenital ichthyoses play a major role and finally result in the pseudopelade-like state. This sequence of events has been established for other inflammatory scalp diseases such as lichen planus and discoid lupus erythematosus. Likewise, it is possible that there is a specific (immunologic?) attack against the hair follicles, similar to the mechanism seen in alopecia areata. As we know from alopecia areata, such a specific attack does not have to manifest itself as erythema.

References

1. Burns FS (1915) A case of generalized keratoderma with unusual involvement of the eyes, and nasal and buccal mucous membranes. J Cutan Dis 33:255–260
2. Dorfman ML, Hershko C, Eisenberg S, Sagher F (1974) Ichthyosiform dermatosis with systemic lipidosis. Arch Dermatol 110:261–266
3. Eramo LR, Esterly NB, Zieserl EJ, Stock EL, Herrmann J (1985) Ichthyosis follicularis with alopecia and photophobia. Arch Dermatol 121:1167–1174
4. Frost P (1978) Less common scaling dermatoses. In: Marks R, Dykes PJ (eds) The ichthyoses. MTP, Lancaster, pp 107–126
5. Happle R (1979) X-linked dominant chondrodysplasia punctata. Review of literature and report of a case. Hum Genet 53:65–73
6. Jagell SF, Holmgren G, Hofer PA (1987) Congenital ichthyosis with alopecia, eclabion, ectropion and mental retardation - a new genetic syndrome. Clin Genet 31:102–108
7. MacLeod JMH (1909) Three cases of "ichthyosis follicularis" associated with baldness. Br J Dermatol 21:165–189
8. Manzke H, Christophers E, Wiedemann HR (1980) Dominant sex-linked inherited chondrodysplasia punctata: a distinct type of chondrodysplasia punctata. Clin Genet 17:97–107
9. Skinner BA, Greist MC, Norins AL (1981) The keratitis, ichthyosis and deafness (KID) syndrome. Arch Dermatol 117:285–289
10. Traupe H, Happle R (1983) Alopecia ichthyotica. A characteristic feature of congenital ichthyosis. Dermatologica 167:225–230
11. Williams ML, Elias PM (1985) Heterogeneity in autosomal recessive ichthyosis. Clinical and biochemical differentiation of lamellar ichthyosis and nonbullous congenital ichthyosiform erythroderma. Arch Dermatol 121:477–488

4.4 The Epidermolytic (Acanthokeratolytic) Ichthyoses

4.4.1 Classification

Just as the term "lamellar ichthyosis" no longer refers to a single entitiy, the group of epidermolytic ichthyoses today comprises at least three different diseases: bullous ichthyotic erythroderma (BIE), ichthyosis bullosa of Siemens (IBS), and ichthyosis hystrix of Curth-Macklin (IHCM). These three diseases

Table 25. Classification of the epidermolytic ichthyoses

Feature	**Diagnosis**		
	Bullous ichthyotic erythroderma of Brocq	Ichthyosis bullosa of Siemens	Ichthyosis hystrix of Curth-Macklin
		Similarities	
Inheritance:	Autosomal dominant	Autosomal dominant	Autosomal dominant
Clinical features:	Keratotic lichenification (rippled aspect)	Keratotic lichenification (rippled aspect)	Keratotic lichenification (rippled aspect)
Histology:	Epidermolytic hyperkeratosis	Epidermolytic hyperkeratosis	Epidermolytic hyperkeratosis
Ultrastructure:	Tonofilament clumping	Tonofilament clumping	Tonofilament clumping
		Differences	
Clinical features:	Ichthyotic erythroderma	No erythroderma	Ichthyotic erythroderma
	Generalized involvement (in most families)	More localized involvement	Generalized involvement
	Blistering	Blistering	No blistering
	Palms and soles free (in most families)	Palms and soles free	Palms and soles affected (not always)
Chemistry:[a]	Low alpha-mannosidase levels in scales and epidermis (two patients)	Normal alpha-mannosidase levels (two patients)	Not done

[a] M. Bergers, Nijmegen, personal communication 1988

share the essential histologic finding of epidermolytic hyperkeratosis (acantho-keratolysis), and all three are inherited as autosomal dominant traits. Clinical and ultrastructural differences enable us, however, to distinguish between the three different cornification disorders (Table 25).

Reading the available literature on patients with epidermolytic hyperkeratosis, one is startled by the variation of disease expression between families, whereas clinical phenotypes are fairly constant within a given family [20, 27]. Each familiy probably has its "own" mutation, and that may account for the clinical and ultrastructural differences. I am inclined to believe that these mutations affect the same gene in all three types. In other words, I assume multiple allelism for the epidermolytic ichthyoses. The situation may well be similar to that of the Duchenne and Becker types of muscular dystrophy.

4.4.2 Bullous Ichthyotic Erythroderma of Brocq

4.4.2.1 Historical Aspects

In 1902, Brocq [8] distinguished a dry from a bullous variant of congenital ichtyosis. About 50 years later, Lapière [21] recognized the peculiar histologic features of this disease and referred to it as "granular degeneration". In the 1960s, Frost and Van Scott [10] introduced the term "epidermolytic hyperkeratosis" for this histologic pattern, which can be found in a variety of hereditary and non-genetic skin disorders. Jung and Schnyder [18] drew attention to the autosomal dominant inheritance of BIE. Dominant transmission of the disease helped to separate BIE from autosomal recessive lamellar ichthyosis.

4.4.2.2 Clinical Features

Directly after birth, the children may present as "enfants brûlé," i. e., they exhibit ichthyotic erythroderma and severe blistering. During the first year of life the blistering and the erythema usually subside, and hystrix-like keratoses develop instead. The axilla, the elbows and the flexural aspect of the knees often are severely affected and show prominent keratotic ridges. On the trunk the hyperkeratosis often gives the skin a lichenified appearance, while spiny, hystrix-like keratoses can project up to 1 cm on the anterior surface of the knees and lower legs (Fig. 48) in some severely affected patients. After removal of these keratoses, a residual erythema is visible even in later life, and blisters develop rather easily after minor trauma. In most families palms and soles are spared (Fig. 49), but there are exceptions to this rule [27]. Patients are prone to develop impetigo and often have an offensive body odor. A daily bath (e. g., with potassium permanganate) usually can control these problems.

In his last publication, appearing posthumously in 1970, Siemens [27] described a familiy with an unusually mild expression of BIE. Typical features were superficial erosions and blisters occuring mainly around the mouth and on the extremities. Scaling was confined to circumscribed areas showing mild kera-

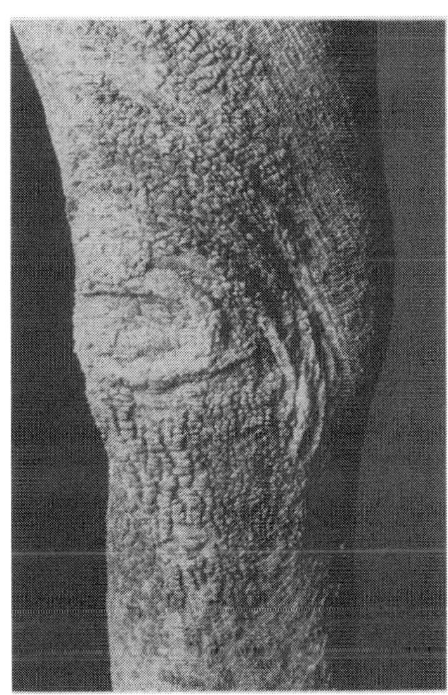

Fig. 48. Bullous ichthyotic erythroderma (BIE). Note hystrix-like hyperkeratoses. (From [29])

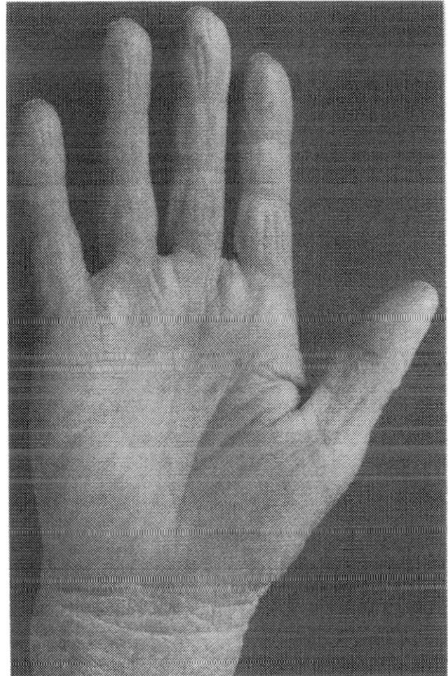

Fig. 49. BIE. In contrast to the Curth-Macklin type, palms and soles usually are spared

totic lichenifications (elbows, neck, axilla). Siemens mentioned that these localized keratotic areas were accompanied by slight erythema and that palms and soles were surprisingly severely affected. I observed a very similar family (father and son) also having clinical features different from the classical course of the condition. The son, a 30-year-old man, consulted us because of a recurrent blistering diesease present since birth. Several grouped small blisters on a red base were seen over the upper leg and lower arms, while inconspicuous yellow keratoses confined to the axilla, the knees, and the flexures of the big joints were noted. A biopsy taken from the knee disclosed the typical features of epidermolytic hyperkeratosis.

4.4.2.3 Histologic and Ultrastructural Features

Histologic examination reveals a basket-weave pattern of orthohyperkeratosis and a huge stratum corneum. Strong PAS-positive deposits can be found in the horny layer. The granular layer is broadened and degenerated (Fig. 50). Coarse keratohyalin granula can be seen. The keratinocytes of the granular layer and of the upper spinous-cell layers show cytoplasmic edema and a perinuclear vacuolization, whereas the basal and suprabasal keratinocytes usually appear normal. Because of the cytoplasmic edema, the boundaries between the keratinocytes appear blurred. These distinctive changes are called "acanthokeratolysis" or "epidermolytic hyperkeratosis". Though erythema is discernible clinically, there are usually only slight to moderate perivascular infiltrates seen in the corium. Blister formation usually occurs at the level of the granular layer. The roof of the

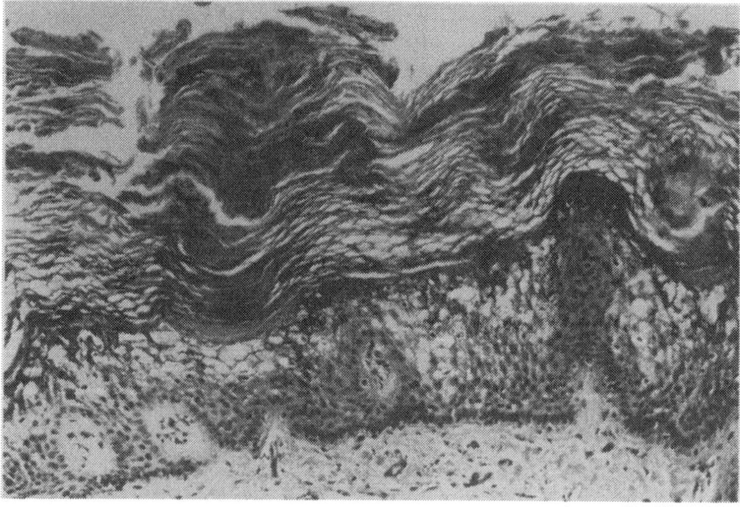

Fig. 50. Histology of BIE. Typical changes of marked epidermolytic hyperkeratosis involving the entire epidermis. Note strong focal PAS-positive staining of the stratum corneum. PAS stain, ×100

blister is formed by the orthohyperkeratotic stratum corneum, the bottom is formed by edematous keratinocytes. At the ultrastructural level, thickened bundles of regular tonofilaments forming ringlike shells around the cell nucleus and irregular clumps of tonofibrils are found (Fig. 51) [2, 20].

4.4.2.4 Biochemical Aspects

The primary biochemical defect which underlies this cornification disorder is unknown. Mali et al. [23] reported on a case with a striking reduction in α-mannosidase activity and suggested that BIE could be a lysosomal storage disease. A second case recently studied at Nijmegen also showed reduced α-mannosidase levels (M. Bergers 1988, personal communication). Holbrook et al. [16] demonstrated a loss of two keratins of the high-molecular-weight class and found an increase of epidermal filaggrin content, suggesting that the abnormal aggregation of tonofibrils in BIE is related to an imbalance of keratin and filaggrin.

4.4.2.5 Genetic Aspects: the Puzzle of Gonadal Mosaicism

Bullous ichthyotic erythroderma follows an autosomal dominant mode of inheritance [18, 20]. A puzzling finding is that in several well-documented cases in the

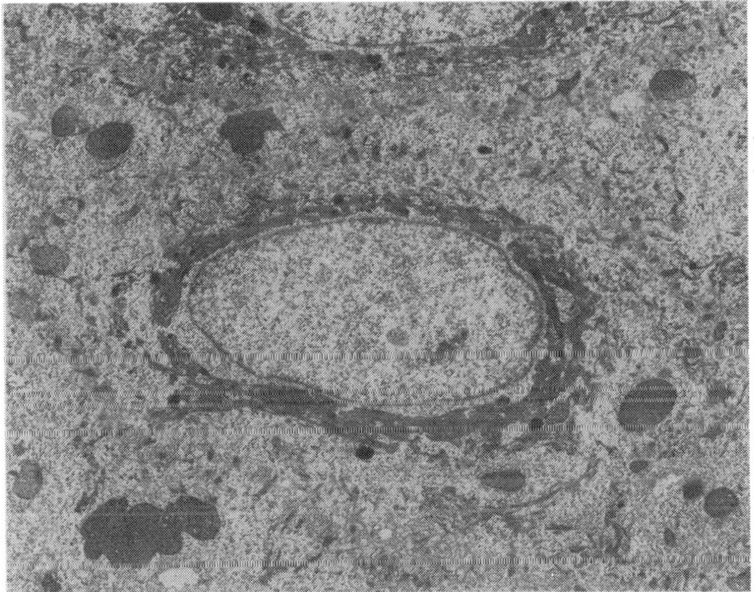

Fig. 51. BIE. Electron micrograph of the upper prickle cell layer. Note the typical shell-like formation of aggregated tonofilaments around the nucleus. In the cell periphery clumps of irregular tonofilaments are seen. These changes result in loss of the normal tonofilament insertion into the desmosomal plates. (Courtesy of Dr. G. Kolde, Münster) ×4200

parent generation, not ichthyosis, but a keratotic nevus with the histologic signs of epidermolytic hyperkeratosis was observed [5, 6, 17]. These epidermolytic nevi show neither blistering nor considerable erythema. Lookingbill et al. [22] reported on a girl with BIE whose father suffered from an epidermolytic nevus comedonicus. Clinically, the father presented with rather inconspicuous keratotic papules on his back.

At first glance, there seems to be in some families an extremely variable expressivity of the disease process, while in the majority of families the disease takes a rather uniform course with little intrafamilial variation of the clinical picture. How can this discrepancy be explained?

It should be noted that the constellation was always that of a localized epidermolytic nevus in the parent and full-blown BIE in the child generation, but never vice versa. Therefore, a somatic mutation occurring during early embryogenesis can account for this strange constellation. It can manifest itself in the parent as a localized epidermolytic nevus. At the same time, such a somatic mutation can also affect the germ line and can result in gonadal mosaicism. Some gametes will carry the defective gene so that offspring can show generalized BIE. This explanation is much more likely than the assumption of variable disease expressivity. Molecular studies in Duchenne muscular dystrophy show that gonadal mosaicism may be much more frequent than previously thought.

A somatic mutation of the BIE/epidermolytic hyperkeratosis gene most certainly accounts for an intriguing disease constellation in two families reported on by Adam and Richards [1]. They observed the presence of epidermolytic hyperkeratosis in a nevoid arrangement following the lines of Blaschko in only one of two monozygotic twins.

From a genetic point of view, BIE is one of the few diseases where we can observe gene action in a localized form (somatic mutation) and in a generalized form (gametic mutation). Other such examples are localized and generalized forms of Darier's disease and neurofibromatosis. One would expect many nevi to have a corresponding generalized disease manifestation. Obviously, this is not the case. Very recently, Happle [13] advanced the concept of lethal genes, suggesting that sporadic skin defects such as nevus flammeus are caused by lethal genes which can survive only in connection with normal cell lines. Hence, only localized expression of these lethal genes can be observed.

Another "localized" epidermolytic disease is palmoplantar keratosis of Vörner. It shares with BIE the same mode of inheritance and the same histologic and ultrastructural features. Interestingly, epidermolytic palmoplantar keratosis and generalized BIE do not run in the same families [12].

4.4.3 Ichthyosis Bullosa of Siemens

4.4.3.1 Historical Aspects

In 1937, Siemens [26] reported on a Dutch family in which six members belonging to three consecutive generations exhibited a peculiar phenotype, ichthyosis bullosa of Siemens, (IBS). Siemens himself compared the blistering in ichthyosis bullosa to that of epidermolysis bullosa simplex and stressed that bullae occured after minor mechanical trauma. The absence of erythroderma and a different distribution of involved skin areas allowed Siemens to separate this entity from BIE of Brocq. In the following decades, no further reports appeared and the condition fell into oblivion. In 1986 we [30] reported on the second family with IBS and recognized the histologic features of this disease as being those of epidermolytic hyperkeratosis. Very recently, a third family with IBS was presented at the 242nd Scientific Meeting of the Dutch Society of Dermatology [28].

4.4.3.2 Clinical Features

The patients suffer from birth from blistering, and from dark-gray hyperkeratoses. In childhood, the hyperkeratoses cover the buttocks, arms, and legs, including the flexural aspects of the extremities (Fig. 52), and the neck. Moreover, circumscribed parts of the axilla with a central sparing and localized hyperkeratoses on the trunk, especially around the navel, can be found. Over the back of the hands, feet, ankle joints and wrists, elbows, and knees, the hyperkeratoses have a lichenified appearance. On the extremities the skin is easily bruised, and especially in summertime bullae occur after minor mechanical trauma. Very often, superficially denuded areas can be noted on the lower aspects of the legs and on the backs of hands and feet (Fig. 53). For this phenomenon Siemens coined the term

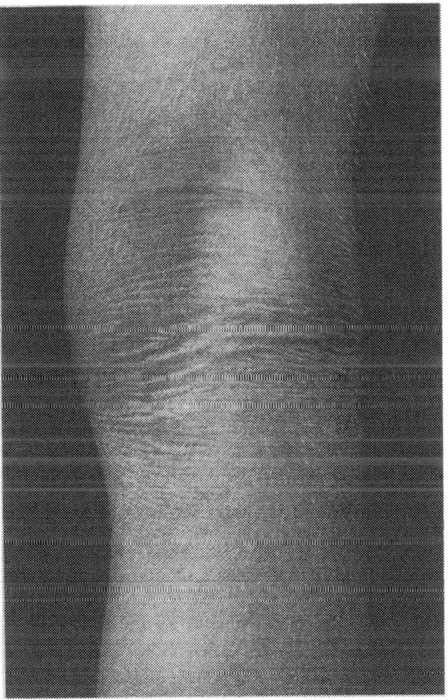

Fig. 52. Ichthyosis bullosa of Siemens (IBS). Involvement of flexures. Note the typical keratotic lichenification

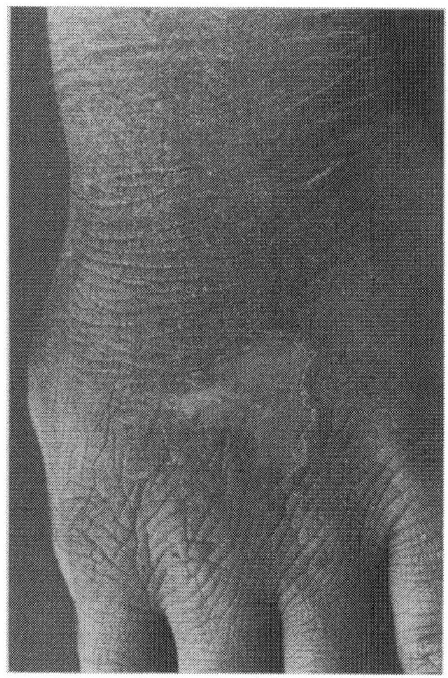

Fig. 53. IBS. Superficially denuded area called "Mauserung" by Siemens on the back of a hand. This is a typical, but not specific sign. (From [30])

"Mauserung" (molting). However, this is not a specific sign, but may also be seen in epidermolytic palmoplantar keratosis of Vörner [12]. In the family we observed, the extent of keratotic involvement becomes less severe in adulthood. With the 31-year-old affected father, hyperkeratosis and keratotic lichenification of the skin were confined to the elbows, knees, and the flexural folds of the big joints, while his daughter still showed widespread involvement. The father stated that blistering had been more severe in childhood, but that bullae still occurred, especially in the summertime, and most often resulted from the combined effect of mechanical trauma and profuse sweating. Spontaneous improvement of the condition during late adolescence can also be inferred from the original account of Siemens [26]. Palms and soles are spared from the hyperkeratotic process. Hyperhidrosis of hands and feet appears to facilitate development of bullae.

4.4.3.3 Histologic and Ultrastructural Features

Histology discloses as the most important finding epidermolytic hyperkeratosis (Fig. 54). Epidermolytic hyperkeratosis is less marked than in BIE and it is important to take a biopsy from a site of maximal clinical involvement (e.g., knees). Otherwise, the typical changes may be missed. The epidermis is moderately thickened and shows plump, confluent rete ridges. Biopsies from fresh blisters show both an intracorneal localization and blisters located at the level of the granular layer [26, 28–30].

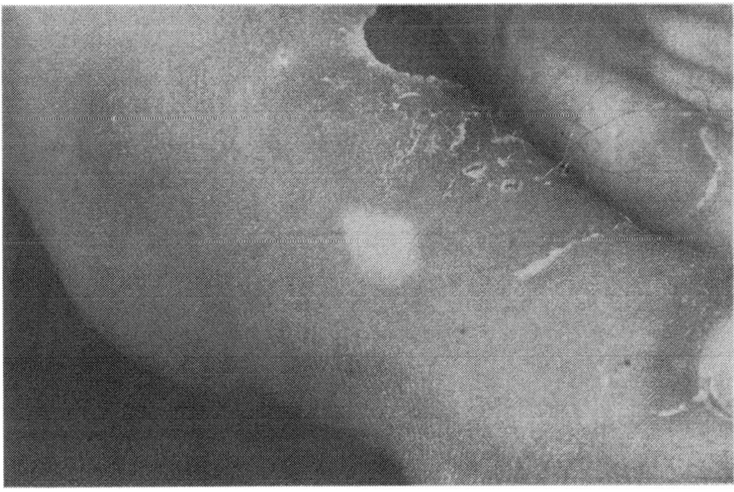

Fig. 54. IBS. Fresh blister induced after minor mechanical trauma over the left big toe

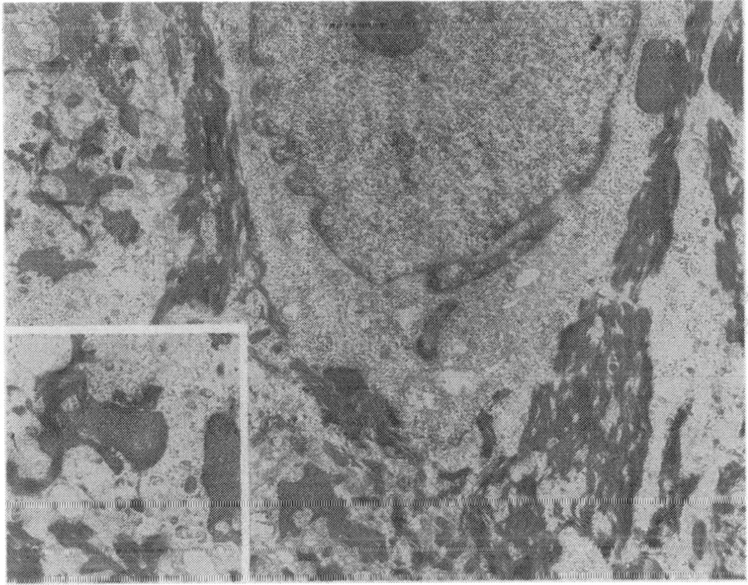

Fig. 55. IBS. Electron micrograph of edematous keratinocytes in the lower granular layer. Note the thickened bundles and irregular clumps of the tonofibrils. ×9500. *Inset:* Higher magnification of the tonofilament clumps showing irregular filamentous material of moderate electron density ×14800. (From [30], courtesy of Dr. Kolde, Münster)

Electron microscopy confirms diagnosis of epidermolytic hyperkeratosis and reveals bulky tonofilament clumps and thickened bundles of tonofibrils (Fig. 55). The presence of epidermolytic hyperkeratosis in ichthyosis bullosa is also confirmed by the recent Dutch observations [28]. Siemens himself did not mention these peculiar changes in his report. Probably he did not recognize them, as the concept of epidermolytic hyperkeratosis or acanthokeratolysis was elaborated only 20 years later.

4.4.4 Ichthyosis Hystrix of Curth and Macklin

4.4.4.1 Historical Aspects

In 1954, Ollendorff-Curth and Macklin [9] reported on a family with an ichthyosis hystrix-like cornification disorder. Seventeen years later, Ollendorff-Curth was able to re-examine the same family [24]. Despite some resemblance to BIE, subtle ultrastructural criteria elaborated by Anton-Lamprecht [3] indicate that ichthyosis hystrix of Curth-Macklin (IHCM) is a distinct subtype of the epidermolytic ichthyoses. The condition is exceedingly rare, and until now only the original family described by Curth and Macklin in 1954 and two other sporadic cases [19, 25] have been reported. Moreover, a family observed by Braun-Falco et al. [7] may also represent ICHM. Without access to electron microscopy and expert evaluation of the findings, IHCM is diagnosed as BIE.

4.4.4.2 Clinical Features

In the family described by Curth and Macklin some affected members presented with generalized involvement of the integument. Symmetrically distributed, hystrix-like keratotic masses covered most of the body, including the flexor surface of the extremities and palms and soles. In other family members, brownish, hyperkeratotic verrucous skin lesions were confined to the elbows, knees, palms, and soles. In childhood, some of the patients suffered from generalized ichthyotic erythroderma while others did not. In the sporadic case reported by Kanerva et al. [19] there was an almost uniform involvement of the entire body, with heavy, papillomatous dark hyperkeratoses but sparing of the palms and soles. In contrast, the family described by Braun-Falco and co-workers [7] showed pronounced palmoplantar keratosis and localized involvement, expecially of the axilla, the groins, the flexural apects of the big joints, and the lateral aspect of the neck and trunk. The case shown in Fig. 56 was observed at the Department of Dermatology in Düsseldorf. Correct diagnosis of IHCM was established by Dr. Anton-Lamprecht of Heidelberg, according to her ultrastructural criteria. I am indebted to Dr. Küster and Dr. Goerz, Düsseldorf, for obtaining these clinical pictures.

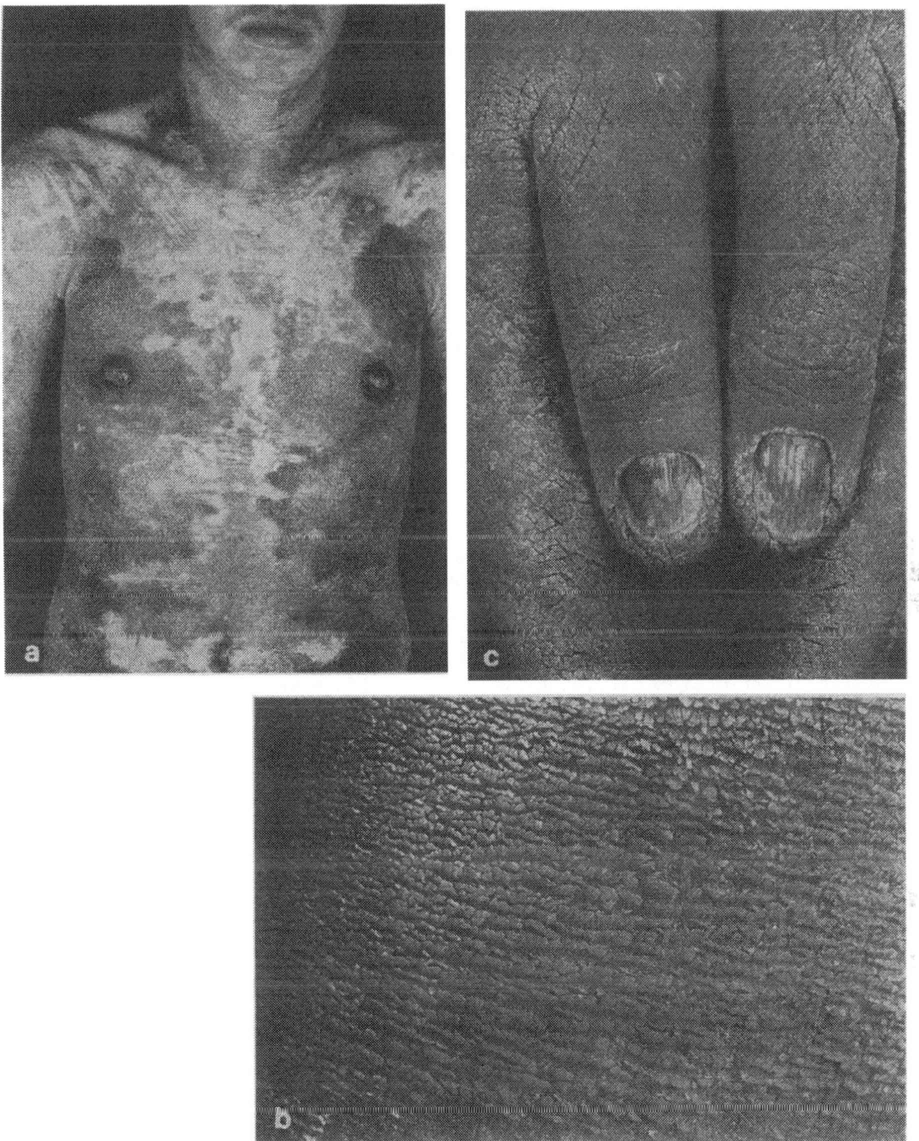

Fig. 56a–c. Ichthyosis hystrix of Curth-Macklin (IHCM). **a** Overview showing the most severe generalized involvement; **b** close-up of horny spikes on the trunk; **c** involvement of the nails. (Courtesy of Dr. Goerz and Dr. Küster, Düsseldorf. Diagnosis of IHCM was established ultrastructurally by Dr. Anton-Lamprecht, Heidelberg)

4.4.4.3 Histologic and Ultrastructural Features

The histologic features are essentially those of epidermolytic hyperkeratosis. There is orthohyperkeratosis, acanthosis, and papillomatosis. The most conspicuous finding is perinuclear vacuolization of the keratinocytes in the granular and upper spinous layers. In some cases the extent of the granular degeneration is similar to that seen in BIE, ichthyosis bullosa, and epidermolytic palmoplantar keratosis. In other cases the granular degeneration is less marked. High magnification with oil immersion shows that some of the keratinocytes are binucleate and that both nuclei are surrounded by a tonofilament shell. In the case studied by Kanerva [19], 10% of the keratinocytes were binucleate, while Anton-Lamprecht found that up to 30% of all keratinocytes above the basal layer contained two nuclei [3].

Electron microscopy permits recognition of the disease [3, 19]. In contrast to BIE, **unbroken** concentric shells of tonofibrils surround the nucleus. The cytoplasm of the keratinocytes shows three rather sharply delineated compartments. In the perinuclear compartment, an abundance of cell organelles such as ribosomes, endoplasmic reticulum, mitochondria, and deformed lamellar bodies (keratinosomes) are found. Moreover, a considerable number of keratinocytes contain conspicuous vacuoles in this perinuclear area. The second compartment is formed by the diagnostic tonofibril shell formation, whereas in an outer cytoplasmic zone again ribosomes, mitochondria, and lamellar bodies can be found. In contrast to BIE, the attachment of the tonofilaments to the desmosomes is not disturbed. This may explain why, also in contrast to BIE, blisters do not occur.

4.4.5 Genetic Counseling of the Epidermolytic Ichthyoses

All three types of epidermolytic ichthyosis share autosomal dominant inheritance. In BIE and IBS the clinical phenotype remains constant through the generations, whereas in the Curth-Macklin type a remarkable variation of disease expression can be seen. The presence of an epidermolytic nevus should not be dimissed as a nongenetic and harmless flaw of beauty. It rather indicates that a somatic mutation of the epidermolytic hyperkeratosis gene has occured that also can involve the germ cell line (gonadal mosaicism) and result in severe full-blown BIE in the next generation. Therefore, parents who have an epidermolytic keratotic nevus should be offered prenatal diagnosis. The characteristic ultrastructural changes found in epidermolytic hyperkeratosis (clumping of tonofilaments, cytolysis of suprabasal cells) permit a safe prenatal diagnosis at 20 weeks of gestation [2, 11, 16].

In IBS the course of the disease is rather mild. As in BIE, prenatal diagnosis should be possible, but I would not advise offering it unless the parents are very concerned. Most likely, the ultrastructural characteristics of IHCM will allow a prenatal diagnosis of this condition as well.

4.4.6 General Comments on Prenatal Diagnosis

The epidermolytic ichthyoses are those that can be best and safely diagnosed prenatally. In this context I want to comment on some general aspects concerning prenatal diagnosis of a cornification disorder. Prenatal diagnosis is a tedious and time-consuming procedure. It requires special skills on the part of the gynecologist who performs fetoscopy and an intimate knowledge not only of the ultrastructural characteristics of the various genetic skin disorders [2], but also of the normal ultrastructure of fetal skin and its regional differences during embryogenesis [14, 15]. Two scientists, Dr. Ingrun Anton-Lamprecht from Heidelberg and Dr. Karen Holbrook from Seattle, paved the way for the significant advances in this field. While Anton-Lamprecht and her co-workers elucidated ultrastructural defects that can be employed as reliable disease markers in many of these diseases [2–4], Holbrook and her group devoted their work to the study of fetal skin ultrastructure [14–16]. Except for the epidermolytic types, the ichthyoses as a group are not ideally suited for prenatal diagnosis by means of electron microscopy [4, 6]. The main reason is that normal keratinization occurs late during embryogenesis, at 24 weeks of gestation [14]. As discussed in Sect. 4.2.4, only two types of lamellar ichthyosis (ELI type B/ichthyosis congenita type II and NELI type B/ichthyosis congenita type IV) can be reliably diagnosed antenatally.

When considering whether to offer prenatal diagnosis in the presence of a keratinization disorder, one should first attempt to establish a diagnosis as precise as possible in at least one affected family member. The second step is to contact one of the specialized centers actually performing this kind of diagnostic procedure well in advance. Currently, I am aware of only four such centers in the world. For practical purpose, the addresses of the directors and the institutional affiliations of these groups are given below:

Prof. Dr. I. Anton-Lamprecht
Direktorin des Instituts für
Ultrastrukturforschung der Haut
Universitäts-Hautklinik
Voßstraße 2
D-6900 Heidelberg
Federal Republic of Germany

Prof. Dr. C. Blanchet-Bardon
Clinique Dermatologique
Hôpital Saint-Louis
2, Place du Dr. A. Fournier
F-75475 Paris, Cedex 10
France

Dr. R. A. J. Eady
Senior Lecturer
Institute of Dermatology
St. John's Hospital for Diseases of the Skin
Homerton Grove
GB - London E 9
Great Britain

Dr. K. A. Holbrook
Head,
Department of Biological
Structure SM-20
University of Washingten School of Medicine
Seattle, WA 98195
United States of America

A full treatment of the ethical issues connected with prenatal diagnosis is beyond the scope of this section. Today, the vast majority of people in Western countries feel that prenatal prevention of a serious genetic disorder is desirable. A minority do not think so. It is important to respect this minority and not to influence these parents. Parents have the right to have children, even if they will be sick. Likewise, the minority objecting to prenatal prevention of genetic diseases must not criticize the majority as being unethical or try to impose their personals views as binding ethical standards. Termination of a pregnancy which is at risk for a serious genetic disease should remain a very personal decision. In practice, many couples will not want to have children at all if prenatal diagnosis is not available. In the future, DNA techniques will permit prenatal diagnosis at a much earlier gestational age. This approach is already available for associated steroid sulfatase deficiency.

References

1. Adam JE, Richards R (1973) Ichthyosis hystrix. Epidermolytic hyperkeratosis; discordant in monozygotic twins. Arch Dermatol 107:278–282
2. Anton-Lamprecht I (1981) Prenatal diagnosis of genetic disorders of the skin by means of electron microscopy. Hum Genet 59:392–405
3. Anton-Lamprecht I, Curth HO, Schnyder UW (1973) Zur Ultrastruktur hereditärer Verhornungsstörungen. II. Ichthyosis hystrix Typ Curth-Macklin. Arch Dermatol Forsch 246:77–91
4. Arnold ML, Anton-Lamprecht I (1985) Problems in prenatal diagnosis of the ichthyosis congenita group. Hum Genet 71:301–311
5. Barker PL, Sachs W (1953) Bullous congenital ichthyosiform erythroderma. Arch Dermatol 67:443–455
6. Blanchet-Bardon C, Nazarro V (1987) Use of morphological markers in carriers as an aid in genetic counselling and prenatal diagnosis. In: Gedde-Dahl T, Wuepper KD (eds) Prenatal diagnosis of heritable skin diseases. Karger, Basel, pp 109–119
7. Braun-Falco O, Schurig V, Meurer M, Klepzig K (1985) Ichthyosis hystrix mit Parakeratose nach Art der kornoiden Lamelle. Hautarzt 36:132–141

8. Brocq L (1902) Erythrodermie congénitale ichthyosiforme avec hyperépidermotrophie. Ann Dermatol Syph (Paris), ser 4, 4:1–31
9. Curth HO, Macklin MT (1954) The genetic basis of various types of ichthyosis in a family group. Am J Hum Genet 6:371–382
10. Frost P, Van Scott EJ (1966) Ichthyosiform dermatoses. Classification based on anatomic and biometric observations. Arch Dermatol 94:113–126
11. Golbus MS, Sagebiel RW, Filly RA, Gindhardt TD, Hall JG (1980) Prenatal diagnosis of congenital bullous ichthyosiform erythroderma (epidermolytic hyperkeratosis) by fetal skin biopsy. N Engl J Med 302:93–95
12. Hamm H, Happle R, Butterfass T, Traupe H (1988) Epidermolytic palmoplantar keratoderma of Vörner: is it the most frequent type of hereditary palmoplantar keratoderma? Dermatologica 177:138–145
13. Happle R (1987) Lethal genes surviving by mosaicism: a possible explanation for sporadic birth defects involving the skin. J Am Acad Dermatol 16:899–906
14. Holbrook KA (1979) Human epidermal embryogenesis. Int J Dermatol 18:329–356
15. Holbrook KA, Odland GF (1980) Regional development of the human epidermis in the first-trimester embryo and the second-trimenster fetus (ages related to the timing of amnioncentesis and fetal biopsy). J Invest Dermatol 80:161–168
16. Holbrook KA, Dale BA, Sybert VP, Sagebiel RWC (1983) Epidermolytic hyperkeratosis: ultrastructure and biochemistry of skin and amniotic fluid cells from two affected fetuses and a newborn infant. J Invest Dermatol 80:222–227
17. Hornstein O (1965) Erythrodermie ichthyosiforme congénitale bulleuse (Brocq). Dermatol Wochenschr 151:1255–1265
18. Jung EG, Schnyder UW (1962) Die "Erythrodermie ichthyosiforme congénitale": ein heterogenes Syndrom. Dermatologica 124:189–191
19. Kanerva L, Karvonen J, Oikarinen A, Lauharanta J, Ruokonen A, Niemi KM (1984) Ichthyosis hystrix (Curth-Macklin). Light- and electron-microscopic studies performed before and after etretinate treatment. Arch Dermatol 120:1218–1223
20. Küchmeister B, Schaeg G, Müller V, Kuhlwein A (1983) Epidermolytic hyperkeratosis in four generations. Histological and electron-microscopical studies and HLA-Types. Z Hautkr 58:1625–1645
21. Lapière S (1953) Les génodermatoses hyperkératosiques de type bulleux. Ann Dermatol Venereol 80:597–614
22. Lookingbill DP, Ladda RL, Cohen C (1984) Generalized epidermolytic hyperkeratosis in the child of a parent with nevus comedonicus. Arch Dermatol 120:223–226
23. Mali JWH, Bergers AMG, Van den Hurk JMA, Mier PD, Van de Staak WJBM (1976) A lysosomal storage disorder of the epidermis characterized by a deficiency of α-mannosidase and an accumulation of mannose-rich materials. Br J Dermatol 95:627–630
24. Ollendorff-Curth H, Allen FH Jr, Schnyder UW, Anton-Lamprecht I (1972) Follow-up of a family group suffering from ichthyosis hystrix type Curth-Macklin. Hum Genet 17:37–48
25. Pinkus H, Nagao S (1970) A case of biphasic ichthyosiform dermatosis. Light- and electron-microscopic study. Arch Klin Exp Dermatol 237:737–748
26. Siemens HW (1937) Dichtung und Wahrheit über die "Ichthyosis bullosa", mit Bemerkungen zur Systemik der Epidermolysen. Arch Dermatol Syph 175:590–608
27. Siemens HW (1970) Über die noch nicht beschriebene, regelmäßig dominante Form der bullösen Erythrodermie ichthyosiforme congénitale. Hautarzt 21:352–355
28. Steijlen P (1988) Ichthyosis bullosa Siemens. Patient demonstration at the 242nd Scientific Meeting of the Dutch Society for Dermatology and Venereology, Nijmegen, Feb. 6
29. Traupe H (1986) Die Ichthyosen: auf dem Weg vom Phän zum Gen. In: Macher E, Czarnetzki B, Knop J (eds) Jahrbuch der Dermatologie 1986. Regensberg and Biermann, Münster, pp 35–48
30. Traupe H, Kolde G, Hamm H, Happle R (1986) Ichthyosis bullosa of Siemens: a unique type of epidermolytic hyperkeratosis. J Am Acad Dermatol 14:1000–1005

5 Associated Congenital Ichthyoses

5.1 The Sjögren-Larsson Syndrome

5.1.1 Historical Aspects

In 1957, Sjögren and Larsson [18] reported on 28 patients belonging to 13 families who all lived in the North Swedish province of Västerbotten. These patients suffered from a syndrome characterized by pronounced congenital ichthyosis, severe mental retardation, and symmetric spastic pyramidal symptoms of the Little type. Sjögren and Larsson demonstrated consanguinity in eight of the 13 families. They concluded that the symptom complex they had observed represented a unique and new genetic disorder inherited as an autosomal recessive trait. Their findings were soon confirmed by many groups reporting cases from all over the world [3-5, 7, 15]. Two years after delineation of the syndrome by Sjögren and Larsson, Greither [4] pointed out that the association of ichthyosis, mental retardation, and spastic paresis of the Little type had already been described 30 years earlier in a very brief case report by Pardo-Castello and Faz [14] in 1932. Nevertheless, the condition rightfully bears the name of Sjögren and Larsson, since their tremendous work established the syndrome as a unique condition. By 1981, more than 120 verified cases of Sjögren-Larsson syndrome (SLS) had been reported [11]. Despite this, SLS is an uncommon disease. In the past 10 years we have taken care of only one girl affected with SLS at the Münster Department of Dermatology. During the same period we observed 40 cases of X-linked recessive ichthyosis. Thus, the incidence is probably less than 1/200000 in Westphalia. The condition is more frequent in Sweden. In the North Swedish province of Västerbotten its incidence is 10.2/100000 inhabitants [11]. It is reasonable to assume that all North Swedish cases are due to the same mutation wich occurred or was carried into this area centuries ago when this highly interrelated population was still very small (founder effect). This explains why the elsewhere rare SLS gene could spread and become so frequent in Västerbotten.

5.1.2 Clinical Features

5.1.2.1 Ichthyosis in the Sjögren-Larsson Syndrome

Ichthyosis in SLS is truly congenital, and generalized hyperkeratosis can be seen at birth. At this time the condition may present with fine scaling only. The typical clinical features develop during the first year of life, after which patients predominantly present with yellowish or dark-brown papillomatous keratosis, giving the skin a lichenified appearance. This verrucous aspect is quite typical (Fig. 57) and is reminiscent of ichthyosis hystrix [4]. It is particularly pronounced on the lateral sides, the back of the neck, the lower abdomen, and the flexures [13]. In addition to the papillomatous keratotic thickening of the skin, thin, adherent scales may also be noted, especially on the lower limbs [13]. Though the

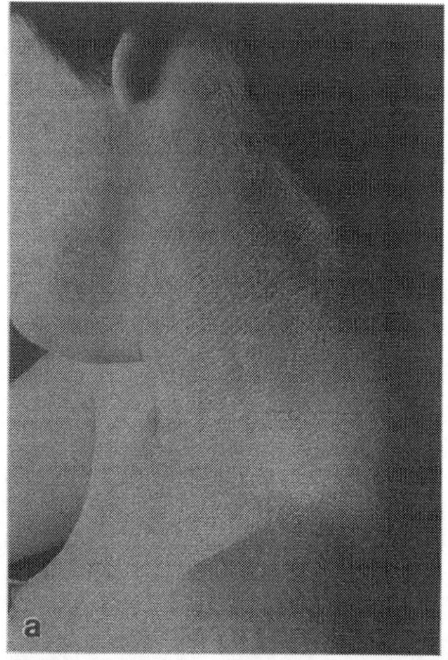

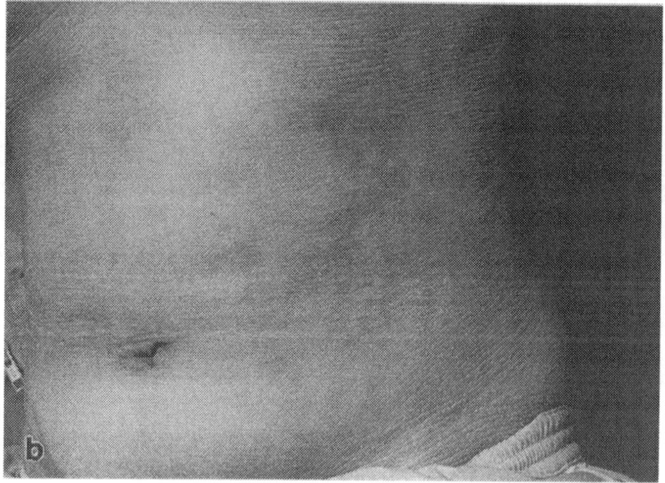

Fig. 57a, b. Typical cutaneous aspect of Sjögren-Larsson syndrome. Note keratotic lichenification (**a**) on neck and (**b**) on lateral sides of the trunk (same patient)

term "congenital ichthyosiform erythroderma" was used by Sjögren and Larsson [18] and later on by several other authors [15] to describe the skin changes, this designation is obviously misleading. It was used for historical reasons as a synonym for ichthyosis congenita. The children are not born with an ichthyotic erythroderma but may exhibit in the neonatal period a slight erythema, mainly over the flexures, which is usually no longer seen in adult life [13]. The outstanding clinical feature of ichthyosis in SLS is the yellowish to dark-brown keratotic lichenification of the skin. These typical skin changes can be noted at the age of a few months, so that the correct diagnosis may be suspected in the neonatal period, while the neurologic and ophthalmologic symptoms become manifest much later [7].

5.1.2.2 Neurologic and Ophthalmologic Findings

Onset of the neurologic manifestations - i.e., pathologic reflexes, muscular hypertonus, paralysis of legs and mental retardation - is usually between 4 and 30 months of age [13]. Some patients develop tetraplegia during childhood, but even in these, the motor handicap of the legs is more severe than that of the arms. After puberty the motor handicap and mental retardation no longer deteriorate with increasing age.

Small glistening dots in the retina, located in the macular region, are the main ophthalmologic finding [3, 10]. In some patients, the ichthyotic changes cause blepharitis, conjunctivitis, and other secondary changes of the cornea. This explains why some patients suffer from photophobia.

5.1.3 Histologic Features

The histologic picture of the skin in SLS is that of a nonspecific benign acanthokeratosis. The disease cannot be distinguished from lamellar ichthyosis on histologic grounds. There is a moderately increased, predominantly orthokeratotic stratum corneum with scattered mild parakeratosis and occasional follicular hyperkeratosis. The epidermis is acanthotic, and usually some papillomatosis can be seen [4, 7, 13]. Epidermal cell turnover in SLS is increased and the ichthyosis can therefore be classified as a hyperproliferation hyperkeratosis [13]. A detailed study of the ultrastructure of SLS skin is lacking, but Anton-Lamprecht [1] emphasized the rare occurrence of lipid vacuoles in the horny layer. Another feature is stiff and very straight bundles of tonofibrils together with normal keratohyalin [1].

5.1.4 Biochemical Aspects

There is some clinical and histopathologic evidence linking the Sjögren-Larsson syndrome to an inborn error of lipid metabolism. Thus, the distinctive macular degeneration termed "glistening dots" is caused by a fatty degeneration of retinal microglia [3]. Complete clearing of the skin manifestation has been claimed in three patients fed a diet in which all of the lipid was given in the form of medium-chain triglycerides [5, 9].

Very recently, Rizzo and co-workers [17] identified a defect of fatty alcohol oxidation. In fibroblasts from four SLS patients they found a marked reduction of fatty alcohol NAD^+ oxireductase (FANADO) to 13% of normal. After inhibition of this enzyme with palmitoyl-coenzyme A, the mean activity of FANADO was decreased to 1% of normal. With regard to the FANADO inhibition data it is conceivable that FANADO is a multi-enzyme complex and that in SLS only a distinct subunit is deficient.

The new findings in SLS support the hypothesis of a fatty alcohol cycle operating in several cell types (fibroblasts, neurons, keratinocytes) [16]. In this cycle FANADO converts fatty alcohol to fatty acids. A block results in the accumulation of fatty alcohols such as hexadecanol. In keratinocytes and neurons the fatty alcohols are then incorporated into lipids which are essential for normal cell membrane functions. FANADO deficiency thus will alter the normal lipid composition of the stratum corneum and the nerve sheaths in SLS. It may well be the biochemical link between the hyperkeratosis and the neurologic degeneration in this neuroichthyosis.

The fascinating findings of Rizzo et al. [17] still have to be confirmed by other groups. Very little is known about the pathobiochemistry of SLS. At the moment it is difficult to explain how a defect in fatty alcohol oxidation interferes with the acitivity of delta-6-desaturase, an enzyme probably implicated in the pathobiochemistry of SLS [6, 8].

In a detailed study of serum fatty acids comprising 11 patients with SLS, healthy controls, and mentally retarded controls Hernell et al. [8] observed a marked decrease of the metabolites derived from linoleic acids in the phospholipids of SLS patients. The total products of delta-6-desaturase were reduced to 3% of that in controls, suggesting a defect of delta-6-desaturase. These findings were recently confirmed. Harper [6] found that in plasma and red blood cells the phospholipids contained low levels of the n-6 series metabolites derived from **cis**-linoleic acid, while the metabolites of the n-3 series derived from alpha-linoleic acid were reduced in red blood cells but raised in plasma. Though fatty acid profiles obviously are altered in SLS, impairment of delta-6-desaturase is not the primary defect. In skin fibroblasts from two SLS patients normal delta-6-desaturase activity was found [2].

5.1.5 Genetic Counseling

SLS is a severe, neurodegenerative skin disorder following an autosomal recessive mode of inheritance. Biochemical recognition of heterozygous gene carriers may be available soon (FANADO testing). As the condition is very uncommon outside of Sweden, the chance that heterozygotes mate is low. Usually, the heterozygous status will become obvious only if parents have an affected child. In these instances, prenatal diagnosis can be attempted and has been successfully performed by fetal skin biopsy in one case [12]. This is quite remarkable, as SLS lacks characteristic histologic or ultrastructural markers [1]. In the case reported, the diagnosis was based on a light-microscopic evaluation of precocious keratinization. It should be noted that in this case the fetal skin biopsy was performed very late (week 23). The parents decided to continue the pregnancy. At 34 weeks of gestation a female infant was spontaneously delivered who had congenital ichthyosis. Whether a safe exclusion diagnosis is possible if fetoscopy is performed at week 20 is not certain. If the FANADO story holds true, antenatal diagnosis may become possible by biochemical means in the near future.

References

1. Anton-Lamprecht I (1978) Ultrastructural criteria for the distinction of different types of inherited ichthyosis. In: Marks R, Dykes PJ (eds) The ichthyoses. MTP, Lancaster, pp 71-87
2. Avigan J, Campbell BD, Yost DA, Hernell O, Holmgren G, Jagell SF (1985) Sjögren-Larsson syndrome: delta^5- and delta^6-fatty acid desaturates in skin fibroblasts. Neurology 35:401-403
3. Daicker B (1972) Zur Kenntnis von Substrat und Bedeutung der sogenannten Schneckenspuren der Retina. Ophthalmologica 165:360-365
4. Greither A (1959) Über das Syndrom: Ichthyosis congenita, Schwachsinn und spastische Störungen vom Typ der Littleschen Krankheit. Hautarzt 10:403-408
5. Guilleminault C, Harpey JP, Lafourcade J (1973) Sjögren-Larsson syndrome. Report of two cases in twins. Neurology 23:367-373
6. Harper JI (1987) Analysis of essential fatty acid metabolism in Sjögren-Larsson syndrome. In: Meneghini CL, Bonifazi E (eds) Proceedings 2nd Congress of the European Society for Pediatric Dermatology, Bari, Oct 2-4, 1987. Pediatr Dermatol News 6:7-9
7. Heijer A, Reed WB (1965) Sjögren-Larsson syndrome. Arch Dermatol 92:545-552
8. Hernell O, Holmgren G, Jagell SF, Johnson SB, Holman RT (1982) Suspected faulty essential fatty acid metabolism in Sjögren-Larsson syndrome. Pediatr Res 16:45-49
9. Hooft C, Kriekemans J, van Acker K, Devos E, Traen S, Verdonck G (1967) Sjögren-Larsson syndrome with exudative enteropathy. Influence of medium-chain triglycerides on the symptomatology. Helv Paediatr Acta 5:447-458
10. Jagell S, Polland W, Sandgren O (1980) Specific changes in the fundus typical for the Sjögren-Larsson syndrome. An ophthalmological study. Acta Ophthalmol (Copenh) 58:321-330
11. Jagell S, Gustavson KH, Holmgren G (1981) Sjögren-Larsson syndrome in Sweden. A clinical, genetic and epidemiological study. Clin Genet 19:233-256
12. Kouseff BG, Matsuoka LY, Stenn KS, Jobbins JC, Mahoney MJ, Hashimoto K (1982) Prenatal diagnosis of Sjögren-Larsson syndrome. J Pediatr 101:998-1001
13. Lidén S, Jagell S (1984) The Sjögren-Larsson syndrome. Int J Dermatol 23:247-253
14. Pardo-Castello V, Faz H (1932) Ichthyosis with Little's disease. Arch Dermatol Syph (Chicago) 26:915
15. Reich H (1972) Sjögren-Larsson-Syndrom. Med Klin 67:909-912
16. Rizzo WB, Craft DA, Dammann AL, Philips MW (1987) Fatty alcohol metabolism in cultured human fibroblasts: evidence for a fatty alcohol cycle. J Biol Chem 262:17412-17419
17. Rizzo WB, Dammann AL, Craft DA (1988) Sjögren-Larsson syndrome. Impaired fatty alcohol oxidation in cultured fibroblasts due to deficient fatty alcohol nicotinamide adenine dinucleotide oxidoreductase activity. J Clin Invest 81:738-744
18. Sjögren T, Larsson T (1957) Oligophrenia in combination with congenital ichthyosis and spastic disorders. Acta Psychiatr Scand 32 [Suppl 113]:1-113

5.2 Ichthyosis and Trichothiodystrophy: the Tay and PIBI(D)S Syndromes

5.2.1 Historical Aspects and Classification

In 1971, Chong Hai Tay [14] of Singapore reported on three children of Chinese descent who suffered from ichthyotic erythroderma, mental and growth retardation, progeria-like facies, and brittle hair. Microscopic examination of the hair shafts disclosed clean transverse fractures (trichoschisis) different from pili torti or other hair defects known at that time. The parents of the three siblings were unaffected and closely related. Tay concluded that this family represented a new recessive disorder. Several years later, American authors [8–10] studied the hair abnormalities of this syndrome in more detail. Using polarization microscopy, they found that the hair shafts exhibited a zebra-like pattern of dark and light bands identical to that seen in the brittle hair, intellectual impairment, decreased fertility and short stature (BIDS) syndrome [3, 7] and established that hair of the Tay syndrome patients also has a decrease in sulfur-containing amino acids (especially cystine) [8–10]. For this sulfur-"deficient" brittle hair Price [10] coined the term "trichothiodystrophy". Jorizzo et al. [8] suggested that the Tay syndrome represented a link to the BIDS syndrome, and in a later publication they introduced the acronym IBIDS for this association [9]. Though the syndrome had already been fully described in 1963 by Salfeld and Lindley [12], it was Tay who recognized it as a distinct clinicogenetic entity. Therefore, the designation "Tay syndrome" is most appropriate [6].

Recently, it was noted that some patients so far regarded as having the Tay syndrome exhibit very severe photosensitivity caused by a DNA repair defect [4, 16]. Moreover, in patients with photosensitivity, ichthyosis is less severe and not present at birth. Hypogonadism is usually lacking and the facial dysmorphism differs from what is seen in Tay-syndrome patients. These differences prompted Rebora and Crovato [11] to separate this group of patients having PIDI(D)S syndrome from those with the Tay and BIDS syndromes (Table 26). From a clinical point of view, this line of thinking appears logical, and therefore the clinical features of Tay and PIDI(D)S syndromes are discussed separately here.

5.2.2 Clinical Features of the Tay Syndrome

Directly after birth, the children present with ichthyotic erythroderma and may be encased in a collodion-like membrane. After a few weeks the erythema sub-

Table 26. Clinical features of the BIDS, Tay, and PIBI(D)S syndromes

	BIDS syndrome	Tay syndrome	PIBI(D)S syndrome
		Similarities	
Hair	Brittle	Brittle	Brittle
Light microscopy	Trichoschisis	Trichchoschisis	Trichoschisis
Polarization microscopy	Tigertail pattern	Tigertail pattern	Tigertail pattern
Nails	Normal?	Dysplastic	Dysplastic
Intelligence	Mild retardation	Mild retardation	Mild retardation
Growth	Short stature	Short stature	Short stature
Immune defense	Frequent infections	Frequent infections	Frequent infections
Hypogonadism	Present	Present	Occasionally present
		Differences	
Ichthyosis	Lacking	Congenital ichthyosis	Ichthyosis of the "vulgaris" type (noncongenital)
Photosensitivity	Lacking	Lacking	Very marked
Facial dysmorphism	Lacking	Progeroid	Unusual facies, but not progeroid

sides. Tay [14] and Happle et al. [6] described in their cases fine, translucent scaling (Fig. 58a), whereas in other patients large, dark yellow-brown, alligator-like hyperkeratoses were reported [8, 9]. The hyperkeratoses cover the trunk and the limbs, but the flexural folds of the extremities may be spared. This may explain why in some cases the ichthyosis was erroneously classified as ichthyosis vulgaris [2, 12]. Palms and soles usually present a thick, fissured keratoderma. Dysplastic nails showing longitudinal ridging as well as horizontal splitting (Fig. 58b) are often observed. Sparse, broken scalp hair is a conspicuous finding (Fig. 58c); light microscopy of such hair discloses trichoschisis (clean transverse fractures), an undulating contour of hair shafts, and folding of hair shafts along their axis, while polarization microscopy reveals the characteristic zigzag (tigertail) pattern of alternating bright and dark zones (Fig. 59). By moving one of the polarizing filters, the position of the dark and bright areas can be exchanged.

Noncutaneous findings include low birth weight, probably related to premature birth because of placental insufficiency, a marked lack of subcutaneous fatty tissue, explaining the progeria-like facies, and short stature. Psychomotor development is delayed and moderate mental retardation is usually found. As a manifestation of hypogonadism, testicular maldescent is frequently noted in boys, while in girls poor sexual maturation may be found. In many cases, an increased proneness to bacterial infections (pyogenic skin infections, pneumo-

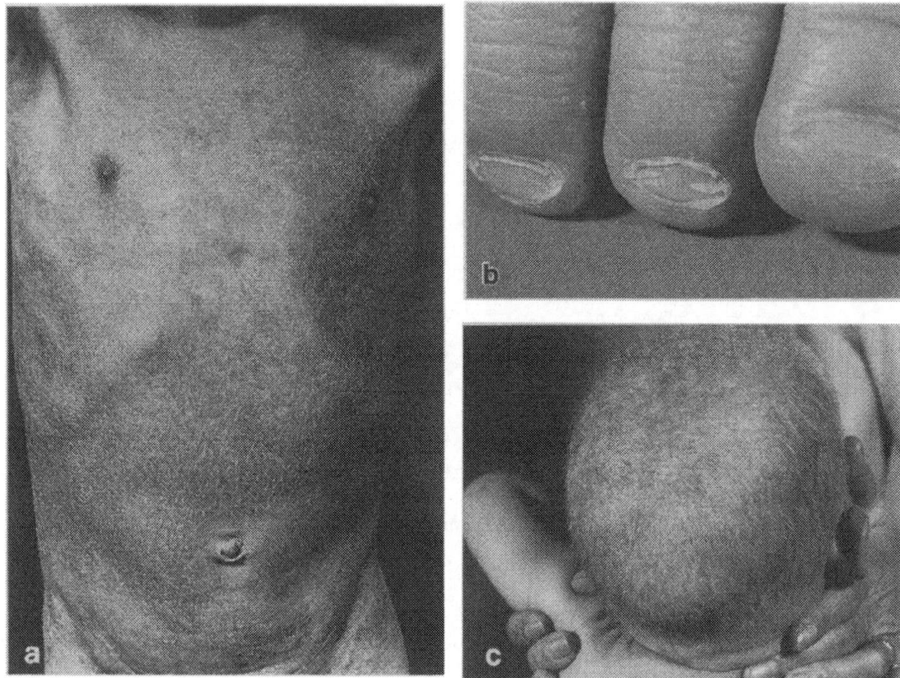

Fig. 58a–c. Aspects of Tay syndrome in a 5-year-old boy. **a** Congenital ichthyosis with rather mild scaling; **b** dysplastic nails showing lamellar splitting; **c** sparse, broken scalp hair. (From [6], courtesy of Dr. Happle, Nijmegen)

nia, otitis, mastitis, sinusitis) is observed, indicating an impaired immune defense.

5.2.3 Clinical Features of the PIBI(D)S Syndrome

The PIBI(D)S syndrome as delineated by Rebora and Crovato [11] shares many features with the Tay syndrome, such as brittle cystine-deficient hair, impaired intelligence, psychomotor retardation, an increased susceptibility to infections, and complications of pregnancy and delivery. It differs from the Tay syndrome by an extreme photosensitivity due to a DNA excision repair defect, by a somewhat different facies, and by a mild, noncongenital ichthyosis [4, 11, 16–18]. There is usually no evidence of hypogonadism. Some patients may exhibit retinal dystrophy and cataracts [11]. Rebora and Crovato emphasize that the children, at first glance, appear to be alert and have an unusually sociable and cuddlesome behavior, making contact easily, even with strangers.

Photosensitivity is certainly the most outstanding feature of the PIBI(D)S syndrome. An exposure of 10–60 min to the sun is enough to induce a severe sunburn [11, 15]. Phototesting shows that the minimal erythema dose to UVB is

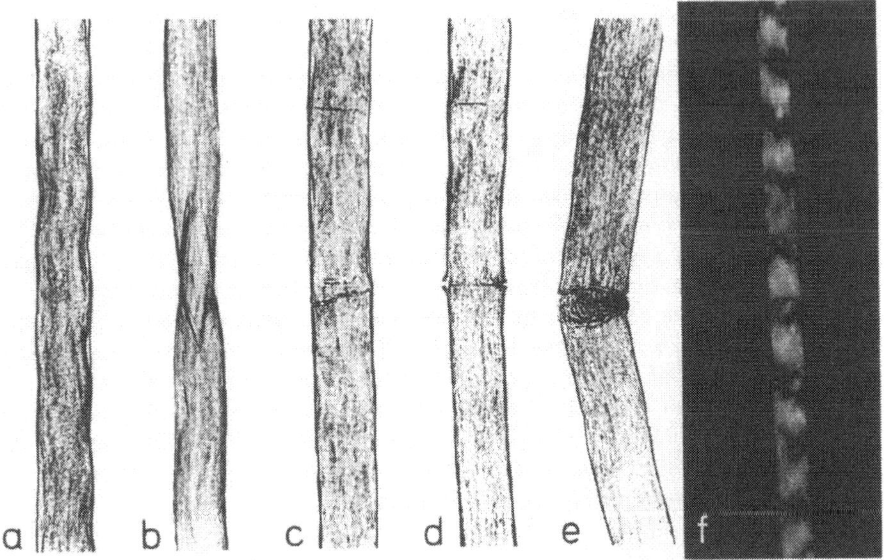

Fig. 59 a–f. Hair abnormalities in the Tay syndrome. **a** Undulating contour of hair shaft, **b** folding of hair shaft along its axis, **c–e** trichoschisis (clean transverse fractures) at various stages of development, **f** polarizing microscopy showing tigertail pattern. (From [6], courtesy of Dr. Happle, Nijmegen)

markedly reduced. With increasing age, the extreme photosensitivity seems to decrease.

5.2.4 Histologic Features of Tay and PIBI(D)S Syndromes

The histologic picture found in the Tay and PIBI(D)S syndromes is that of a nonspecific benign acanthokeratosis [2, 8–11]. There is a moderately increased orthokeratotic stratum corneum, a thin granular layer, moderate acanthosis, and mild papillomatosis. Furthermore, slight perivascular inflammatory changes can be noted. These histologic changes, reminiscent of ichthyosis vulgaris, are the same in both the Tay and PIBI(D)S syndromes. Ultrastructural examinations are lacking, and therefore we do not know whether the Tay and the PIBI(D)S syndromes differ in this repect.

5.2.5 Biochemical Aspects

The primary biochemical defects of the various trichothiodystrophy syndromes are unknown. Though terms like "sulfur-deficient brittle hair" or "trichothiodystrophy"suggest a true deficiency of sulfur-containing amino acids, this is not true. The abnormal hair of trichothiodystrophy patients usually contains about

45% less cystine and 35% less proline than found in normal hair [5, 17]. The circulating blood levels for the various animo acids are normal. In one patient with PIBI(D)S syndrome the in vitro uptake of cystine into hair follicles was normal. Thus, the popular hypothesis of a defective transport mechanism for sulfur-containing amino acids may not be true, at least not in the PIBI(D)S syndrome [15]. Two-dimensional gel electrophoresis of the proteins of abnormal hair discloses a loss of high-sulfur protein and the replacement of this fraction by components of similar molecular weight but lower cystine content [5, 17]. The loss of high-sulfur proteins affects the structure of the hair matrix. This may explain the alternating birefringence observed on polarizing microscopy.

Very recently, the nature of the extreme photosensitivity in PIBI(D)S patients was elucidated at the molecular level [16, 18]. By complementation studies Stefanini et al. [13] were able to show that PIBI(D)S patients have a DNA excision repair defect which is identical to the defect of complementation group D of xeroderma pigmentosum. Surprisingly, even in later life, PIBI(D)S patients do not develop the typical signs and symptoms of xeroderma pigmentosum and do not show an increased incidence of skin tumors.

5.2.6 Genetic Aspects and Counseling

The genetics of the three trichothiodystrophy syndromes is poorly understood. Price et al. [10] suggested that trichothiodystrophy is caused by a singular gene defect having a broad and variable clinical spectrum. In contrast, Happle et al. [6] suggested that the BIDS syndrome and the Tay syndrome are caused by different genes and assumed genetic heterogeneity for these syndromes. Because of the long list of similarities between the BIDS syndrome and the Tay syndrome, I assume that we are dealing with multiple allelism.

The genetic relationship between the PIBI(D)S syndrome and the classical Tay syndrome is even more difficult to determine. Trichothiodystrophy is usually not a feature of the xeroderma pigmentosum group-D mutation. Therefore, I assume that the PIBI(D)S phenotype is caused by a deletion mutation, affecting both the gene for xeroderma pigmentosum group D and a neighboring gene responsible for ichthyosis and trichothiodystrophy (the Tay syndrome gene). The remaining main difference between the PIBI(D)S and the Tay syndrome would then be that in PIBI(D)S the ichthyosis is noncongenital and less severe than in the Tay syndrome. This situation would be very similar to that of associated steroid sulfatase deficiency in which ichthyosis is also sometimes less pronounced than in patients with isolated X-linked recessive ichthyosis. A contiguous gene syndrome can account for the striking facial dysmorphism, too.

As far as genetic counseling is concerned, there is convincing evidence that both the Tay syndrome and the PIBI(D)S syndrome are inherited as autosomal recessive traits [6, 11]. Successful prenatal diagnosis of the Tay syndrome has been reported recently by Blanchet-Bardon [1] – however, at a late gestational age. By ultrasound-guided fetoscopy, she was able to obtain scalp biopsies from the affected fetus and to demonstrate the typical hair shaft abnormality. In patients with PIBI(D)S syndrome a molecular approach to prenatal diagnosis should be possible by DNA repair studies in the near future. The clinical expressivity of the Tay syndrome and PIBI(D)S syndrome can vary considerably. Some patients are only mildly affected in later life. This should be borne in mind when the question of prenatal diagnosis is raised.

References

1. Blanchet-Bardon C (1987) Prenatal diagnosis in Tay syndrome. Workshop on prenatal diagnosis. In: 17th World Congress of Dermatology, Berlin, May 24–29
2. Braun-Falco O, Ring J, Butenand D, Selzle D, Landthaler M (1981) Ichthyosis vulgaris, Minderwuchs, Haardysplasie, Zahnanomalien, Immundefekte, psychosomatische Retardation and Resorptionsstörungen. Kasuistischer Bericht über zwei Geschwister. Hautarzt 33:67–74
3. Brown AC, Belser RB, Crounse RG, Wehr BF (1970) A congenital hair defect. Trichoschisis with alternating birefringence and low sulfur content. J Invest Dermatol 54:496–509
4. Crovato F, Rebora A (1985) PIBI(D)S syndrome: a new entity with defect of the deoxyribonucleic acid excision repair system. J Am Acad Dermatol 13:683–686
5. Gillespie JM, Marshall RL (1983) A comparison of the proteins of normal and trichothiodystrophic human hair. J Invest Dermatol 80:195–202
6. Happle R, Traupe H, Gröbe H, Bonsmann G (1984) The Tay syndrome (congenital ichthyosis with trichothiodystrophy). Eur J Pediatr 141:147–152
7. Jackson CE, Weiss L, Watson JHL (1974) "Brittle" hair with short stature, intellectual impairment and decreased fertility: an autosomal recessive syndrome in an Amish kindred. Pediatrics 54:201–207
8. Jorizzo JL, Crounse RG, Wheeler CE (1980) Lamellar ichthyosis, dwarfism, mental retardation, and hair shaft abnormalities. A link between the ichthyosis-associated and BIDS syndromes. J Am Acad Dermatol 2:309–317
9. Jorizzo JL, Atherton DJ, Crounse RG, Wells RS (1982) Ichthyosis, brittle hair, impaired intelligence, decreased fertility and short stature (IBIDS syndrome). Br J Dermatol 106:705–710
10. Price VH, Odom RB, Ward WH, Jones FT (1980) Trichothiodystrophy. Sulfur-deficient brittle hair as a marker for a neuro-ectodermal symptom complex. Arch Dermatol 116:1375–1384
11. Rebora A, Crovato F (1987) PIBI(D)S syndrome-trichothiodystrophy with xeroderma pigmentosum (group D) mutation. J Am Acad Dermatol 16:940–947
12. Salfeld K. Lindley MJ (1963) Zur Frage der Merkmalskombination bei Ichthyosis vulgaris mit Bambushaarbildung und ektodermaler Dysplasie. Dermatol Wochenschr 147:118–128
13. Stefanini M, Lagomarsini P, Arlett CF, Marionini S. Borrone C, Crovato F, Trevisan G, Cordone G, Nuzzo F (1986) Xeroderma pigmentosum (complementation group D) mutation is present in patients affected by trichothiodystrophy with photosensitivity. Hum Genet 74:107–112
14. Tay CH (1971) Ichthyosiform erythroderma, hair shaft abnormalities, and mental and growth retardation. A new recessive disorder. Arch Dermatol 104:4–13
15. Van Neste D, Boré P (1983) Trichothiodystrophie: une étude morphologique et biochimique. Ann Dermatol Venereol 110:409–417
16. Van Neste D, Caulier B, Thomas P. Vasseur F (1985) PIBIDS: Tay's syndrome and xeroderma pigmentosum (letter). J Am Acad Dermatol 12:372–373
17. Van Neste D, Gillespie M, Marshall R (1987) Heterogeneity of trichothiodystrophy: preliminary biochemical results. In: Happle R, Grosshans E (eds) Pediatric dermatology. Springer, Berlin Heidelberg New York Tokyo, pp 170–174
18. Yong SL, Cleaver JE, Tullis GD, Johnston MM (1984) Is trichothiodystrophy part of the xeroderma pigmentosum spectrum? Am J Hum Genet 36:82

5.3 The Comèl-Netherton Syndrome

5.3.1 Historical Aspects

In 1949, the Italian dermatologist Comèl [7] from Pisa delineated a new type of congenital ichthyosis. He reported on a 23-year-old woman suffering from an ichthyosis-like dermatosis characterized by migratory, serpiginous skin lesions showing double-edged scales. Comèl recognized that this was a new skin disorder and coined the term "ichthyosis linearis circumflexa". Nine years later, Netherton [22] described a 4-year-old girl suffering from congenital ichthyotic erythroderma and a characteristic hair shaft abnormality which he called "bamboo hair". In 1964 Wilkinson and his associates [30] reported a similar case and introduced the term "trichorrhexis invaginata" for the peculiar hair shaft abnormality. Furthermore, they suggested that atopic diathesis is an additional symptom and referred to the association of congenital ichthyosis, trichorrhexis invaginata, and atopic diathesis as "Netherton's syndrome". In 1968, Schnyder and Wiegand [23] first described trichorrhexis invaginata in two patients suffering from ichthyosis linearis circumflexa. Over the next few years, it became obvious that in most cases reported as Netherton's syndrome the ichthyosis corresponded to ichthyosis linearis circumflexa (ILC) as described by Comèl, while only a very few cases showed generalized involvement with congenital ichthyotic erythroderma (CIE) [19]. For historical reasons, I think it most appropriate to refer to the syndrome of congenital ichthyosis with trichorrhexis invaginata as the "Comèl-Netherton syndrome". The nature of the ichthyosis in this syndrome has been the subject of a considerable debate, raising the question of whether the Comèl-Netherton syndrome is a heterogeneous condition [1, 15, 19]. We recently argued that the Comèl-Netherton syndrome can encompass a broad clinical spectrum and should be viewed as a singular disease [27, 28]. Moreover, I strongly suspect that the peeling-skin syndrome type B is identical with the Comèl-Netherton syndrome. This issue is discussed below in Sect. 6.5.4.

Incidence

The Comèl-Netherton syndrome is a rare disease. By 1984 a total of 58 cases had been reported [27]. Over the past 10 years Dr. Happle and I have observed six cases at the Münster Department [28]. This would mean a minimal incidence of 1/50000 in Westphalia. I am much indebted to Dr. Happle, who established the correct diagnosis of the syndrome in several patients, including two cases previously considered to be examples of Leiner's disease or erythrodermic lamellar ichthyosis. I learned how important it is to routinely perform a microscopic examination of shaven (not plucked!) hair in patients with ichthyotic erythroderma.

5.3.2 Clinical Features

In most cases reported, the cutaneous manifestation of the syndrome corresponds to that of ILC [12, 19, 27] (Fig. 60). On the trunk and the extremities erythematous, circinate, anular, and serpiginous patches often bordered by distinctive, double-edged scales can be seen [6, 8, 10, 17]. The remaining unaffected skin, especially in the antecubital and popliteal areas, usually is lichenified. Frequently, there is a distincitive perioral erythema, not seen in other ichthyoses [8]. During childhood, scalp hair is brittle and breaks easily. In later life, the characteristic hair shaft abnormality of trichorrhexis invaginata (Fig. 61) can be confined to the eyebrows or may even be absent [1, 19]. Parents very often give a history of a more generalized erythematous involvement at birth and in the first year of life, indicating evolution of congenital ichthyotic erythroderma into ichthyosis linearis circumflexa (ILC) [4, 8].

According to the literature, ILC is the prevailing type of cutaneous manifestation present in about 80%–90% of patients with Comèl-Netherton syndrome [5, 12, 19, 27]. Our own experience with the syndrome is quite different. Of six patients we observed, five exhibited congenital ichthyotic erythroderma and only one 12-year-old boy presented with ichthyosis linearis circumflexa (Table 27). In this boy, the disease was said to have started as CIE as well. In our experience, erythema can be very marked in CIE patients with the syndrome. It is reasonable to assume that quite a number of patients considered to have typical erythroder-

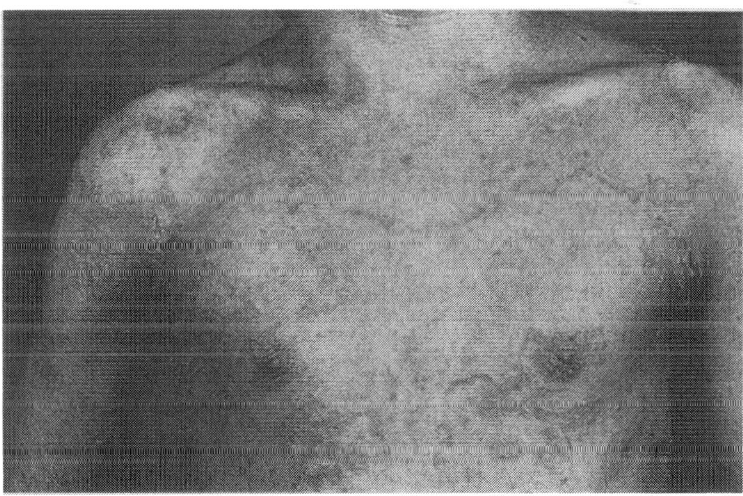

Fig. 60. Comèl-Netherton syndrome. Ichthyosis linearis circumflexa in a 12-year-old boy. Typical aspect with serpiginous lesions

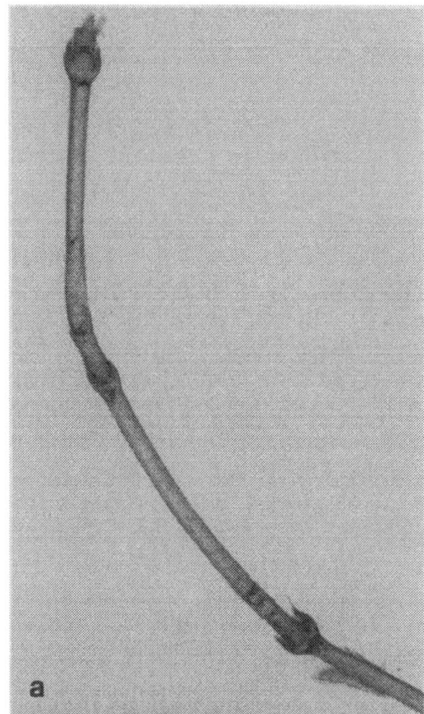

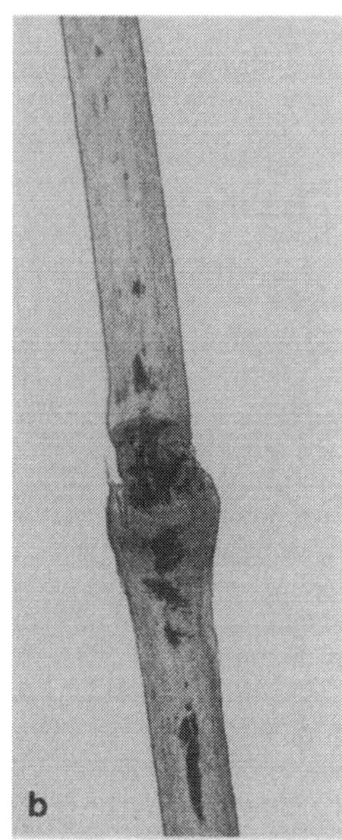

Fig. 61 a, b. Trichorrhexis invaginata. **a** Multiple bamboo nodules in a single hair shaft (overview); **b** typical aspect in another hair

mic lamellar ichthyosis (ELI) or Leiner's disease actually are unrecognized Comèl-Netherton cases. As in ELI, the hyperkertoses are fine, but often have an exfoliative appearance and can be peeled off easily (Fig. 62). In one CIE child we observed a loss of the (outer) nail plate (Fig. 63). Due to a considerable transepidermal water loss the children often experience hypernatremic dehydration and hypothermia in the neonatal period [11, 13, 27, 28].

Noncutaneous Findings

Both clinical variants of the Comèl-Netherton syndrome share a number of noncutaneous disease manifestations (Table 28). In our experience, this noncutaneous involvement of the gene defect is more severe in those patients in whom CIE is present. In several children with the CIE phenotype the disease took a fatal course because of a severe immune deficiency [8, 28]. In patients with the ILC phenotype, impetigo and a generalized lymphadenopathy may be seen as manifestations of this immune deficiency, while patients with the congenital ichthyotic erythroderma (CIE) phenotype often suffer from severe and recurrent bronchopneumonia and sepsis. In the ILC patients gastrointestinal involvement (enteropathy) may become obvious only after ingestion of nuts, causing diarrhea and a worsening of the skin condition [1, 10], whereas in the CIE patients pro-

Table 27. Clinical findings in our own series of Comèl-Netherton syndrome patients

Patient no, clinical phenotype	Sex	Age	Hypernatremic dehydration as a neonate	Failure to thrive	Growth retardation	Enteropathy	Immune defect	Remarks
1, ILC	M	12 years	No	No	Mild	No	Recurrent skin infektions	Born with CIE
2, CIE	F	6 months	Yes	Severe weight loss soon after birth	Marked	Severe malnutrition	Pseudomonas sepsis	Died at 10 months
3, CIE	M	2 months	?	Severe weight loss soon after birth	Marked	Severe malnutrition	Recurrent broncho-pneumonia	Extreme anemia; died at age 9.5 months
4, CIE	M	8 years	Yes	Slow to gain weight	Mild	No	No	Initially diagnosed as ELI
5, CIE	M	1 year	Yes	Slow to gain weight	Mild	No	No	Brother of patient 4
6, CIE	M	20 years	?	No	No	No	Recurrent skin infections	Initially diagnosed as Leiner's disease

ILC, Ichthyosis linearis circumflexa; CIE, congenital ichthyotic erythroderma; ELI, erythrodermic lamellar ichthyosis

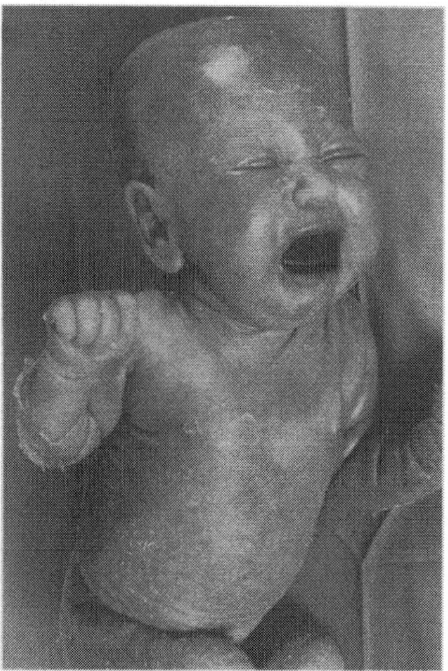

Fig. 62. Comèl-Netherton syndrome. Congenital ichthyotic erythroderma in a 6-month-old girl. The fine translucent scales can be peeled off easily. Note striking resemblance to peeling-skin syndrome type B. Correct diagnosis was confirmed by presence of trichorrhexis invaginata in this case

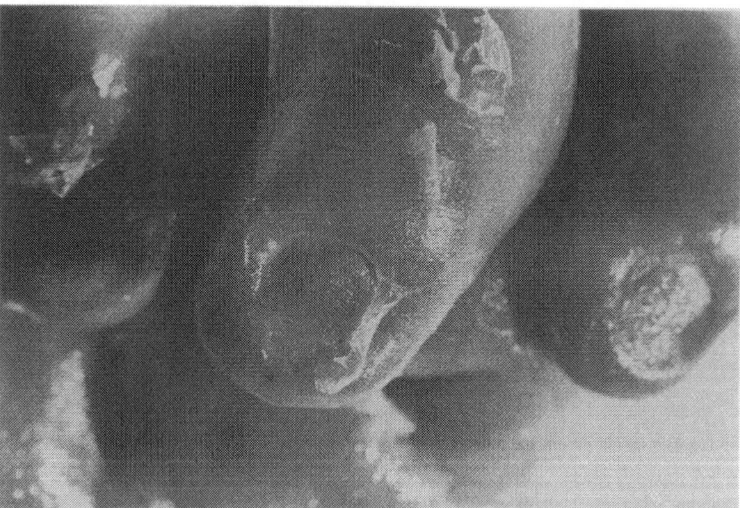

Fig. 63. Unusual loss of the outer nail plate resembling anonychia in a severely affected 8-week-old boy with the CIE phenotype

Table 28. Severity of noncutaneous symptoms in Comèl-Netherton syndrome[a]

Symptoms	ILC phenotype	CIE phenotype
Hypernatremic dehydration	Lacking	Mild to extreme
Failure to thrive	Lacking or mild	Mild to extreme
Growth retardation	Mild	Mild to marked
Enteropathy	Mild	Mild to extreme
Immune defect	Mild	Marked to extreme

[a] This table is based on the analysis of 58 cases in the literature and six of our own observations

nounced malnutrition is often seen. According to Caputo, deterioration of the skin status after intake of nuts is a constant phenomenon in the Comèl-Netherton syndrome and may be employed as a challenge test having great diagnostic value (Dr. R. Caputo, personal communication, Bari 1987). Children with the severe CIE type often do not gain weight and do not grow. In the ILC children these problems are much less serious, though a retarded bone age and short stature may also be noted [12, 13].

As a general rule, hypotrichosis is more pronounced in the CIE variant, though even these patients may show normal scalp hair in later life. Cambazard et al. [5] recently described a 5-year-old girl with the CIE phenotype displaying notable parietal-occipital alopecia in a manner seen in punks or Iroquois Indians. Due to the marked inflammation, patients with the CIE phenotype often experience periods of oozing and occasionally even present with superficial blisters [5, 21].

Though in many papers, especially the early ones, atopic diathesis is mentioned, this should be regarded as an inconstant sign of the syndrome. The term "atopic diathesis" in itself is vague. The disease may have a striking resemblance to atopic dermatitits, especially in the ILC patients. I had the opportunity to follow one such patient over many years, and even when he was not being treated with etretinate or emollients he had periods when he was totally free of the typical serpiginous and gyrate skin lesions, but showed only dry skin and lichenification, especially over the flexural aspects of the limbs. Other authors consider the intolerance to certain foods such as nuts, eggs, or fish a sign of an atopic reaction [8, 10, 30]. Whether the incidence of atopic asthma bronchiale exceeds that of normal controls is not certain. In my opinion, atopic dermatitis is not a constituent of the Comèl-Netherton syndrome; rather, the disease may look similar to atopic dermatitis and to the hyper-IgE syndrome.

It should be noted that extreme levels of IgE are usually found, up to 10000 IU, and that the specific IgE levels may show very high RAST classes against a multitude of antigens. The determination of the total IgE can be helpful for differential diagnosis from other types of congenital ichthyosis in which the IgE levels are normal or only slightly raised. However, excessive IgE values do not prove an atopic diathesis.

5.3.3 Histologic and Ultrastructural Features

Histology discloses the same features in patients with the ILC variant and in those with the CIE phenotype. The most characteristic changes, such as the deposition of a strongly eosinophilic material in the stratum corneum, are more pronounced in the CIE patients [20], whereas in the ILC patients these distinctive changes may be seen only when the biopsy is taken from the edge of an active border of a migrating skin lesion [18]. On conventional hematoxylin/eosin staining a markedly parakeratotic stratum corneum, often containing masses of pyknotic granulocytes, is seen (Fig. 64). The granular layer is usually diminished, and may be lacking completely in those parts of the biopsy which clinically correspond to the active borders of the specimen.

Comèl [7] reported a detachment of the stratum corneum from the underlying epidermis. Such a subcorneal cleft formation is a frequent finding [14, 18]. The malpighian layer is increased and usually there is considerable papillomatosis. Marked inflammatory infiltrates in the perivascular position are present in the papillary dermis. Especially in the CIE patients, there is marked exocytosis (inflammatory cells invading the epidermis), and considerable spongiosis of the epidermis may result. Furthermore, the keratinocytes of the upper prickle-cell layer can be vacuolated. PAS staining shows large masses of an eosinophilic amorphous material replacing the normal stratum corneum [18, 31].

Electron microscopy discloses the presence of round cytoplasmic bodies in the keratinocytes of the granular and prickle-cell layer with a diameter varying

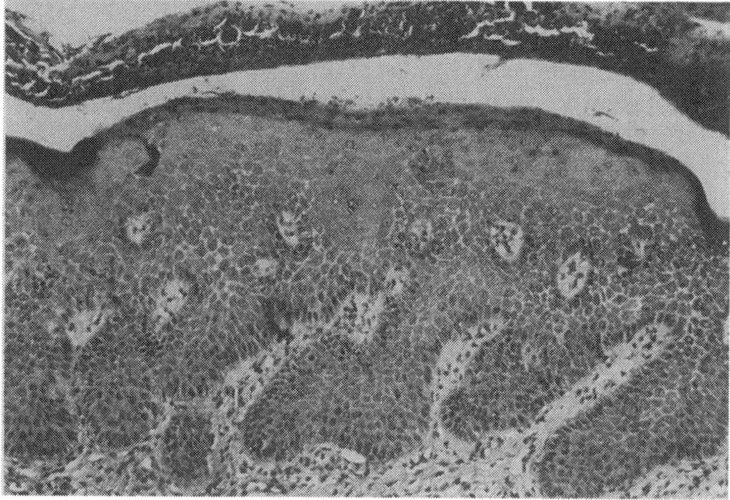

Fig. 64. Histology of the Comèl-Netherton syndrome (CIE child, same as in Fig. 57). Note masses of pyknotic granulocytes in the parakeratotic stratum corneum and intracorneal cleft formation. The upper prickle-cell layer shows marked degenerative and necrolytic changes with blurred cell boundaries, contrasting with the acanthotic lowermost portion of the epidermis. HE, ×100

from 0.3 to 10 μm [9, 26, 32]. These inclusion bodies are most likely lysosomes. Their numerous presence in the Comèl-Netherton syndrome is not a specific, but nevertheless a very useful ultrastructural finding not reported so far in other types of ichthyosis. Moreover, there is a marked decrease of the desmosome-tonofilament system and a lack of lamellar bodies (keratinosomes) [9]. As in autosomal dominant ichthyosis vulgaris, the keratohyalin granules may be absent, reflecting the loss of a granular layer seen on routine histology. Understandably, filaggrin staining will also be negative. The horny layer is replaced by parakeratotic cells connected by a few desmosomes. These parakeratotic cells are filled with an amorphous substance that is also discharged to the extracellular spaces [9, 32].

A recent immunohistochemical study illustrates similarities, but also differences between the inflammatory process in atopic dermatitis and that in the Comèl-Netherton syndrome. Using a panel of monoclonal antibodies, Arico and associates [3] studied a man with ILC. As in atopic dermatitis [29], they found an increase of CD1+ dendritic Langerhans/indeterminate cells in the epidermis. However, the papillary infiltrate was composed mainly of CD3+ and CD8+ cells having cytotoxic functions, while in atopic dermatitis a predominance of T-helper cells (CD4+ cells) can be expected [29]. The discontinuous arrangement of CD5+ cells near the dermo-epidermal junction was a conspicuous finding so far not observed in other keratinization disorders [3].

5.3.4 Pathogenesis of Trichorrhexis Invaginata

Light-microscopic investigations show that trichorrhexis invaginata can be detected in scalp biopsies [2, 20, 24]. Transmission-electron microscopy reveals that formation of the bamboo nodule is not visible below the level of the keratogeneous zone [16]. Normally, SH groups disappear just above the keratogeneous zone and S-S linkages appear in the hair shaft [25]. In trichorrhexis invaginata hairs, this physiologic conversion of SH to S-S groups seems to be disturbed and a significant amount of SH groups can still be found in the cortex cells. In terms of pathophysiology, this means a diminished number of cross-linkages of the keratin structure and a weaker coherence of cortical cells. It is conceivable that due to the upward force of the growing hair shaft, these soft sections of the hair shaft are put under pressure and, when driven upward, fold around the more stable section of the hair and thus form the typical bamboo nodules.

5.3.5 Biochemical Aspects

The biochemical basis of the Comèl-Netherton syndrome is unknown. Intermittent aminoaciduria is a nonspecific and variable finding often reported [6, 12, 20]. As in psoriasis, urinary polyamine levels are elevated compared with those in normal individuals [31]. Furthermore, the activities of acid phosphatase, beta-glucuronidase, and transglutaminase seem to be increased in the scales of these patients [31]. Similar elevations may be found in psoriatic scales.

5.3.6 Remarks on Therapy

Therapy poses a number of problems that are peculiar to the Comèl-Netherton syndrome. In the neonatal period, great care has to be given to fluid balance. The children are prone to develop hypernatremic dehydration [11, 13, 28] because they lose considerable amounts of water via the inflamed skin. In some children, an extreme weight loss can be observed soon after birth. The malnutrition problem can be so severe that they slowly become cachectic and finally die of an additional sepsis (cases 2 and 3 of our series). There is no known effective remedy for this problem. It is possible that the malnutrition/malabsorption problem is related to inflammatory bowel changes caused by the fundamental immune defect/dysregulation which is a typical feature of the disease. If this is so, then temporary immunosuppressive therapy (e.g., cyclosporin A) may be the appropriate answer. Though I have no personal experience with this kind of therapy, I would advise at least trying cyclosporin A when encountering a severe malnutrition problem in such a patient. The drug was not yet available when we took care of those children in whom the disease was fatal.

As far as skin care is concerned, it is important to use bland emollients only and to avoid active ingredients such as salicylic acid and urea (at least in the first years of life). The impaired barrier function of the skin results in an unusual penetration of active substances which may exert serious systemic side effects. If retinoids are to be used, the dosage has to be lower than in other cornification disorders (see Sect. 7.2). Photochemotherapy (PUVA) seems to be an effective way to control the cutaneous lesions [21], but I feel uneasy about possible side effects after long-term treatment (PUVA lentigines, cancer risk).

5.3.7 Genetic Aspects and Counseling

Today it is clear that the Comèl-Netherton syndrome is inherited as an autosomal recessive trait, though initially X-linked dominant inheritance had also been discussed [8, 30]. According to the literature, there is a preponderance of women [5, 11, 27]. This is an artifact, however, since the predominance of the female sex is seen in the mildly affected ILC cases, while in the more severe CIE cases, more men than women are affected [5, 27, 28]. In 1984, I performed an extensive review of the literature [27]. Of 58 verified cases published at that time, 51 displayed the ILC and seven the CIE phenotype [27]. In the ILC group the sex ratio (F/M) was 1.4 (30 women, 21 men). In the CIE group the sex ratio was 0.75 (three women, four men) [27]. It is interesting that in contrast to the predominance of the ILC type in the literature (87%), in our own series of six patients only one patient belonged to the ILC group, while five patients (one girl, four boys) belonged to the more severe CIE group. Two of these patients (one girl, one boy) died at the age of 10 months because of problems related to the disease (severe malnutrition, pronounced immune deficiency). Comparing our own data with those in the literature, the following conclusions can be drawn:

1. Patients with the more severe CIE phenotype are often not diagnosed as having Comèl-Netherton syndrome and are hence significantly underrepresented in the literature.
2. In general, the disease takes a more severe course in boys than in girls.
3. Though the sex ratio deviates from the expected 1:1 in the two phenotypic subsets of the disease (more women and girls in the ILC groups, more men and boys in the CIE group), there is no reason to believe that this is true of the disease as a whole.
4. The sex ratio data do not support X-linked dominant inheritance, but are compatible with an autosomal recessive mode of transmission.

The notion that the two clinical phenotypes are caused by only one gene defect finds further support in the observation of both ILC and CIE variants among sibs [4, 6, 8, 17]. Given the fatal course the disease may take, prenatal diagnosis would be desirable. Unfortunately, a safe prenatal exclusion diagnosis is not possible [2].

References

1. Altman J, Stroud J (1969) Netherton's syndrome and ichthyosis linearis circumflexa. Arch Dermatol 100:550–558
2. Anton-Lamprecht I (1989) Pränatale Diagnostik von Genodermatosen. 35th Meeting of the German Dermatological Society, 27 April–May 1988, Munich. Hautarzt 39 [Suppl VIII]: 16–20
3. Arico M, Di Leonardo S, Pravata G, Noto G, Brignole G (1987) Netherton's syndrome in a male. An immunohistochemical study. In: Meneghini CL, Bonifazi E (eds) Proceedings 2nd Congress European Society for Pediatric Dermatology. Pediatr Dermatol News 6:267–271
4. Broberg A, Suurküla M (1987) A case of Netherton's syndrome with a defective yeast opsonization in serum. In: Meneghini CL, Bonifazi E (eds) Proceedings 2nd Congress European Society for Pediatric Dermatology. Pediatr Dermatol News 6:31–33
5. Cambazard F, Thivolet M, Ferrier MC, Mauduit G, Chouvet B, Hermier M (1986) Le syndrome Iroquois: une variante du syndrome de Netherton? Ann Dermatol Venereol 113:941–945
6. Caputo R, Vanotti P, Bertani E (1984) Netherton's syndrome in two adult brothers. Arch Dermatol 120:220–222
7. Comèl M (1949) Ichthyosis linearis circumflexa. Dermatologica 98:122–136
8. Dupré A, Bonafé JL, Carrère S (1978) Ichthyose linéaire circonflexe de Comèl et syndrome de Netherton. Conception Générale. A propos de 4 observations. Ann Dermatol Venereol 105:49–54
9. Frenk E, Mevorah B (1972) Ichthyosis linearis circumflexa Comèl with trichorrhexis invaginata (Netherton's syndrome). An ultrastructural study of the skin changes. Arch Dermatol Forsch 245:42–49
10. Gianotti F (1969) La maladie de Netherton. Étude de deux cas et des rapports avec les génodermatoses érythématodesquamatives circinées variables. Ann Dermatol Venereol 96:147–156
11. Greene SL, Muller SA (1985) Netherton's syndrome. Report of a case and review of the literature. J Am Acad Dermatol 13:329–337
12. Greig D, Wishart J (1982) Growth abnormality in Netherton's syndrome. Aust J Dermatol 23:27–30

13. Jones SK, Thomson LM, Surbrugg SK, Weston WL (1986) Neonatal hypernatraemia in two siblings with Netherton's syndrome. Br J Dermatol 114:741–743
14. Hersle K (1972) Netherton's disease and ichthyosis linearis circumflexa. Report of a case and review of the literature. Acta Derm Venereol (Stockh) 52:298–302
15. Hurwitz S, Kirsch N, McGuire J (1971) Reevaluation of ichthyosis and hair shaft abnormalities. Arch Dermatol 103:266–271
16. Ito M, Ito K, Hashimoto K (1984) Pathogenesis of trichorrhexis invaginata (bamboo hair). J Invest Dermatol 83:1–6
17. Kassis V, Nielsen JM, Klem-Thomsen H, Dahl-Christensen J, Wadskov S (1986) Familial Netherton's disease. Cutis 37:175–178
18. Mevorah B, Frenk E (1974) Ichthyosis linearis circumflexa Comèl with trichorrhexis invaginata (Netherton's syndrome). A light-microscopical study of skin changes. Dermatologica 149:193–200
19. Mevorah B, Frenk E, Brooke EM (1974) Ichthyosis linearis circumflexa Comèl. A clinicostatistical approach to its relationship with Netherton's syndrome. Dermatologica 149:201–209
20. Michalowski R, Urban J, Kucharska D (1978) Netherton-Syndrom mit Alopezie und Prolinurie. Hautarzt 29:205–208
21. Nagata T (1980) Netherton's syndrome which responded to photochemotherapy. Dermatologica 161:51–56
22. Netherton EW (1958) A unique case of trichorrhexis nodosa – "bamboo hairs." Arch Dermatol 78:483–487
23. Schnyder UW, Wiegand K (1968) Haaranomalien bei Ichthyosis linearis circumflexa Comèl. Hautarzt 19:494–499
24. Stevanovic DV (1969) Multiple defects of the hair shaft in Netherton's disease. Association with ichthyosis linearis circumflexa. Br J Dermatol 81:851–857
25. Taneda A, Ogana H, Hashimoto K (1980) The histochemical demonstration of protein-bound sulfhydryl groups and disulfide bands in human hair by a new staining method (DACM staining). J Invest Dermatol 75:365–369
26. Thorne EG, Zelickson AS, Mottaz JH, Katz HI, Deaton BH (1975) Netherton's syndrome. An electron microscopic study. Arch Dermatol Res 253:177–183
27. Traupe H (1984) Neuere Untersuchungen zur Klinik, Genetik, Histologie und Therapie der Ichthyosen. Thesis (Habilitationsschrift), University of Münster, pp 241–266
28. Traupe H, Happle R (1987) The clinical spectrum of the Comèl-Netherton syndrome. Second Congress of the European Society for Pediatric Dermatology, 2–4 Oct 1987, Bari.
29. Uno H, Hanifin JM (1980) Langerhans cells in acute and chronic epidermal lesions of atopic dermatitits, observed by L-dopa histofluorescence glycol methacrylate thin sections, and electron microscopy. J Invest Dermatol 75:52–60
30. Wilkinson RD, Curtis GH, Hawk WS (1964) Netherton's disease. Arch Dermatol 89:46–54
31. Yoshiike T, Manabe M, Negi M, Ogawa H (1985) Ichthyosis linearis circumflexa: morphological and biochemical studies. Br J Dermatol 112:277–283
32. Zina A, Bundino S (1979) Ichthyosis linearis circumflexa Comèl and Netherton's syndrome; an ultrastructural study. Dermatologica 158:404–412

5.4 X-Linked Dominant Ichthyosis

5.4.1 Historical Aspects and Nomenclature

X-linked dominant ichthyosis is a multisystem disorder involving skin, bones, and eyes [4–8]. The condition also is often called "X-linked dominant chondrodysplasia punctata" [5, 8, 16, 17]. How the disease is named depends of course, on how it is looked at. For a dermatologist, ichthyotic erythroderma at birth evolving into a nonerythematous ichthyosis with linear skin lesions is the hallmark of the condition, while a pediatrician may attach more importance to the mild chondrodysplasia punctata. I prefer the designation "X-linked dominant ichthyosis" (XDI).

Historically, however, isolation of XDI as a distinct entity has to be seen in the context of splitting the chondrodysplasia punctata group. In 1971, Spranger and associates [20] recognized the genetic heterogeneity of chondrodysplasia punctata and distinguished the autosomal recessive rhizomelic type from the less severe Conradi-Hünermann type, for which an autosomal dominant inheritance pattern was assumed. Children affected with the rhizomelic type usually die within the first year of life, while those showing the Conradi-Hünermann type have a much better prognosis. In the years 1977–1979, Rudolf Happle [4, 5, 7, 8] delineated XDI as a third distinct variant of chondrodysplasia punctata, characterized by a mosaic pattern of skin lesions. As in incontinentia pigmenti, the disease occurred exclusively in the female sex and the cutaneous changes showed a similar linear distribution pattern with widespread atrophic lesions, pigmentary disturbances and ichthyosis. Because of the striking resemblance of the peculiar distribution pattern to that seen in incontinentia pigmenti and focal dermal hypoplasia, Happle argued that he was dealing with a further X-linked dominant gene defect and interpreted the linear cutaneous involvement as an example of X-chromosome inactivation [4, 5, 7, 8]. This concept was soon confirmed by other groups, corroborating the existance of a third X-linked dominant type of chondrodysplasia punctata [11, 16, 17].

In the meantime, many cases previously considered to be examples of the autosomal dominant Conradi-Hünermann type have been shown to belong to the X-linked dominant type [5, 16]. Very recently, several cases published years ago as Conradi-Hünermann syndrome without skin involvement were recognized as examples of Warfarin embryopathy [10]. Thus, the existance of an autosomal dominant variant of chondrodysplasia punctata is so far not established beyond doubt.

5.4.2 Clinical Features

5.4.2.1 Cutaneous Findings

At birth, the affected girls suffer from severe ichthyotic erythroderma. The erythema is usually generalized, whereas the thick, adherent hyperkeratoses follow a linear pattern [2, 7, 11]. The ichthyotic erythroderma clears up after a few months. In an older child, systematized atrophoderma (Fig. 65), mainly involving the hair follicles, pigmentary disturbances and ichthyosis are noted. The hyperkeratoses are usually arranged in a mosaic-like pattern (Fig. 66) following the lines of Blaschko and are more pronounced in the atrophic areas [7]. A patchy to more universal involvement, affecting for example the entire volar forearm may also be seen [7, 16]. In the adult patients, patchy areas of cicatricial alopecia (alopecia ichthyotica; Fig. 67) are a constant feature and sometimes may even be the only manifestation seen in mildly affected female conductors [16]. Hair obtained from the marginal zone of alopecia ichthyotica in these patients exhibits on light microscopy a number of nonspecific alterations, such as variations of the shaft diameter and twisting of the hair shaft, similar to pili torti. Trichorrhexis nodosa is another nonspecific finding [7, 16]. Similar hair shaft abnormalities can be seen in other ichthyoses featuring alopecia ichthyotica [21] (see Sect. 4.3). In XDI eyebrows and eyelashes are often sparse, showing an undirected growth [5, 15, 16]. Many patients show minor nail anomalies, for example flattening of the nail plates (platonychia) or splitting into layers (onychoschisis) [3, 7].

5.4.2.2 Noncutaneous Findings

There are a number of typical noncutaneous findings (Table 29). Stippled calcifications of the area of enchondral bone formation (Fig. 68) are the characteristic skeletal manifestation of all chondrodysplasia punctata types. The stippled epiphyses are visible at birth and during the first years of life on roentgenographic examination. After puberty, the punctate calcifications often are no longer discernible. A short stature and asymmetric shortening of legs, giving rise to moderate or severe kyphoskoliosis, are the most obvious skeletal anomalies in later life. [5, 16, 17]. Unilateral hexadactyly [11, 16] and severe dysplasia of hip joints [8, 15] can also be noted in some cases. Moreover, most patients show an asymmetric facial appearance which is due to hypoplasia of one side, a flattened nose bridge, and frontal bossing.

Cataracts are observed in about two thirds of the cases [6]. They are usually asymmetric, often unilateral, and may be confined to one quadrant of the eye as a manifestation of functional X-chromosome mosaicism. Even when the cataracts are bilateral, they tend to be far more severe on one of the two eyes. There is no psychomotor retardation. The patients have an average intelligence and life expectancy is normal.

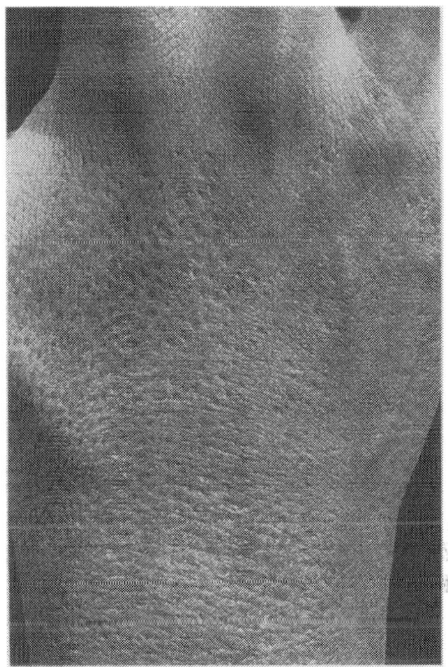

Fig. 65. X-linked dominant ichthyosis in an older child. Note follicular atrophoderma

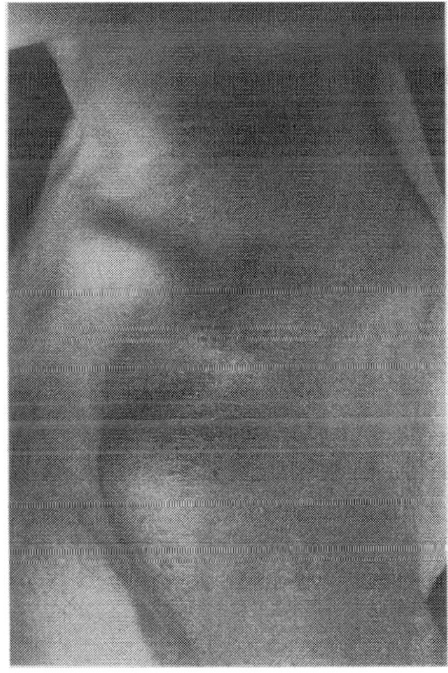

Fig. 66. X-linked dominant ichthyosis at adult age. The hyperkeratoses are distributed in a linear, blotchy pattern. (From [5], courtesy of Dr. R. Happle, Nijmegen)

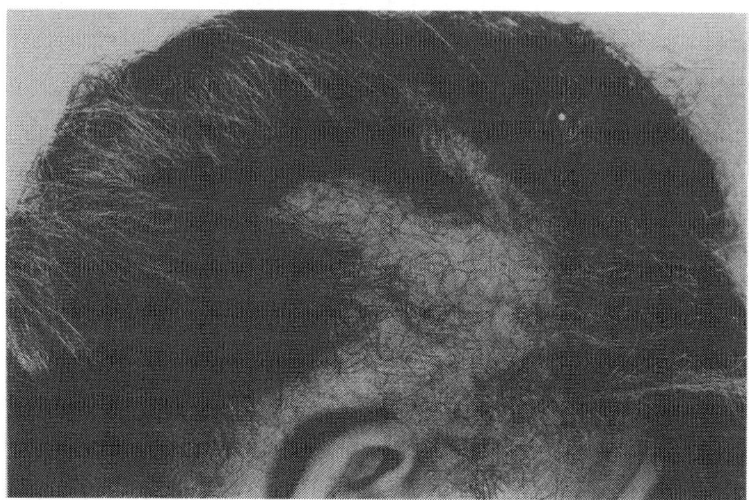

Fig. 67. Alopecia ichthyotica in an adult patient with X-linked dominant ichthyosis. (From [9], courtesy of Dr. R. Happle, Nijmegen)

Table 29. Main clinical features of X-linked dominant ichthyosis

Skin	Bones	Face	Eye	Life expectancy
Ichthyotic erythroderma at birth, resolving within a few months	Stippled calcifications (no longer visible in adult life)	Asymmetric appearance	Cataracts in ⅔ of patients, often unilateral and confined to a quadrant of the eye	Normal
Linear arrangement of both hyperkeratoses and pigmentary disturbances (if the latter present)	Short stature	Flattened nose bridge		
Follicular atrophoderma	Asymmetrical shortening of legs	Frontal bossing		
Cicatricial alopecia	Kyphoscoliosis			

5.4.3 Histologic and Ultrastructural Features

The histologic features of XDI resemble those of autosomal dominant ichtyosis vulgaris. Routine histology discloses a moderately increased orthohyperkeratotic stratum corneum, a diminished granular layer, slight acanthosis, and slight peri-

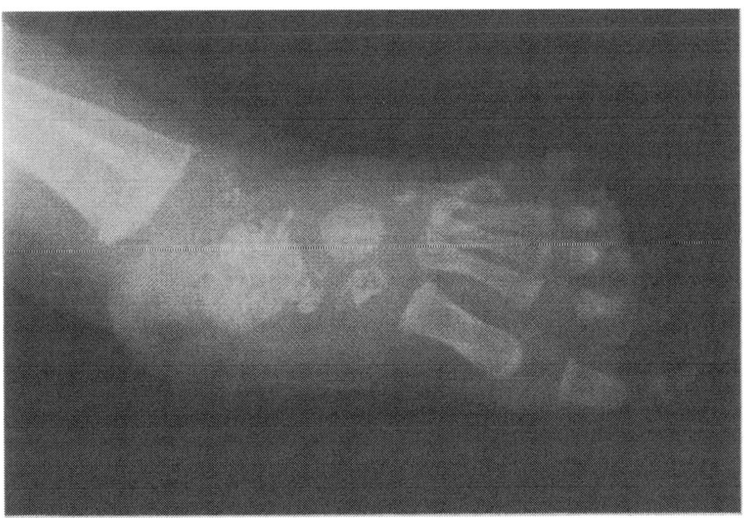

Fig. 68. XDI. Stippled calcifications in a newborn. (Courtesy of Dr. R. Happle, Nijmegen)

vascular infiltrates in the upper dermis. In the newborn an extreme follicular hyperkeratosis can be very striking [5, 12]. Interestingly, histochemical staining for calcium (von Kossa's stain) reveals calcifications within the epidermis [12]; these are more pronounced in the hair follicles.

In the older child the calcium depositions can often no longer be visualized by histochemistry. However, electron microscopy shows a large number of cytoplasmic vacuoles (Fig. 69) containing electron-dense stellate bodies [12] in the keratinocytes of the granular layer. It is reasonable to assume that these electron-dense stellate bodies represent calcium crystals. The vacuolization of keratinocytes in the granular layer is a further striking feature [12]. Electron microscopy also discloses the presence of normally structured keratohyalin granules and thus permits an unequivocal ultrastructural distinction from autosomal dominant ichthyosis vulgaris [12]. A significant reduction in the number of Langerhans' cells which undergo degeneration is a surprising ultrastructural finding of XDI [13]. The mechanism causing the degeneration of Langerhans cells is unknown. As the Langerhans' cells contain numerous hydrolytic enzymes, it has been speculated that the release of these enzymes from damaged Langerhans' cells may cause the characteristic vacuolization of the granular keratinocytes and be related to the epidermal calcifications [13].

5.4.4 Homology in the Mouse

X linked dominant ichthyosis is one of the few human genetic disorders for which a homologous animal model exists [9]. In 1973, Phillips et al. [19] reported a murine mutant which they called "bare patches" (bpa). The skin lesions found in this mouse (linear pigmentary disturbances, linear arrangement of hyperkera-

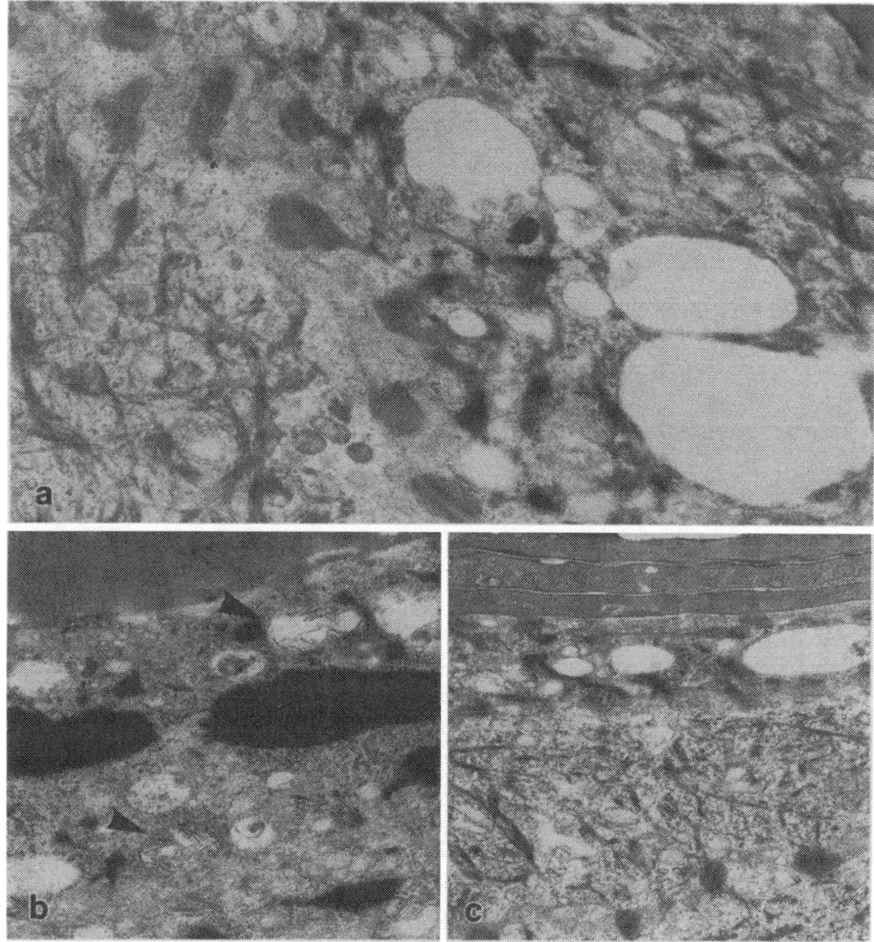

Fig. 69a–c. X-linked dominant ichthyosis. Electron micrograph. **a** Typical vacuolization of the keratinocytes in the granular layer. × 20300. **b** Two vacuoles contain characteristic needle-like inclusions *(arrows)*. × 15800. **c** Survey of the lower horny layer and the epidermis. Note regular keratinization of the corneocytes and vacuolization of the granular layer. × 13400. (Courtesy of Dr. G. Kolde, Münster)

toses, linear absence of hair) correspond to the cutaneous manifestation of XDI in humans. In a detailed study, Happle et al. [9] were able to demonstrate a similar homology, not only for the cutaneous but also for the skeletal and ocular manifestations. Furthermore, breeding experiments have shown that the bpa mouse is caused by an X-linked dominant gene which is lethal for male embryos [19]. The genes for X-linked dominant ichthyosis and the bpa mouse are obviously homologous. This genetic homology confirms a concept elaborated by Ohno [18] that during the evolution of mammals, the original X-chromosome of a common ancestor has been preserved (hypothesis of the "conservative" X-chromosome).

5.4.5 Genetic Counseling

XDI is caused by an X-linked dominant gene which is lethal for male embryos. As a consequence, only girls can be affected. After the neonatal period the expression of the gene defect is usually rather mild. Therefore, the question of prenatal diagnosis should be approached with caution. As always, parents should not be influenced in their personal decision. Because of the typical unilateral limb defect antenatal diagnosis may be possible by ultrasound even today.

In the near future a precise mapping of the XDI gene on the X-chromosome can be expected, and this gene assignment should theoretically allow prenatal diagnosis using flanking cDNA probes. The primary biochemical defect of XDI is unknown, but the Happle group [1] recently reported a striking reduction of cathepsin B-like activity in the scales of affected patients. How this finding relates to the disturbed calcium metabolism in the disorder is still unclear. In the eighth edition of his *Catalog of Mendelian Inheritance in Man,* McKusick [14] still discusses XDI under the same entry (number 30295) as X-linked recessive chondrodysplasia punctata. This may evoke the wrong impression, as if the two diseases could be allelic. This possibility can be rejected out of hand. The ichthyosis in the X-linked recessive type of chondrodysplasia punctata is X-linked recessive ichthyosis with underlying steroid sulfatase deficiency (see Sect. 3.2, Associated Steroid Sulfatase Deficiency). In contrast, patients with XDI have normal steroid sulfatase activity. Their type of ichthyosis is completely different. In XDI ichthyosis is related to a generalized defect of calcium metabolism, causing – among other things – intraepidermal calcifications. Moreover, the steroid sulfatase gene escapes X-inactivation, while the locus for XDI fully participates in X-inactivation.

References

1. Bergers M, Mier PD, van Dooren-Grebe R, Traupe H, Happle R (1988) Enzymatic diagnosis of congenital disorders of keratinization. 18th annual meeting of the European Society for Dermatological Research, June 19–22, 1988, Munich
2. Bodian EL (1966) Skin manifestations of Conradi's disease (chondrodystrophia congenita punctata). Arch Dermatol 94:743–748
3. Goerttler E (1979) Chondrodysplasia punctata Typ Conradi-Hünermann. Z Hautkr 54:676–677
4. Happle R (1979) X-linked dominant ichthyosis. Clin Genet 15:239–240
5. Happle R (1979) X-linked dominant chondrodysplasia punctata. Review of literature and report of a case. Hum Genet 53:65–73
6. Happle R (1981) Cataracts as a marker of genetic heterogeneity in chondrodysplasia punctata. Clin Genet 19:64–66
7. Happle R, Kästner H (1979 X-gekoppelt dominante Chondrodysplasia punctata. Ein osteokutanes Syndrom. Hautarzt 30:590–594
8. Happle R, Matthiass HH, Macher E (1977) Sex-linked chondrodysplasia punctata? Clin Genet 11:73–76
9. Happle R, Phillips RJS, Roessner A, Jünemann G (1983) Homologous genes for X-linked chondrodysplasia punctata in man and mouse. Hum Genet 63:24–27

10. Hosenfeld D, Wiedemann HR (1987) Chondrodysplasia punctata im Erwachsenenalter als Cumarinembryopathie erkannt. 6. Symposium Klinische Genetik in der Pädiatrie. Juli 3-5 1987, Bad Homburg
11. Joosten R, Habedank M (1979) Sex-linked type of chondrodysplasia punctata due to a new mutation. Acta Paediatr Belg 32:275-278
12. Kolde G, Happle R (1984) Histologic and ultrastructural features of the ichthyotic skin in X-linked dominant chondrodysplasia punctata. Acta Derm Venereol (Stockh) 64:389-394
13. Kolde G, Happle R (1985) Langerhans-cell degeneration in X-linked dominant ichthyosis. A quantitative and ultrastructural study. Arch Dermatol Res 277:245-247
14. McKusick VA (1988) Mendelian inheritance in man. In: Catalogs of autosomal dominant, autosomal recessive, and X-linked phenotypes, 8th edn Johns Hopkinks University Press, Baltimore, pp 1263-1264
15. Maleville J, Alt J, Grosshans E (1969) Atrophodermie folliculaire, pseudopelade, kératose pilaire des sourcils et état ichthyosique. Bull Soc Fr Dermatol Syphiligr 76:85-86
16. Manzke H, Christophers E, Wiedemann HR (1980) Dominant sex-linked inherited chondrodysplasia punctata: a distinct type of chondrodysplasia punctata. Clin Genet 15:97-107
17. Mueller RF, Crowle PM, Jones RAK, Davison BCC (1985) X-linked dominant chondrodysplasia punctata: a case report and family studies. Am J Med Genet 20:137-144
18. Ohno S (1967) Ancient linkage groups and frozen accidents. Nature 244:259-262
19. Phillips RJS, Hawker SH, Moseley HJ (1973) Bare patches, a new sex-linked gene in the mouse, associated with a high production of XO females. I. A preliminary report of breeding experiments. Genet Res 22:91-99
20. Spranger JW, Opitz JM, Bidder U (1971) Heterogeneity of chondrodysplasia punctata. Hum Genet 11:190-212
21. Traupe H, Happle R (1983) Alopecia ichthyotica. A characteristic feature of congenital ichtyosis. Dermatologica 167:225-230

6 Recently Recognized Ichthyoses

In this chapter a number of uncommon ichthyoses are discussed, that were only recently recognized as distinct entities. My criterion for inclusion of a given disorder in this group is that at least three independent reports confirm the particular condition. An exception to this guideline is made for congenital migratory ichthyosis with neurologic and ophthalmologic abnormalities (Sect. 6.7) because of the constellation of symptoms in this disorder. Autosomal dominant lamellar ichthyosis and ichthyosis bullosa of Siemens are discussed elsewhere (Sects. 4.2.2 and 4.4.3). The KID syndrome is not an ichthyosis, but rather represents a unique type of erythrokertoderma. Nevertheless, it may be regarded as an ichthyosis-like condition and also is included here. In Sect. 6.8 a large number of ichthyoses of uncertain status are described. Some of these represent "university hospital syndromes" (fortuitous associations), while others may emerge as distinct entities in the future.

6.1 Dorfman's Syndrome: Neutral Lipid Storage Disease with Ichthyotic Erythroderma

6.1.1 Historical Aspects

In 1974, Maurice L. Dorfman and his associates [4] delineated a new type of congenital ichthyosis characterized by ichthyotic erythroderma, severe fatty changes of the liver, and variable neurologic and ocular involvement. The biochemical hallmark of this syndrome was nonmembrane-bound lipid accumulations in the granulocytes of the peripheral blood (Fig. 70) and in granulocyte precursors in the bone marrow [4]. Lipid-containing vacuoles in the granulocytes had previously been described in 1953 by Jordans [6] seen in two brothers

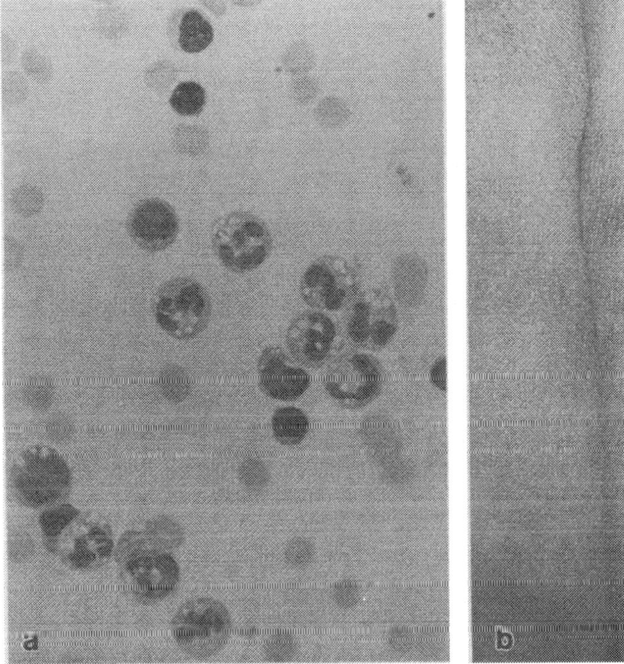

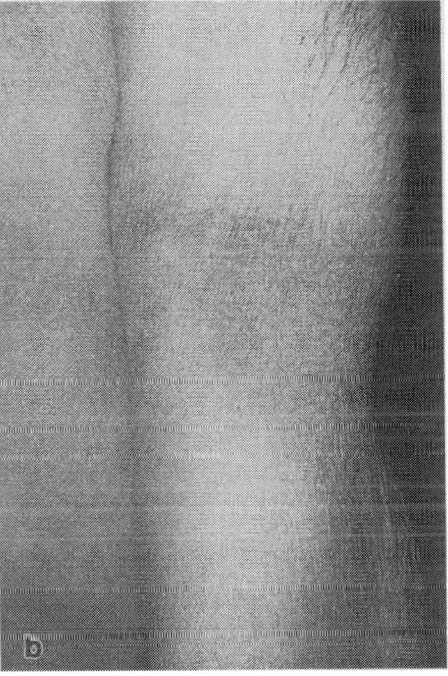

Fig. 70 a, b. Dorfman's syndrome. **a** Multiple lipid vacuoles in virtually every granulocyte and monocyte, but not in small lymphocytes in a Wright-stained buffy coat preparation (From [11], courtesy of Dr. Mary Williams, San Francisco). **b** Fine scaling, lichenification and mild underlying erythroderma. (From [12], courtesy of Dr. Mary Williams, San Francisco)

suffering from progressive muscular dystrophy, and are hence often referred to as "Jordans' anomaly." In 1966, Rozenszajn et al. [9] reported on four cases of Jordans' anomaly in an Iraqui family. Two of these patients were also studied in Dorfman's series [4].

The unique constellation of clinical and biochemical findings present in the four patients they described allowed Dorfman and co-workers [4] to recognize the disease as a distinct type of congenital ichthyosis. The important findings of Dorfman et al. were soon confirmed [2, 7]. So far, 17 patients belonging to ten different families have been reported [8, 10, 12, 14]. Chanarin et al. [2] introduced the term "neutral lipid storage disease" for the condition. They demonstrated that lipid vacuoles were present in fibroblasts even after several subcultures and that these lipid inclusions contained excessive amounts of triglycerides. Today, two different types of neutral lipid storage diseases are distinguished: (a) Dorfman's syndrome, featuring ichthyosis, and (b) a special type of carnitine deficiency in which ichthyosis is not present [1, 10].

6.1.2 Clinical Features

6.1.2.1 Cutaneous Findings

At birth, mild ichthyotic erythroderma is present. At least one child was born as a collodion baby [14]. In some patients, the erythema is visible also in later life, whereas in others it subsides. The scaling is generalized, and fine, white hyperkertoses cover the entire body, including the flexures (Fig. 70b) and the face, producing tautness or even mild ectropion [4, 84, 10, 12, 14]. Palms and soles are also involved. Due to the hyperkeratosis, the skin may have a lichenified appearance [44]. The nails occasionally show longitudinal ridging, and in older patients alopecia ichthyotica may develop [44].

Table 30. Possible noncutaneous findings in Dorfman's syndrome (neutral lipid storage disease with ichthyotic erythroderma)

Nerves	Muscle	Liver	Eye	Other
Neurosensory deafness	Muscular weakness	Fatty degeneration	Bilateral cataracts	Abnormal electrocardiogram
Horizontal nystagmus	Abnormal electromycogram	Elevated liver enzymes	Strabism	Gluten-sensitive enteropathy
Ataxia		Hepatosplenomegaly	Retinal dysfunction	Diabetes mellitus

6.1.2.2 Noncutaneous Findings

There is a multitude of possible noncutaneous manifestations (Table 30), involving the eyes, muscles, nerves, liver, and possibly also the gastrointestinal tract [1-5, 7, 8, 10]. This organ involvement can vary considerably in severity [14] and may be progressive with increasing age [12]. Bilateral nuclear cataracts can be present in infancy or develop during adult life. Despite elevated serum muscle enzymes, there is usually only mild muscular weakness. In some patients muscular involvement is progressive [12]. The patient reported on by Miranda et al. [7] had a weakness of eyelid closure and was unable to raise his head from a lying position. The neurologic impairment is likewise variable and can include ataxia, bilateral neurosensory hearing loss, and a fine horizontal nystagmus. Psychomotor development seems to be normal and patients have an average intellectual endowment. Liver biopsies disclose a severe fatty degeneration [4, 10, 14], whereas serum transaminases need not be increased. One patient suffered from severe steatorrhea which may have been related to the numerous lipid inclusions found in his gastric and rectal mucosa [7]. According to Miranda et al. [7], the gastrointestinal symptoms, and to a lesser degree muscular weakness, respond to a gluten-free diet.

6.1.3 Histologic and Ultrastructural Features of the Skin

Routine histology reveals a nonspecific benign acanthokeratosis and does not permit distinction from other types of nonbullous congenital ichthyosis [4, 12]. There usually is an increased orthohyperkeratotic stratum corneum, which may show scattered foci of parakeratosis. The granular layer is variable and may be reduced in parts of the biopsy but markedly increased in other parts. The epidermis is broadened. There are slight perivascular infiltrates in the upper dermis. A foamy cytoplasm of the keratinocytes in the basal and granular layer may be recognized at higher magnification if specifically searched for. Special lipid stains reveal prominent lipid droplets in the keratinocytes of the basal and granular layers and allow a clear-cut distinction from lamellar ichthyosis [5, 10, 14]. Electron microscopy discloses a peculiar abnormality of the lamellar body (keratinosomes). multilaminated spherules that are distorted and replace the normal internal disk structure of the lamellar bodies [5] can be seen. At the stratum granulosum/stratum corneum interface these spherules disperse into electron-lucent slits [5].

6.1.4 Genetic Counseling

Dorfman's syndrome is inherited as an autosomal recessive trait [8, 10, 12]. Until now, only patients with an Arabic ethnic background have been reported [10, 12, 14]. A recent case from Sicily can be attributed to the Arab domination of Sicily during the seventh century [8]. This raises the question of whether all cases might be due to a common mutation many centuries ago. Recognition of heterozygous gene carriers may sometimes be possible by demonstration of the typical lipid vacuoles in circulating eosinophils [8, 12]. In at least one family this test was negative, however [14]. It is important to note that the characteristic lipid inclusions have to be specifically looked for in both affected patients and possible gene carriers. If an automated blood cell count is done, a "normal" result will be handed out erroneously [10, 12, 14]. The primary biochemical defect of the syndrome is still unknown. Angelini et al. [1] demonstrated a specific defect in long-chain fatty acid oxidation, but other groups were not able to confirm their finding [3, 7, 13]. The lipid stored in fibrolasts is triglyceride and has an unremarkable fatty acid profile [13]. A primary defect of fatty acid uptake, oversynthesis, or impaired β-oxidation could be excluded [13]. Di Donato et al. [3] found a specific defect in the degradation of endocellularly synthesized triglycerides, while degradation of exogeneously supplied neutral lipids was not impaired. Surprisingly, lipid scale studies demonstrated that scales contain a normal amount of triglycerides but have increased n-alkane levels [5]. Prenatal diagnosis is not yet available, but given the usually mild course of the disease it may not be necessary.

References

1. Angelini C, Phillipart M, Borrone C, Bresolin N, Lucke S (1980) Multisystem triglyceride storage disorder with impaired long-chain fatty oxidation. Ann Neurol 7:5–10
2. Chanarin I, Patel A, Slavin G, Wills EJ, Andrews TM, Stewart G (1975) Neutral lipid storage disease: a new disorder of lipid metabolism. Br Med J 1:553–555
3. Di Donato S, Garavaglia B, Strisciuglio P, Borrone C, Andria G (1988) Multisystem triglyceride storage disease is due to a specific defect in the degradation of endocellularly synthesized triglycerides. Neurology 38:1107–1110
4. Dorfman ML, Hershko C, Eisenberg S, Sagher F (1974) Ichthyosiform dermatosis with systemic lipidosis. Arch Dermatol 110:261–266
5. Elias PM, Williams ML (1985) Neutral lipid storage disease with ichthyosis, defective lamellar body content and intracellular dispersion. Arch Dermatol 121:1000–1008
6. Jordans GH (1953) The familial occurence of fat-containing vacuoles in the leukocytes diagnosed in two brothers suffering from dystrophia musculorum progressiva. Acta Med Scand 146:419–424
7. Miranda A, Di Mauro S, Estwood A, Hays A, Johnson WG, Olate M, Whitlock R, Mayeux R, Rowland LP (1979) Lipid storage myopathy, ichthyosis and steatorrhea. Muscle Nerve 2:1–13
8. Musumeci S, D'Agata A, Romano C, Patané R, Cutrone D (1988) Ichthyosis and neutral lipid storage disease. Am J Med Genet 29:377–382
9. Rozenszajn L, Klajman A, Yaffe D, Efrati PC (1966) Jordans' abnormality in white blood cells. Report of a case. Blood 28:258–265
10. Venencie PY, Armengaud D, Foldès C, Vieillefond A, Coulombel L, Hadchouel M (1988) Ichthyosis and neutral lipid storage disease (Dorfman-Chanarin syndrome). Pediatr Dermatol 5:173–177
11. Williams ML, Elias PM (1987) Genetically transmitted generalized disorders of cornification. The ichthyoses. Dermatol Clin 5:155–178
12. Williams ML, Koch TK, O'Donnell JJ, Frost PH, Epstein LB, Grizzard WS, Epstein CJ (1985) Ichthyosis and neutral lipid storage disease. Am J Med Genet 20:711–726
13. Williams ML, Monger DJ, Rutherfold SL, Hincenbergs M, Rehfeld SJ, Grunfeld C (1988) Neutral lipid storage disease with ichthyosis: lipid content and metabolism of fibroblasts. J Inherited Metab Dis 11:131–143
14. Wolf R, Zaritzky A, Pollack S (1988) Value of looking at leukocytes in every case of ichthyosis. Dermatologica 177:237–240

6.2 Hystrix-like Ichthyosis with Deafness: the HID Syndrome

6.2.1 Historical Aspects and Nomenclature

In 1977, the Schnyder/Anton-Lamprecht group [1, 2, 6, 7] described one 17-year-old patient suffering from ichthyosis hystrix with severe neurosensory hearing loss bordering on deafness. Because of peculiar ultrastructural features not found in any other cornification disorder [1, 2] they suggested that this patient suffered from a distinct type of ichthyosis. Three cases reported from France [4], a case presentation at the 34th meeting of the German Dermatological Society in Zürich in 1985 [5], and an observation of our own (unpublished) corroborate the existence of this syndrome as an independent entity. A handy name for this condition is so far lacking. The Heidelberg group [6, 7] named it "ichthyosis hystrix gravior type Rheydt", after the city of origin of the first patient. This designation is not very mnemonic and does not allude to deafness, which is a cardinal symptom of the disease. I suggest calling it "hystrix-like ichthyosis with deafness (HID) syndrome".

6.2.2 Clinical Features

Shortly after birth, red patches develop on the skin and evolve into ichthyotic erythroderma accompanied by hystrix-like hyperkeratoses. The dark-gray keratotic masses involve the entire body, including the face and the flexural surface of the extremities (Fig. 71). The skin of patients is prone to bacterial (impetigo) and mycotic infections, especially to generalized candidosis [4–6]. Palms and soles are mildly affected. Gilardi and Schnyder [5] observed mucosal involvement with several patches of leukoplakia in their case. Alopecia ichthyotica, absence of eyebrows and eyelashes, and dystrophic nails can be further findings [4]. Except for the onychotic nails, the skin lesions do not suggest a mycotic infection, but there usually is widespread fungal involvement. Both dermatophytes and Candida albicans can be cultured from almost everywhere on the skin when swabs are taken [4, 5].

Etretinate treatment results in a spectacular clearing of the hyperkeratotic skin lesions, though the underlying erythema persists [4, 5]. Badillet et al. [4] stressed that treatment with retinoids also had a dramatic effect on the mycotic infections which considerably improved under etretinate therapy. The reason for this may be that the chemical composition of scales provides excellent conditions for fungal growth in this particular disease.

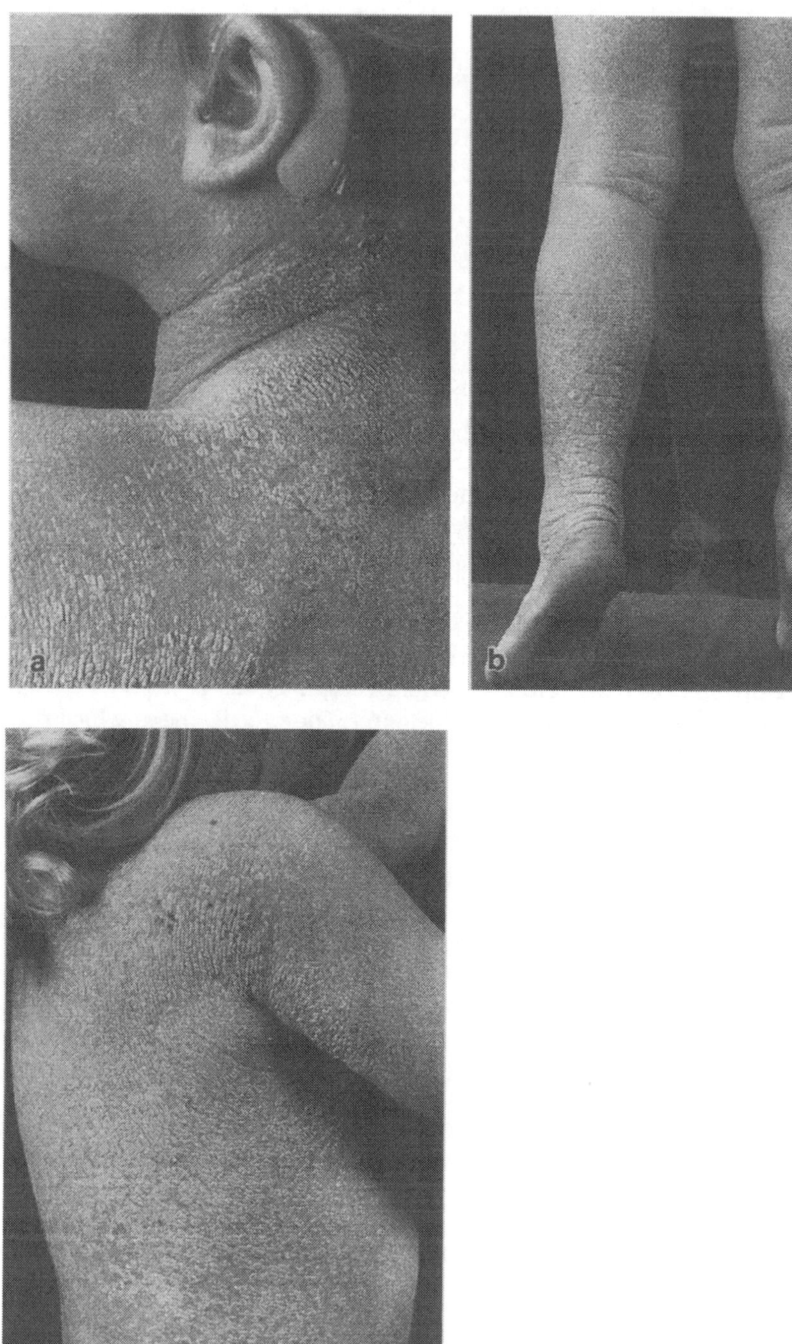

Fig. 71a–c. HID syndrome in a 3-year-old girl. **a** Note hystrix-like ichthyosis and hearing aid prescribed for severe bilateral hearing loss. **b** The hyperkeratoses also involve the flexures, while palms and soles are only mildly affected. **c** Marked involvement of the trunk allows exclusion of the KID syndrome

A bilateral inner hearing loss (neurosensory deafness) is a cardinal feature of the HID syndrome. It is very severe and borders on total deafness, but is nonprogressive during later life. A superficial, punctate keratitis was present in some cases.

6.2.3 Histologic and Ultrastructural Features

Histology reveals a nonspecific benign acanthokeratosis and is very similar to that of lamellar ichthyosis [4–6]. The markedly broadened stratum corneum is usually orthokeratotic but may show scattered foci of parakeratosis. The epidermis is acanthotic and a sawtooth-like papillomatosis can be observed. The granular layer is of normal size or even increased. Keratinocytes often are vacuolized; the cell nucleus is then surrounded by an empty halo, and the remaining cytoplasm contains keratohyalin granules in a ringlike formation. Such altered keratinocytes, reminiscent of a "birds eye" [5] can be seen in clusters in the upper prickle-cell layer and granular layer, while the remaining epidermis looks normal. In the dermis, moderate perivascular infiltrates can be noted.

Electron microscopy permits clear-cut recognition of the HID syndrome [1, 2, 4, 5]. It discloses blown-up cells with a large central nucleus in the granular layer. There is a marked reduction of tonofibrils, few keratohyalin granules, and an abnormal production of membrane-bound granules containing mucous substances [2]. The content of these mucous-containing granules is discharged to the intercellular space, which is almost completely filled with this homogenous material [2, 5].

6.2.4 Differential Diagnosis

The main differential diagnosis of the HID syndrome is the keratitis with ichthyosis-like hyperkeratosis and deafness (KID) syndrome. Though there are some similarities (Table 31) between the HID syndrome and the KID syndrome, it is important to note that the latter condition is a localized keratinization disorder (hence an erythrokeratoderma and not an ichthyosis) and is associated with severe vascularizing keratitis, while in the HID syndrome keratitis is punctate and much less severe, if at all present. Keratitis is a very nonspecific sign found in several types of congenital ichthyoses; it does not in itself warrant lumping the so-affected HID cases with the KID syndrome. The HID syndrome has very distinctive ultrastructural features. In the KID syndrome, ultrastructural investigations give essentially normal results.

Baden and Bronstein [3] recently reported on a patient suffering from ichthyotic erythroderma and deafness in whom the ichthyosis was rather mild and not hystrix-like. In addition, this patient displayed albinoid retinas, a diminished vibratory sense in the legs, and marked pes cavus. Thus, the overall clinical picture was somewhat different from the HID syndrome.

Bullous ichthyotic erythroderma can also present as a hystrix-like ichthyosis. This diagnosis is ruled out easily because of the completely different histologic

Table 31. Differential diagnosis between the HID and KID syndromes

Feature	HID syndrome	KID syndrome
	Similarities	
Ear involvement	Bilateral hearing loss (neurosensory "deafness")	Bilateral hearing loss (neurosensory "deafness")
Cutaneous immune defense	Proneness to mycotic and bacterial skin infections	Proneness to mycotic and bacterial skin infections
Alopecia	Cicatrical alopecia possible	Cicatrical alopecia possible
	Differences	
Course of disease	Shortly after birth multiple red patches appear and develop into ichthyotic erythroderma	Children may be born with full-blown ichthyotic erythroderma which spontaneously resolves soon
	At the age of 1 year full blown ichthyotic erythroderma; afterwards, static course	At the age of 1 year reoccurrence of hyperkeratotic patches; progressive spreading until puberty
Cutaneous involvement	Entire body affected, including the trunk	Hyperkeratoses confined to predilection sites; trunk always spared
Palms and soles	Mildly affected	Severely affected with typical aspect
Eyes	No vascularizing keratitis, but punctate keratitis possible	Vascularizing keratitis (possible)
Electron microscopy	Reduction of tonofibrils, overproduction of mucous material	Essentially normal; glycogen storage in various tissues, but not epidermis

and ultrastructural features. In our own patient I initially considered ichthyosis hystrix of Curth-Macklin.

6.2.5 Genetic Counseling

So far, all cases reported have been sporadic and no definite mode of inheritance has yet emerged. X-linked recessive inheritance can be excluded, as the condition has occurred in both sexes. Both autosomal recessive and autosomal dominant inheritance are possible. The disease is very disfiguring. Therefore, prenatal diagnosis would be desirable. It may not be possible by electron microscopy, since the condition is not truly congenital but just starts at birth.

References

1. Anton-Lamprecht I (1976) Biologic compensation for missing protective function of the skin due to congenital lack of tonofibrils. J Invest Dermatol 66:259
2. Anton-Lamprecht I (1978) Ultrastructural criteria for the distinction of different types of inherited ichthyoses. In: Marks R, Dykes PJ (eds) The ichthyoses. MTP press, Lancaster, pp 71-87
3. Baden HP, Bronstein BR (1988) Ichthyosiform dermatosis and deafness. Report of a case and review of the literature. Arch Dermatol 124:102 106
4. Badillet C, Blanchet-Bardon C, Cabral O, Puissant A (1982) Étude mycologique de trois cas d'erythrodermie avec keratite et surdité (ichthyose de Rheydt). Bull Soc Mycol Med (Paris) 11:191-198
5. Gilardi S, Schnyder UW (1985) Ichthyosis hystrix gravior Typus Rheydt (Ichthyosis hystrix gravior mit Taubheit). In: Eichmann A (ed) Dia-Klinik (case presentation). 34. Tagung der Deutschen Dermatologischen Gesellschaft, 20-24 March 1985, Zürich. Springer, Berlin Heidelberg New York Tokyo, pp 54-55
6. Gülzow J, Anton-Lamprecht I (1977) Ichthyosis hystrix gravior Typus Rheydt: ein otologisch-dermatologisches Syndrom. Laryng Rhinol Otol (Stuttg) 56:949-955
7. Schnyder UW (1977) Ichthyosis hystrix Typus Rheydt (Ichthyosis hystrix gravior mit praktischer Taubheit). Z Hautkr 52:763-766

6.3 Not an Ichthyosis at All: the Keratitis, Ichthyosis-like Hyperkeratosis, and Deafness (KID) Syndrome

6.3.1 Historical Aspects and Nomenclature

In 1915, the American dermatologist Frederick S. Burns [3] delineated the keratitis, ichthyosis-like hyperkeratosis, and deafness (KID) syndrome in full detail. He described a 16-year-old boy who was partially blind, totally deaf, and displayed a peculiar type of hyperkeratotic involvement localized to the head and the limbs with bizarre, sharply outlined lesions over the face. The disease had started at the age of 1 year and progressed until the age of about 10 years. During the following years the conditions remained unchanged. Though Burns presented his case at the 38th Meeting of the American Dermatological Association in May 1914, the syndrome he described soon fell into oblivion.

More than 50 years later the condition was rediscovered by U. W. Schnyder [16], who reported on a very similar patient who was suffering, however, from additional cerebral damage. Schnyder [16] regarded this skin disorder as a new type of erythrokeratoderma. His observation prompted a number of groups to report similar cases [1, 2, 15] and helped a great deal to establish the condition as a distinct cornification disorder. There was and still is, however, some uncertainty about the proper classification of this syndrome. If one sticks to the classic definition of ichthyosis as a genetic cornification disorder with **universal** involvement, then the KID syndrome does not qualify as an ichthyosis, but rather represents an erythrokeratoderma [13]. Unfortunately, a number of groups reported the condition under misleading labels such as "atypical ichthyosiform erythroderma" [15] or "ichthyosiform dermatosis" [1]. In the Anglo-American literature the attribute "ichthyosiform" is liberally used in a very ambiguous way for all kinds of different scaling disorders, including the ichthyoses, though "ichthyosiform" means ichthyosis-like and not ichthyotic. In 1981, Skinner et al. [17] misclassified the disorder as ichthyosis and coined the acronym KID (keratitis, ichthyosis, and deafness) syndrome. Though the KID syndrome is not an ichthyosis at all, this designation has been very successful [7]. It is now deeply entrenched in the medical literature [6–9]. To prevent further confusion the acronym "KID" should be retained. However, I suggest redefining the "I" in this acronym as standing for "ichthyosis-like hyperkeratosis".

6.3.2 Clinical Features

At birth, affected children present with erythroderma which usually disappears after a few days [6, 7, 14]. In most cases hyperkeratotic plaques with underlying erythema develop at the age of 1 year, in some cases even earlier. Küster et al.

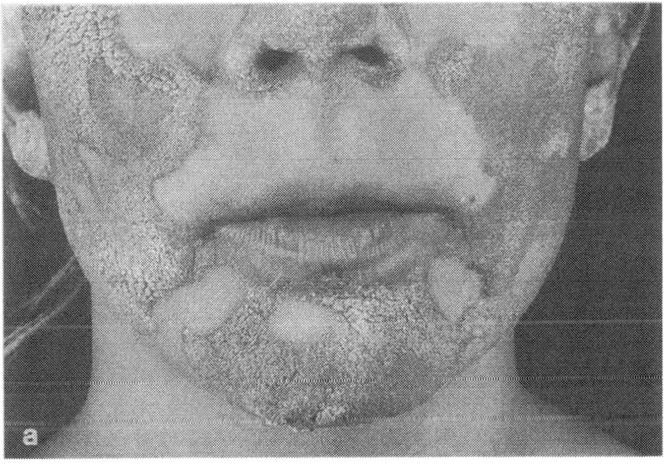

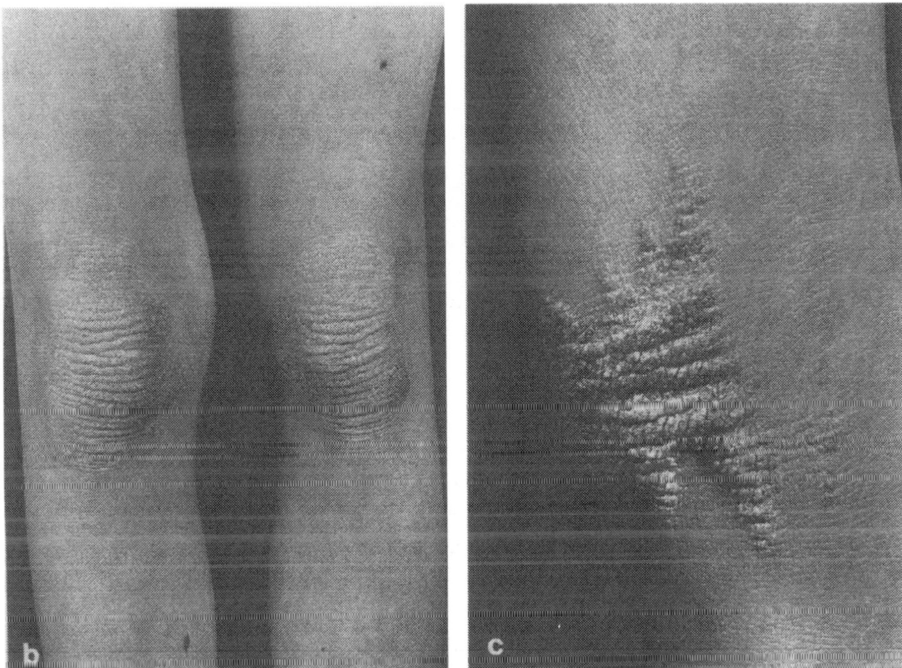

Fig. 72a–c. KID syndrome in a 5-year-old-boy. **a** Typical facial involvement with bizarre, sharply outlined verrucous hyperkeratotic plaques; **b** marked hyperkeratotic lesions over the knees; **c** typical localized verrucous lesion over the hollow of the knee. In contrast to the HID syndrome, there is no involvement of the trunk. (Courtesy of Dr. Küster, and Dr. Plewig, Düsseldorf)

[10] emphasized that two clinical subsets of the KID syndrome can be distinguished: One subset is characterized by very localized involvement mainly affecting a few predilection sites (face, elbows, knees, palms, and soles) [4, 10, 16], as depicted in Fig. 72, while in other cases [9, 17] the cutaneous involvement and the eye involvement are more severe and severe scarring alopecia can be noted. However, all patients share some signs such as the bizarre, sharply demarcated erythematous-squamous plaques over the face, similar verrucous plaques with a rippled hyperkeratosis over the normal predilection sites, and the peculiar palmoplantar keratoderma with a leather-like aspect [4]. The nails often show leukonychia or are dysplastic. In many patients recalcitrant bacterial and mycotic infections occur (reviewed in [7]). Chronic mucocutaneous candidosis may pose a special problem.

6.3.2.1 KID Syndrome and Skin Cancer

Several patients suffering from the KID syndrome have developed squamous cell carcinoma [1, 6, 11]. Obviously, the condition harbors an unusual risk for developing epithelial cancer. Leukoplakia, which is usually considered an obligate precancerosis, was already mentioned in the first report of the syndrome by Burns [3]. In a recent case observed in France multiple squamous cell carcinomas of the skin were found. This French patient died of general metastasis at the age of 37 years [6].

6.3.2.2 Noncutaneous Findings

Bilateral neurosensory deafness and vascularizing keratitis are essential features of the syndrome. The hearing loss is congenital, whereas vascularizing keratitis develops during the course of the disease. Its expression can be variable. It is preceded by photophobia. The keratitis can eventually lead to total blindness [7]. Physical growth and psychomotor development are unaffected. Patients have an average intellectual endowment.

6.3.3 Histologic Features

Histology reveals the picture of a nonspecific benign acanthokeratosis. Follicular plugging can be striking. The stratum corneum is markedly increased and usually orthohyperkeratotic. The granular layer is broadened in most, but not all cases [14]. Several authors describe a distinctive vacuolization of the granular layer [7, 9, 14]. In the case of Jurecka et al. [9], the PAS stain showed a pathologic storage of glycogen in various types of tissues (nerves, smooth muscle, connective tissue) but not within the epidermis. A recent study failed to confirm this finding [6]. Detailed ultrastructural studies are so far lacking, but two reports indicate that there are no gross abnormalities of tonofibrils, keratohyalin granules, or lamellar bodies [7, 9]. This may be taken as a further argument that the HID and KID syndromes are distinct entities.

6.3.4 Treatment

General treatment modalities are discussed in Chap. 7. However, special care has to be given to the prevention of skin cancer in these patients. Early excision of suspect lesions is recommended. Retinoids such as etretinate may have a place in the prevention of epithelial neoplasias in this disorder. As far as scaling is concerned, etretinate is beneficial and gives acceptable results, though palmar hyperkeratoses do not improve very much [6]. Treatment with isotretinoin has been associated with an exacerbation of corneal vascularization in one patient [8]. Therefore, a close ophthalmologic follow-up under retinoid therapy may be advisable [8].

6.3.5 Genetic Counseling

Most cases of the KID syndrome have been sporadic. Hence, the mode of inheritance is still unclear, but there is some evidence pointing to autosomal dominant inheritance. In one family, father-to-daughter transmission was reported [6]. On the other hand, the KID syndrome has also been observed in two siblings who had unaffected parents [12]. Because of the possibility of gonadal mosaicism, the existence of one such family does not exclude dominant transmission. The sex ratio is normal. Males do not tend to be more severely affected than females. Therefore, X-linked recessive and X-linked dominant modes of inheritance are rather unlikely. The general paucity of familial cases may be taken as a clue that this syndrome is caused by a dominant gene and that most cases represent de novo mutations. Differential diagnosis from the HID syndrome is important and is discussed in Sect. 6.2.

Because of the severity of the disorder, prenatal diagnosis would be desirable but is not available so far. In the absence of characteristic ultrastructural changes, and with respect to the delayed onset of the definite hyperkeratotic involvement, the usual fetoscopic ultrastructural approach to prenatal diagnosis may not be feasible. We will probably have to wait for elucidation of the primary biochemical defect before prenatal diagnosis becomes possible. With respect to the findings of Jurecka et al. [9], the search for such a primary defect should also include deficiencies in carbohydrate metabolism. Very recently, Gebhart et al. [5] suggested that an established disorder of carbohydrate metabolism, namely Pompe's disease, might be associated with ichthyosis [5]. However, the signs and symptoms of the KID syndrome do not match any of the known glycogen-storage diseases. Moreover, it is not yet clear whether the cases of Gebhart et al. [5] represent a chance association between autosomal dominant ichthyosis vulgaris and Pompe's disease, or whether scaling is related to the alpha-1,4 glucosidase deficiency.

References

1. Baden HP, Alper JV (1977) Ichthyosiform dermatosis, keratitis and deafness. Arch Dermatol 113:1701-1704
2. Beare JM, Froggatt NP, Kernohan DC, Allen IV (1972) Atypical erythrokeratodermia with deafness, physical retardation and peripheral neuropathy. Br J Dermatol 87:308-314
3. Burns FS (1915) A case of generalized congenital keratoderma with unusual involvement of the eyes, ears, and nasal and buccous membranes. J Cutan Dis 33:255-260
4. Cram DL, Resneck JS, Jackson B (1979) A congenital ichthyosiform syndrome with deafness and keratitis. Arch Dermatol 115:467-471
5. Gebhart W, Mainitz M, Jurecka W, Niebauer G, Paschke E, Stöckler S, Sluga E (1988) Ichthyosiforme Schuppung bei α-1,4 Glukosidase-Mangel. Hautarzt 39:228-232
6. Grob JJ, Breton A, Bonafe JL, Sauvan-Ferdani M, Bonerandi JJ (1987) Keratitis, ichthyosis, and deafness (KID) syndrome. Vertical transmission and death from multiple squamous cell carcinomas. Arch Dermatol 123:777-782
7. Harms M, Gilardi S, Levy PM, Saurat JH (1984) KID syndrome (keratitis, ichthyosis, and deafness) and chronic mucocutaneous candidiasis: case report and review of the literature. Pediatr Dermatol 2:1-7
8. Hazen PG, Carney JM, Lanfston RHS, Meisler DM (1986) Corneal effect of isotretinoin: possible exacerbation of corneal neovascularization in a patient with the keratitis, ichthyosis, deafness ("KID") syndrome. J Am Acad Dermatol 14:141-142
9. Jurecka W, Aberer E, Mainitz M, Jürgensen O (1985) Keratitis, ichthyosis, and deafness syndrome with glycogen storage. Arch Dermatol 121:799-801
10. Küster W, Lamprecht A, Goecke TU, Anton-Lamprecht I, Kind P, Goerz G (1986) Erythrokeratodermia with hearing impairment (KID syndrome). ESDR symposium on genodermatoses and genetics of skin diseases, February 6-8, 1986, Oslo.
11. Lancaster L, Fournet BLF (1969) Carcinoma of the tongue in a child. Report of a case. J Oral Surg 27:269-270
12. Legrand I, Litoux P, Quere M, Stalder JF, Ertus M (1982) Un syndrome rare oculo-auriculo-cutané (syndrome de Burns). J Fr Ophthalmol 5:441-445
13. Marghescu S, Wolff HH, Braun-Falco O (1982) Kongenitale Erythrokeratodermie mit Taubheit Schnyder. Hautarzt 33:416-419
14. Oikarinen A, Käär L, Ruokonen A (1980) A congenital ichthyosiform syndrome with deafness and elevated serum steroid disulphate levels. Acta Derm Venereol (Stockh) 60:503-507
15. Rycroft RJG, Moynahan EJ, Wells RS (1976) Atypical ichthyosiform erythroderma, deafness and keratitis. A report of two cases. Br J Dermatol 94:211-217
16. Schnyder UW, Wissler H, Wendt GG (1968) Eine weitere Form von atypischer Erythrokeratodermie mit Schwerhörigkeit und cerebraler Schädigung. Helv Paediatr Acta 23:220-230
17. Skinner BA, Greist MC, Norins AL (1981) The keratitis ichthyosis, and deafness (KID) syndrome. Arch Dermatol 117:285-289

6.4 The Ichthyosis Follicularis, Atrichia, and Photophobia (IFAP) Syndrome

6.4.1 Historical Aspects and Nomenclature

At the end of the past century the designation "ichthyosis follicularis" was quite popular and was used as an umbrella term for a variety of skin diseases such as keratosis pilaris, Darier's disease, pityriasis rubra pilaris, and ichthyosis vulgaris. Therefore, this term has fallen into miscredit. There is, however, at least one entity which may be regarded as true follicular ichthyosis: The "ichthyosis follicularis, atrichia, and photophobia (IFAP) syndrome," first described by MacLeod in 1909 [6].

6.4.2 Clinical Features

MacLeod [6] reported on a familiy in which three of five boys presented a distinct skin disease characterized by extensive noninflammatory spiny follicular hyperkeratoses, atrichia, and severe photophobia. Some 50 years later, Zeligman and Fleisher [9] described two unrelated boys suffering from the same syndrome. Recently, Eramo and co-workers [2] reported on two other unrelated boys and delineated this condition from other syndromes featuring keratosis follicularis and alopecia. We recently observed a further boy and can confirm that the IFAP syndrome is a distinct entity [4]. Including our patient, eight boys but no girls with the IFAP syndrome have been reported so far. This may be a first clue for an X-linked recessive type of inheritance [2, 4].

The congenital absence of hair (congenital atrichia) is the most striking clinical feature of the IFAP syndrome (Fig. 73). The boy we observed was born as a mildly affected collodion baby and presented with generalized follicular keratosis over the entire body including the scalp. Follicular hyperkeratosis was very prominent, however, over the knees. In addition to the follicular involvement, mild generalized scaling with underlying erythema was noticed. The follicular involvement had improved in our case very much during the first year of life and was no longer very marked when we first saw this child. In most of the previously reported cases it was more severe, and thornlike projections giving the skin the feeling of a "nutmeg grater" are described [2, 9]. Sensitivity to light (photophobia) is the third cardinal feature of the IFAP syndrome. The boy we observed also showed a transient, but marked disturbance of nail growth, whereas in the other cases dysplastic nails were not reported. The teeth are normal in the IFAP syndrome, and sweating and hearing are likewise not impaired.

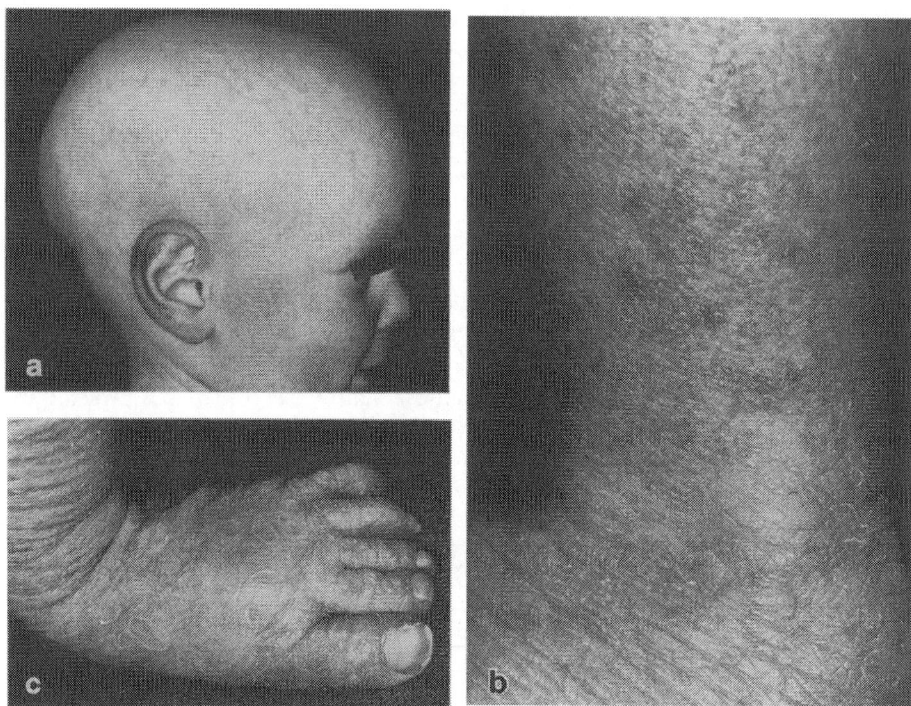

Fig. 73a–c. Ichthyosis follicularis, atrichia, and photophobia (IFAP) syndrome in a 2-year-old boy. **a** Striking congenital atrichia, **b** follicular hyperkeratosis, **c** mild congenital ichthyosis

In two boys (case 1 of Eramo et al. and our own observation) the condition was accompanied by a severe retardation of growth and motor development, by asthma bronchiale, and by a proneness to infections. Generalized seizures with accompanying high fevers and severe ophthalmologic problems (progressive corneal vascularization) can also occur. Torticollis was a striking feature in the cases of MacLeod [6] and Eramo et al [2], but it is not a constant sign.

6.4.3 Histologic Features

Skin biopsies taken from the legs (ichthyosis) disclose a benign acanthokeratosis and hyperkeratosis of the follicular openings. The granular layer is well preserved [2, 4, 6]. Therefore, autosomal dominant ichthyosis vulgaris and the epidermolytic types of ichthyosis can be excluded. Biopsies from the scalp reveal numerous atrophic hair follicles with their bulbs located within a thinned dermis and show the absence of sebaceous glands [4, 9].

6.4.4 Genetic Counseling

As discussed above, X-linked recessive inheritance is the most likely type of transmission. So far, nothing is known about the primary biochemical defects underlying the IFAP syndrome. Since a number of features (torticollis, growth and motor development retardation, proneness to infections) have been observed in only a few cases, it is tempting to speculate that these cases could represent a complex contiguous gene syndrome, as is the case in associated steroid sulfatase deficiency. Prenatal diagnosis is so far not available.

6.4.5 Clues for Differential Diagnosis

The IFAP syndrome represents a link between the heterogenous group of ichthyoses and the heterogeneous group of atrichias [8]. On clinical and histological grounds, the IFAP syndrome can easily be distinguished from simple keratosis pilaris, autosomal dominant ichthyosis vulgaris, and all other types of ichthyosis. Difficulties in differential diagnosis may arise when it comes to the group of syndromes that feature keratosis follicularis. I regard keratosis follicularis spinulosa decalvans (KFSD) of Siemens and keratosis pilaris rubra atrophicans faciei essentially as clinical variants of the same X-linked gene defect (allelic forms). Because the IFAP syndrome and KFSD share follicular keratosis and alopecia they may be mistaken for each other. However, in the IFAP syndrome the hyperkeratotic involvement is congenital and there is true congenital atrichia, wheras in KFSD the follicular hyperkeratoses are not present at birth. Moreover, alopecia is neither universal nor congenital, but patchy. It gradually develops as a result of follicular atrophoderma and hence presents the histologic features of pseudopelade.

Within the heterogenous group of atrichias a number of uncommon ectodermal dysplasias featuring universal alopecia, nail abnormalities, and "dry skin" have been described [3]. In most of these cases a detailed study of the cutaneous phenotype (sufficient dermatologic description, skin histology, etc.) is lacking and a meaningful discussion of a differential diagnosis is not possible [3, 8]. However, in 1969, Morris et al. [7] reported on a skin condition resembling the IFAP syndrome in some respects: They observed a boy suffering from generalized spiny hyperkeratosis, congenital atrichia, a bilateral sensorineural hearing deficit, and severe hypohidrosis. There was marked hyperkeratosis involving the palms and soles. Britton and associates [1] reported on an identical case also presenting follicular keratosis, atrichia, and deafness. These two cases may represent a distinct syndrome, because the follicular keratosis affects the nose in a striking manner not seen in the IFAP syndrome or in KFSD. Ichthyosis was not present in these two patients.

Hazell and Marks [5] reported on four patients with keratosis follicularis and pseudoacanthosis nigricans under the term "follicular ichthyosis". The clinical details given in their report are scarce. Their patients displayed follicular hyperkeratosis, but no generalized scaling, and hence did not suffer from ichthyosis. However, these patients probably represent a unique cornification disorder that should be classified within the framework of the syndromes featuring keratosis pilaris.

References

1. Britton H, Lustig J, Thompson BJ, Meyer S, Esterly NB (1978) Keratosis follicularis spinulosa decalvans. An infant with failure to thrive, deafness and recurrent infections. Arch Dermatol 114:761-764
2. Eramo LR, Esterly NB, Zieserl EJ, Stock EL, Herrmann J (1985) Ichthyosis follicularis with alopecia and photophobia. Arch Dermatol 121:1167-1174
3. Freire-Maia N, Pinheiro M (1984) Ectodermal dysplasias: a clinical and genetic study. Liss, New York
4. Hamm H, Meinecke P, Traupe H (1989) The ichthyosis follicularis, atrichia, and photophobia syndrome: a distinct entity. 5th International Congress of Pediatric Dermatology, July 11-15, 1989, Milan
5. Hazell M, Marks R (1984) Follicular ichthyosis. Br J Dermatol 111:101-109
6. MacLeod JMH (1909) Three cases of "ichthyosis follicularis" associated with baldness. Br J Dermatol 21:165-189
7. Morris J, Ackerman AB, Koblenzer PJ (1969) Generalized spiny hyperkeratosis. A previously undescribed syndrome. Arch Dermatol 100:692-698
8. Vogt BR, Traupe H, Hamm H (1988) Congenital atrichia with nail dystrophy, abnormal facies, and retarded psychomotor development in two siblings: a new autosomal recessive syndrome? Pediatr Dermatol 5:236-242
9. Zeligman I, Fleisher L (1959) Ichthyosis follicularis. Arch Dermatol 80:413-420

6.5 Peeling-Skin Syndrome: Clinical and Morphological Evidence for Two Types

6.5.1 Historical Aspects

In 1921, Fox [4] very briefly reported a case of life-long, noninflammatory skin shedding under the label "keratolysis exfoliativa congenita". Three years later, Wile [11] described an unusual type of congenital ichthyotic erythroderma occuring in three family members. He emphasized consanguinity, peeling of areas of skin, and pruritis as cardinal features of this condition. In 1982, Levy and Goldsmith [8] reported a further case and reinvestigated one of the original patients studied by Wile. They affirmed that this disease is a distinct type of congenital ichthyosis and introduced the name "peeling-skin syndrome". It is quite obvious that the condition Wile [11] and Levy and Goldsmith [8] delineated is different from that of Fox. Unfortunately, the designation Levy and Goldsmith chose had already been used by Kurban and Azar [7], who referred to four cases similar to those of Fox as "continual skin peeling". In the past few years both conditions have been reported as "peeling-skin syndrome" [3, 5, 9] or as "continual peeling-skin syndrome" [1, 10]. To complicate things further, both conditions are regarded as ichthyosis, and both are probably inherited as autosomal recessive traits. Therefore, I suggest distinguishing between the peeling-skin syndrome, type A (cases similar to that of Fox) and the peeling-skin syndrome, type B (cases similar to those of Wile).

6.5.2 Peeling-Skin Syndrome, Type A

Kurban and Azar [7] described this syndrome in four siblings. Abdel-Hafez and associates [1] reported two further consanguinous families with three affected siblings each. Isolated cases were observed by Bechet [2], by Heid et al. [6], and by Silverman et al. [10]. The onset of first symptoms seems to be variable. In some cases type A is congenital, whereas in others the disease starts at 3–6 years of age. There is a generalized peeling of the skin in thin, superficial flakes of differing size and shape [1, 10], involving the entire body suface including the face. The peeling is asymptomatic and noninflammatory. It does not show marked seasonal variations. Polarizing microscopy revealed a tiger-tail pattern in the case of Heid, which is otherwise considered to be typical of the trichothiodystrophy syndromes. Apparently, the case of Heid is so far the only one investigated in this respect.

Histology discloses orthohyperkeratosis and a normal epidermis. On light microscopy the splitting is seen either within the lower part of the stratum corneum or directly above the well-preserved granular layer [1, 10]. Ultrastructural studies provide clear evidence that the actual separation occurs within the stratum corneum [1, 10]. In the case studied by Silverman et al. [10], this separation surprisingly took place within the cytoplasm of corneocytes and not - as would be expected - between adjacent cells. The plasma membrane of the separating cell remained firmly attached to the adjacent underlying cell. Moreover, Silverman et al. [10] demonstrated unique intercellular electron-dense globular deposits in the corneocytes of their patient.

6.5.3 Peeling-Skin Syndrome, Type B

Familial cases have been reported by Wile [11] (three siblings) and Hacham-Zahdeh and Holubar [5] (two siblings). Sporadic cases were observed by Levy and Goldsmith [8], Dicken [3], and Mevorah et al. [9]. Congenital ichthyotic erythroderma (CIE) is present at birth. In some patients the erythema later subsides, but an erythematous background usually persists. Typically, erythematous scaling, migratory patches (Fig. 74) appear anywhere on the body except on palms and soles. The erythematous skin lesions have an exfoliative character. When grasped with a finger, the peripheral collarette can easily be peeled back. Moderate rubbing of the skin induces peeling. The disease can be accompanied by considerable pruritis. The gross appearance of the hair is normal, but there are periods when it can be pulled out easily. Laboratory findings disclose markedly elevated levels of total IgE [5, 8, 9]. An aminoaciduria is found in some cases. Short stature and retarded bone age can be additional features [1, 4], and some patients are susceptible to skin infections.

Histologic examination discloses a psoriasiform picture characterized by parakeratosis, a lacking granular layer, considerable acanthosis, and a chronic perivascular infiltrate in the dermis. The split occurs directly above the granular layer or directly above the acanthotic epidermis lacking a granular layer. According to Levy and Goldsmith [8], the granular layer is replaced by a regenerating parakeratotic stratum corneum 24 h after stripping, although the granular layer is still present in freshly stripped lesions. Mevorah and co-workers [9] studied in their patient the ultrastructure in detail and observed the presence of numerous oval, electron-dense, irregularly vacuolated bodies up to 800 nm in length in the keratinocytes of the granular layer. In many areas the stratum corneum was detached from the underlying noncornified epidermis. In contrast to type A, this detachment always occured intercellularly.

6.5.4 Is Peeling-Skin Syndrome, Type B, Identical to the Comèl-Netherton Syndrome?

The clinical, histologic, and ultrastructural differences between type A and type B of the peeling-skin syndrome are so profound that there can be no doubt that we are dealing with two entirely separate conditions. Type B shows a number of

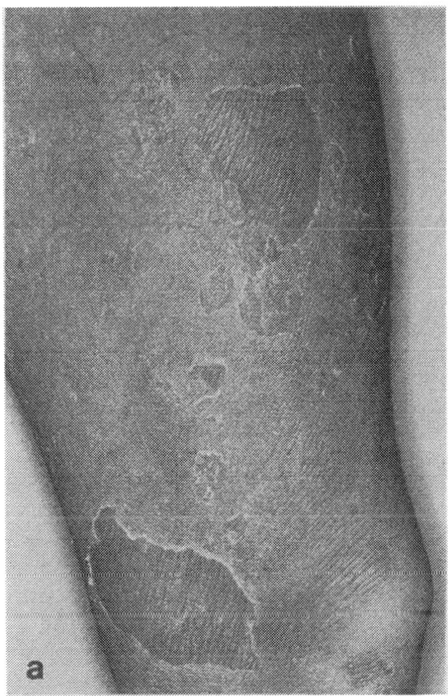

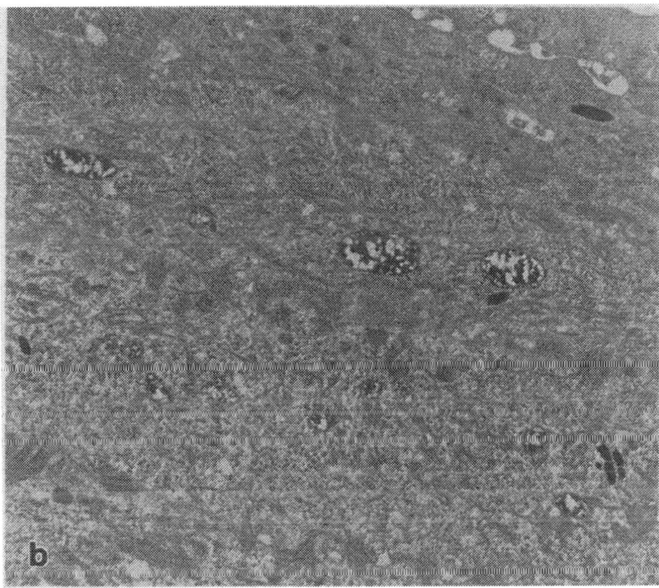

Fig. 74a, b. Peeling-skin syndrome, type B. **a** Clinical aspect with erythematous and scaling migratory patches edged by horny collarette, evolving on a background of diffusely thickened skin. **b** Electron micrograph. At the level of the granular layer oval, electron-dense vacuolated bodies are present. ×20000. (From [9], courtesy of Dr. B. Mevorah, Lausanne)

Table 32. Similarities between the peeling-skin syndrome, type B, and the Comèl-Netherton syndrome, suggesting a genetic relationship

Shared cutaneous features:	Congenital ichthyotic erythroderma Polycyclic skin lesions in later life Peeling of skin Pruritus Alopecia
Shared possible associations:	Short stature Retarded bone age Proneness to (skin) infections
Shared histologic features:	Psoriasiform histology Granular layer frequently absent Detachment of the stratum corneum from the epidermis
Shared laboratory findings:	Elevated IgE levels Aminoaciduria in some cases

striking similarities to the Comèl-Netherton syndrome (Table 32), though this is not stated in the literature. I am aware that the typical hair shaft abnormailty (trichorrhexis invaginata) is not (no longer?) present in the peeling-skin syndrome, type B. Interestingly, the patients of Wile [11] displayed alopecia at a young age, as can be seen from the photographs in his publication. When reinvestigated by Levy and Goldsmith [8], alopecia was no longer present. A similar improvement is typical of the Comèl-Netherton syndrome. I think the list of similarities between the peeling-skin syndrome, type B, and the Comèl-Netherton syndrome is impressive and suggests a genetic relationship between the two syndromes (multiple allelism or variable disease expression).

References

1. Abdel-Hafez K, Safer AM, Selim MM, Rehak A (1983) Familial continual skin peeling. Dermatologica 166:23-31
2. Bechet PE (1938) Deciduous skin. Arch Dermatol Syph (Chicago) 37:267-271
3. Dicken CH (1985) Peeling skin syndrome. J Am Acad Dermatol 13:158-160
4. Fox H (1921) skin shedding (keratolysis exfoliativa congenita): report of a case. Arch Dermatol Syph (Chicago) 3:202
5. Hacham-Zahdeh S, Holubar K (1985) Skin peeling syndrome in a Kurdish family. Arch Dermatol 121:545-546
6. Heid E, Harbit RB, Lazrak B (1983) Desquamation familiale continue. Ann Derm Venereol 110:141-143
7. Kurban AK, Azar HA (1969) Familial continual skin peeling. Br J Dermatol 81:191-195
8. Levy SB, Goldsmith LA (1982) The peeling skin syndrome. J Am Acad Dermatol 7:606-613
9. Mevorah B, Frenk E, Saurat JH, Siegenthaler G (1987) Peeling skin syndrome: a clinical, ultrastructural and biochemical study. Br J Dermatol 116:117-125
10. Silverman AK, Ellis CN, Beais TF, Woo TY (1986) Continual skin peeling syndrome. An electron-microscopic study. Arch Dermatol 122:71-75
11. Wile UJ (1924) Familial study of three unusual cases of congenital ichthyosiform erythroderma. Arch Dermatol Syph (Chicago) 4:487-498

6.6 Autosomal Dominant Congenital Ichthyosis and Keratoderma Hereditaria Mutilans of Vohwinkel

In 1929, Vohwinkel [5] described keratoderma hereditaria mutilans (KHM) as a distinct type of palmoplantar keratosis (PPK). The disease is characterized by diffuse palmoplantar hyperkeratoses having a "honeycombed" appearance. Moreover, it features constricting bands around the distal fingers and toe joints. The keratotic constrictions can be very severe and may result in loss of fingers and toes, especially of the fifth and fourth digits. Another abnormality consistently associated with KHM is linear circumscribed keratotic lesions on the elbows and knees [2–4]. Moreover, some patients have a mild ichthyosis [1, 3, 6]. We (H. Hamm and H. Traupe 1988, unpublished) have seen a further patient with KHM and mild generalized ichthyosis (Fig. 75), but the classic mutilations were absent in our case. Apparently, constrictions of the digits are not an obligate feature of KHM. Histologic studies in our case disclosed a scattered parakeratosis associated with a preserved granular layer. These histologic features are, of course, nonspecific, but they resemble those found in autosomal dominant lamellar ichthyosis.

KHM is an established autosomal dominant trait. In the patients observed by Camisa and Rossana [1] and in our own patient, ichthyosis and PPK co-segregated through several generations. Thus, we are dealing here with a further example of congenital ichthyosis transmitted as a dominant trait. The presence of concomitant KMH makes differential diagnosis from autosomal dominant lamellar ichthyosis easy. From a conceptual point of view, three different explanations can be given for the association of ichthyosis and KMH in these cases:

1. We are dealing with a contiguous gene syndrome implying a translocation or deletion mutation that has affected two neighboring gene loci, one for ichthyosis, and one for KMH.
2. Ichthyosis together with KHM is a distinct entity in itself.
3. Mild congenital ichthyosis is an inconstant feature of the condition and caused by the same metabolic defect as KHM.

At the moment all three explanations are possible. Because ichthyosis in these patients is mild and seems to be somewhat variable, I favor the hypothesis that ichthyosis is an inconstant sign of KHM.

References

1. Camisa C, Rossanna C (1984) Variant of keratodermia hereditaria mutilans (Vohwinkel's syndrome). Treatment with orally administered isotretinoin. Arch Dermatol 120:1323–1328

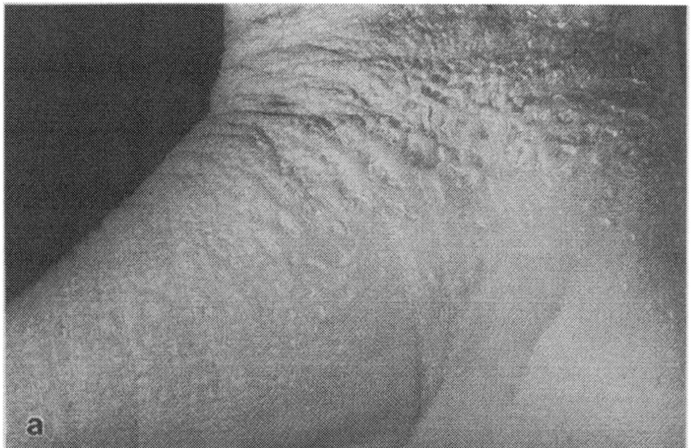

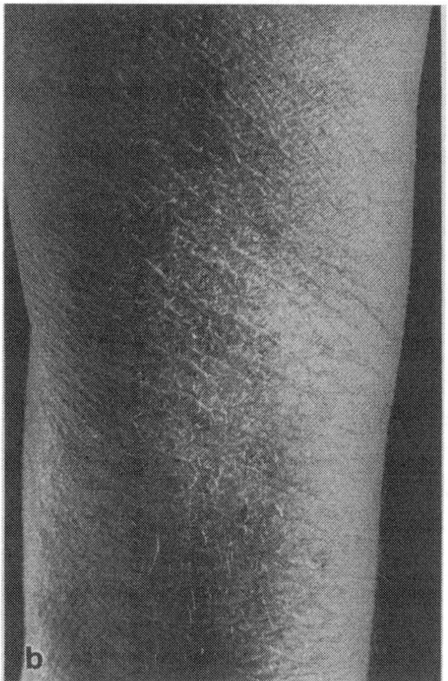

Fig. 75 a, b. Congenital ichthyosis with keratoderma hereditaria mutilans. **a** Typical aspect showing honeycombed palmar hyperkeratosis; **b** mild congenital ichthyosis

2. Chang Sing Pong AFI, Oranje AP, Vuzevki VD, Stolz E (1981) Successful treatment of keratoderma hereditaria mutilans with an aromatic retinoid. Arch Dermatol 117:225–228
3. Gibbs RC, Frank SB (1966) Keratoderma hereditaria mutilans (Vohwinkel): differentiating features of conditions with constriction of digits. Arch Dermatol 94:619–625
4. Goldfarb MT, Woo TY, Rasmussen JE (1985) Keratoderma hereditaria mutilans (Vohwinkel's syndrome): a trial of isotretinoin. Pediatr Dermatol 2:216–218
5. Vohwinkel KH (1929) Keratoma hereditarium mutilans. Arch Dermatol Syph (Berl) 158:354–364
6. Wirz F (1930) Keratoma hereditarium mutilans. Arch Dermatol Syph (Berl) 159:311–312

6.7 Congenital Migratory Ichthyosis with Neurologic and Ophthalmologic Abnormalities

In 1985, Zunich and associates [1] reported on two unrelated children displaying an identical complex phenotype. Though no further cases have been described so far, I believe that these two children represent a distinct syndrome. Clinically, the ichthyosis has some resemblance to the peeling-skin syndrome, type B. As in peeling-skin syndrome, type B, there was congenital ichthyotic erythroderma, pruritus, migratory scaling, and regions where the upper layer of the stratum corneum was detached and peeled off. However, in addition to these cutaneous features, both children exhibited facial dysmorphism, retinal colobomas, and abnormalities in spacing, size, and number of teeth. Brachydactyly and a broad second toe were noted. The neurologic involvement was characterized by a conductive hearing loss, psychomotor delay, wide-based gait, and autistic mannerisms. Moreover, both children developed seizures which were triggered by fever. Histologic studies disclosed orthohyperkeratosis, a well-preserved granular layer, and acanthosis with plump, confluent rete ridges. An ultrastructural examination revealed a shell-like formation of tonofilaments attached to keratohyalin granules around the nucleus, a finding reminiscent of epidermolytic hyperkeratosis. Dermal nerves showed a disorganization of myelin.

The constellation of clinical and ultrastructural findings in these two children is unique. All other types of neuroichthyosis can be excluded immediately. Since the cases of Zunich were not familial, nothing can be said about the inheritance pattern. In the first case, pregnancy of the mother had been complicated by aflatoxin exposure.

References

1. Zunich J, Esterly NB, Holbrook KA, Kaye CI (1985) Congenital migratory ichthyosiform dermatosis with neurologic and ophthalmologic abnormalities. Arch Dermatol 121:1149–1156

6.8 Ichthyoses of Uncertain Status

Today, we can differentiate between more than 20 different types of ichthyosis discussed in detail in this book. Moreover, there are at least 20 reports dealing with isolated cases or with a single family suffering from ichthyosis different in some respects from the well-established ichthyosis types. Some of these reports, especially the earlier ones, do not meet the minimal criteria for delineating a new type of ichthyosis. Clinical details are often insufficient and adequate histologic examinations are lacking. I am aware that some of the cases reported in this chapter may not represent unique conditions, but rather "university hospital syndromes." However, other case and family reports discussed below certainly concern true emerging syndromes. For detailed information the reader will have to consult the original reference.

6.8.1 Unestablished Ichthyoses with Bone Disease

Koller and associates [11] described a two-generation family in which six members were affected with a syndrome characterized by diaphyseal cortical thickening of the long bones, bowed legs, a tendency to fracture, and ichthyosis. Moreover, the patients had muscle weakness and a wagging gait. Roentgenograms disclosed marked cortical thickening of the diaphysis and narrowing of the marrow channel. The ichthyosis was also inherited as an autosomal dominant trait and was described as ichthyosis vulgaris. While the article gives a good description of the radiographic findings, the ichthyosis is ill defined. According to the authors, the skeletal dysplasia in the family reported does not fit in with any reported type of osteogenesis imperfecta or with any previously described sclerotic bone dysplasias.

Baraitser et al. [2] described a brother and sister featuring distal arthrogryposis, facial immobility, and generalized ichthyosis under the label of recessively inherited windmill-vane camptodactyly-ichthyosis syndrome. Originally, their patients were considered to have the Freeman-Sheldon syndrome. From the pictures accompanying this report it can be concluded that the ichthyosis is very mild. Because the parents are said to be unaffected by both ichthyosis and the bone dysplasia, the assertion that this is an autosomal recessive syndrome, is probably true. No histologic or ultrastructural studies were performed.

Dowd and Munro [4] reported on a 58-year-old man who had suffered from ichthyosis since birth with gross, well-demarcated, warty hyperkeratoses on the limbs, total alopecia since the age of 10 days, and leukonychia. Moreover, he was noted to have widespread keratosis pilaris with cutaneous horns over the extensor aspects of the elbows and hyperkeratotic lesions over the buttocks, hands, and feet. On radiologic grounds, an osteopetrosis was diagnosed. Histologic studies of the skin ruled out epidermolytic hyperkeratosis and showed a nonspecific benign acanthokeratosis in addition to follicular plugging.

6.8.2 Unestablished Ichthyoses in Association with Alopecia or Hair Shaft Abnormalities

Hammerstein et al. [8] reported mild congenital ichthyosis in three of four sibs born to consanguinous parents. In the remaining family members the ichthyosis did not occur. Patchy alopecia was seen, and the hair was unruly. Microscopic examination of the hair shafts disclosed irregular twisting along its axes, often referred to as "pili torti". The histologic findings were described in detail and were very striking: there was orthohyperkeratosis and follicular plugging, and the granular layer was either absent or extremely reduced. Moreover, the epidermis was more or less atrophic. Large, bandlike corneal opacities (fibrinoid degeneration of the cornea with a band-shaped keratopathy) were a further symptom.

Comment: The ophthalmologic and cutaneous alterations in this family are well documented and quite puzzling. The histologic findings reported would be expected in autosomal dominant ichthyosis vulgaris but not in a congenital ichthyosis. Onset of the disease process at birth and autosomal recessive inheritance exclude dominant ichthyosis vulgaris. I conclude that this family represents a distinct entity.

Yesudian and Srinivas [25] described unusual hair shaft abnormalities in two siblings suffering from autosomal recessive lamellar ichthyosis. The hair abnormalities may be described as trichoptilosis, i.e., the hair is cut longitudinally. Similar hair alterations have been described in the Comel-Netherton syndrome. The histologic features reported in these cases (parakeratosis and a thin granular layer) would also be compatible with this diagnosis, but clear-cut evidence for trichorrhexis invaginata was not observed.

Braun-Falco and Landthaler [3] described an 18-year-old woman suffering from ichthyosis vulgaris, deafness, pili torti, and dental anomalies. Both parents and three sibs of the patient were also deaf but showed no skin alterations. The hair shaft abnormalities were well documented but are not very specific. The cutaneous features and a histologic examination supported the diagnosis of autosomal dominant ichthyosis vulgaris. A number of clinical findings, such as premature loss of teeth, twisted hair ("pili torti"), and ichthyosis vulgaris, were observed in one patient only. They may have been associated by pure chance.

Jagell et al. [10] reported on a family with severe lamellar ichthyosis, alopecia ichthyotica, eclabion, ectropion, and mental retardation without neurologic symptoms or retinal changes. Their claim that this is a new genetic syndrome is not well founded, since eclabion, ectropion, and alopecia ichthyotica are frequently observed in lamellar ichthyosis.

Menni et al. [15] reported on two brothers suffering from lamellar ichthyosis and unusual hair shaft abnormalities. The main findings in their two cases were transverse fissures of the hair shaft and a "muff-like" detachment of the cuticle. The clinical details in this report were insufficient and a detailed histologic examination was not carried out.

6.8.3 Unestablished Ichthyoses with Neurologic Involvement

Kopec and Levine [12] reported generalized ichthyosis and multiple connective tissue nevi in a patient suffering from Down's syndrome (trisomy 21). The hyperkeratotic process in this patient involved the entire body surface, including palms and soles. Nevertheless, the scaling was mild and was described as resembling ichthyosis vulgaris or X-linked recessive ichthyosis. However, onset of the hyperkeratoses was delayed, occuring first at the age of 20 years. Histologic examination revealed the absence of a granular layer and epidermal atrophy. These histologic features are usually found in autosomal dominant ichthyosis vulgaris.

Dykes and associates [5] reported in detail on two brothers belonging to a large family in which affected members displayed ichthyosis, hepatosplenomegaly and signs of cerebellar degeneration. Clinically and histologically the ichthyosis was similar to autosomal dominant ichthyosis vulgaris, but a pedigree analysis excluded this possibility. An X-linked recessive ichthyosis was ruled out by steroid sulfatase testing. Cerebellar ataxia was a problem in two older brothers. When this family was reported, neutral lipid storage disease was not yet a well-established type of ichthyosis. The neurologic findings and hepatosplenomegaly would fit in with neutral lipid storage disease (Dorfman's syndrome). Likewise the pedigree of this family would be compatible with an autosomal recessive gene, despite a preponderence of affected males.

Gebhart et al. [6] recently reported on two patients suffering from infantile and juvenile types of alpha-1,4 glucosidase deficiency (Pompe's disease) with clinical and microscopic findings resembling those of ichthyosis vulgaris. Glycogen accumulations were demonstrated even in the cytoplasm of keratinocytes, suggesting a correlation between this pathologic storage process and the ichthyosis. On routine histology the ichthyosis would have been classified as ichthyosis vulgaris, since the granular layer was lacking and the epidermis atrophic. Electron-microscopic studies disclosed areas showing atypical, crumbly and spongy keratohyalin, whereas in other areas keratohyalin granules were apparently completely absent. The ultrastructural findings support a diagnosis of dominant ichthyosis vulgaris. The relationship to the glycogen storage is so far unclear.

6.8.4 Unestablished Ichthyoses and Renal Impairment

Goyer et al. [7] reported a very large family in which 23 of 78 examined members showed features of either renal disease, hearing loss, or ichthyosis. While the hearing loss and the nephropathy were well studied, the cutaneous alterations were only briefly mentioned. It is possible that this family represents the association of the autosomal dominant type of Alport's syndrome (hereditary nephritis and deafness) with autosomal dominant ichthyosis vulgaris. On the other hand, it should be kept in mind that renal dysfunction can cause acquired ichthyosis-like changes clinically mimicking ichthyosis vulgaris.

In 1973, Passwell and co-workers [16] described a family in which seven members exhibited congenital ichthyotic erythroderma and renal glycosuria. A close look at the pedigree, however, shows that ichthyosis was transmitted as an autosomal recessive trait, while glycosuria behaved as an autosomal dominant trait in the family. Further features in this family were mental retardation and short stature. The skin over the dorsum of hands and feet was described as being atrophic.

In 1975, Passwell and associates [17] described a different family in which autosomal recessive lamellar ichthyosis was associated with mental retardation, dwarfism, and renal impairment. Histologic examinations supported the diagnosis of congenital ichthyosis in this family. The constellation of findings was unusual. When this report appeared, neutral lipid storage disease had not yet been delineated. It should be included in the differential diagnosis today.

6.8.5 Miscellaneous

Pincus et al. [18] reported on a 4.5-year-old boy who suffered from an erythrodermic type of ichthyosis, accompanied by hyperimmunoglobulinemia E, recurrent infections, and defective neutrophil chemotaxis. Moreover, there was striking alopecia and the nails were dystrophic. Histologic examinations revealed marked hyperkeratosis, focal parakeratosis, and thickening of the granular layer. Polarizing microscopy of the hair was not done, and routine microscopy of the hair was lacking. Possibly, their patient suffered from the Comèl-Netherton syndrome.

In 1984, Marghescu and associates [14] described a 57-year-old woman suffering from congenital reticular ichthyotic erythroderma. This patient displayed unique cutaneous and ultrastructural features not found in other cornification disorders. At birth she apparently suffered from congenital ichthyotic erythroderma, which later evolved into a mosaic distribution of normal and erythrokeratotic and pigmented skin. These erythrokeratotic and pigmented skin lesions formed patch and bandlike areas and were arranged in a reticular pattern. On histologic examination the normal-appearing skin showed a regular epidermis and orthokeratosis, while biopsies from the affected areas disclosed parakeratosis, a vacuolization of the epidermis as in epidermolytic hyperkeratosis, and amyloid depositions in the papillary dermis. On electron microscopy the normal skin showed again a regular keratinization, whereas in the affected skin a peculiar three-dimensional network of fine filaments, forming perinuclear shells, was observed. These ultrastructural alterations and a high number of binucleate cells were reminiscent of the electron-microscopic features of ichthyosis hystrix of Curth-Macklin. However, subtle ultrastructural differences (three-dimensional network of filaments) indicated that in this patient the perinuclear shell formation was probably due to glycoproteins, and not to tonofilaments. Clinically, the most unique aspect of this dermatosis was the mosaic, yet generalized distribution of normal and erythrokeratotic skin, which did not follow the lines of Blaschko but was arranged in a reticular pattern. A genetic explanation for this unique distribution pattern is difficult, but I imagine that a very early somatic mutation resulting in two genetically different cell lines is most likely. It is tempting to speculate that this dermatosis is a further example of a lethal gene that can survive only by mosaicism.

Lahmar and associates [13] described a Tunesian boy suffering from lamellar ichthyosis associated with a spastic syndrome of the lower extremities. The absence of mental retardation distinguished this type of ichthyosis from the more common Sjögren-Larsson syndrome. On electron microscopy a large number of keratinocytes were seen to contain big vacuoles, often measuring up to the size of the nuclei. These vacuoles were well limited and partially lined by a membrane. Interestingly, etretinate treatment altered the appearance of the keratinocytes in the transition zone.

After treatment with retinoids, the keratinocytes of the granular layer showed pronounced intracellular edema, resulting in cells that looked empty (phantom cells). Since the ultrastructure of the Sjögren-Larsson syndrome has never been described in detail, it is difficult to decide whether this patient really represents a distinct entity.

Hazell and Marks [9] described patients with keratosis follicularis under the misleading term "follicular ichthyosis". Though these cases may represent a distinct cornification disorder, the condition they described should not be classified as ichthyosis, because the hyperkeratosis was not generalized, but confined to hair follicles.

Ruzicka and associates [19] described a 15-year-old girl suffering from erythrodermic lamellar ichthyosis, neurosensory deafness, severe mental retardation, dental aplasia, brachydactyly, clinodactyly, accessory cervical ribs, and carcinoma of the thyroid. The cutaneous alterations correspond to the erythrodermic type of lamellar ichthyosis (ELI type A). Apart from her skin condition, perhaps the most striking feature is that at the age of 14 she already suffered from a thyroid carcinoma. I assume that this case is a further example of a contiguous gene syndrome involving the gene for erythrodermic lamellar ichthyosis type A and other neighboring genes.

Stormorken et al. [21] reported a family in which in three generations of affected members suffered from thrombocytopathia, muscle fatigue, asplenia, miosis, migraine, dyslexia, and ichthyosis. The most striking feature was a prolonged bleeding time which could be related to a platelet dysfunction. Apparently, this condition was inherited as an autosomal dominant trait. While a number of the peculiar features (platelet dysfunction, muscle weakness, asplenia) were studied in some detail, this cannot be said of the ichthyosis. Clinically, the ichthyosis resembled ichthyosis vulgaris, but histologic and ultrastructural studies were not performed. It is difficult to imagine how this multifaceted syndrome could be caused by a single biochemical defect. Once again, a contiguous gene syndrome featuring autosomal dominant ichthyosis vulgaris in association with other conditions is more likely.

Sidransky and associates [20] reported a family in which ichthyosis vulgaris was transmitted through three generations and was associated with full cheeks and sparse eyebrows. The ichthyosis in the family was not studied. Because of insufficient clinical and histologic details and because of lacking ultrastructural examinations the claim of Sidransky et al. that this family represents a new type of dominant ichthyosis vulgaris is hardly justified [22]. Ichthyosis vulgaris is known to be frequently associated with atopic dermatitis [23]. Sparse lateral eyebrows are a common feature of this frequent polygenic condition. Full cheeks until puberty are the only feature that was unusual in the family of Sidransky.

In 1984 we [24] reported on a 26-year-old Pakistani suffering from atypical ichthyosis vulgaris and from very severe hypogenitalism and hypogonadism. This patient (case 2 of [24]) clinically resembled X-linked recessive ichthyosis, but there was no steroid sulfatase deficiency. Moreover, pedigree data did not indicate X-linked inheritance. In my opinion, this patient represents a so far unclassifiable distinct type of ichthyosis vulgaris that can be distinguished from both X-linked recessive ichthyosis and an autosomal dominant ichthyosis vulgaris on biochemical and ultrastructural grounds.

In 1941, Bäfverstedt [1] described a solitary case of generalized hystrix-like hyperkeratosis accompanied by mental retardation and epilepsy. Blistering was not a feature of this condition. Apparently, the histologic features were those of a nonspecific benign acanthokeratosis. However, when Bäfverstedt first described his case epidermolytic hyperkeratosis had not yet been described as a distinct histologic pattern. Probably he would not have recognized epidermolytic hyperkeratosis, even if present. The relationship of this case to other types of hystrix-like ichthyosis, for example the HID syndrome and ichthyosis hystrix of Curth-Macklin, remains, unclear.

References

1. Bäfverstedt B (1941) Fall von genereller, naevusartiger Hyperkeratose, Imbecillität, Epilepsie. Acta Derm Venereol (Stockh) 22:207–212
2. Baraitser M, Burn J, Fixsen J (1983) A recessively inherited windmill-vane camptodactyly/ichthyosis syndrome. J Med Genet 20:125–127
3. Braun-Falco O, Landthaler M (1978) Ichthyosis vulgaris, Taubheit, Pili torti und Zahnanomalien. Hautarzt 29:276–280
4. Dowd PM, Munro DD (1983) Ichthyosis and osteopetrosis. J R Soc Med 76:423–426
5. Dykes PJ, Marks R, Harper PS (1979) A syndrome of ichthyosis, hepatosplenomegaly and cerebellar degeneration. Br J Dermatol 100:585–590
6. Gebhart W, Mainitz M, Jurecka W, Niebauer G, Paschke E, Stöckler S, Sluga E (1988) Ichthyosiforme Schuppung bei α-1,4 Glukosidase-Mangel. Hautarzt 39:228–232
7. Goyer RA, Reynolds J Jr, Burke J, Burholder P (1968) Hereditary renal disease with neurosensory hearing loss, prolinuria and ichthyosis. Am J Med Sci 256:166–179
8. Hammerstein W, Meiers HG, Haensch R (1975) Die Hornhautveränderungen bei Ichthyosen. Albrecht v. Graefes Arch Klin Exp Ophthal 195:161–173
9. Hazell M, Marks R (1984) Follicular ichthyosis. Br J Dermatol 111:101–109
10. Jagell SF, Holmgren G, Hofer PA (1987) Congenital ichthyosis with alopecia, eclabion, ectropion and mental retardation – a new genetic syndrome. Clin Genet 31:102–108
11. Koller ME, Maurseth K, Haneberg B, Aarskog D (1979) A familial syndrome of diaphyseal cortical thickening of the long bones, bowed legs, tendency to fracture and ichthyosis. Pediatr Radiol 8:179–182

12. Kopec AV, Levine N (1979) Generalized connective tissue nevi and ichthyosis in Down's syndrome. Arch Dermatol 115:623-624
13. Lahmar L, Frenk E, Gharbi R, Walzer C (1984) Ichthyose généralisée associée a un syndrome spastique des membres inférieurs, une variante de syndrome de Sjögren-Larsson? Étude en microscopie optique et électronique de l'ichthyose et de son évolution sous traitement oral à l'étrétinate. Ann Dermatol Venereol 111:885-892
14. Marghescu S, Anton-Lamprecht I, Rudolph PO, Kaste R (1984) Kongenitale retikuläre ichthyosiforme Erythrodermie. Hautarzt 35:522-529
15. Menni S, Piccinno R, Crosti C, Sala F (1985) Two cases of lamellar ichthyosis with unusual hair shaft abnormalities. Dermatologica 171:180-182
16. Passwell J, Zipperkowski L, Katznelson D, Szeinberg A, Crispin M, Pollak S, Goodman R, Bat-Miriam M, Cohen BE (1973) A syndrome characterized by congenital ichthyosis with atrophy, mental retardation, dwarfism, and generalized aminoaciduria. J Pediatr 82:466-471
17. Passwell JH, Goodman RM, Ziprkowski M, Cohen BE (1975) Congenital ichthyosis, mental retardation, dwarfism and renal impairment: a new syndrome. Clin Genet 8:59-65
18. Pincus SH, Thomas IT, Clark RA, Ochs HD (1975) Defective neutrophil chemotaxis with variant ichthyosis, hyperimmunoglobulinemia E, and recurrent infections. J Pediatr 6:908-911
19. Ruzicka T, Goerz G, Anton-Lamprecht I (1981) Syndrome of ichthyosis congenita, neurosensory deafness, oligophrenia, dental aplasia, brachydactyly, clinodactyly, accessory cervical ribs and carcinoma of the thyroid. Dermatologica 162:124-136
20. Sidransky E, Feinstein A, Goodman RM (1987) Ichthyosis-cheek-eyebrow (ICE) syndrome: a new autosomal dominant disorder. Clin Genet 31:137-142
21. Stormorken H, Sjaastad O, Langslet A, Sulg I, Egge K, Diderichsen J (1985) A new syndrome: thrombocytopathia, muscle fatigue, asplenia, miosis, migraine, dyslexia and ichthyosis. Clin Genet 28:367-374
22. Traupe H (1987) Letter. What is the ichtyosis in the so-called ichthyosis-cheek-eyebrow (ICE) syndrome? Clin Genet 32:418
23. Traupe H, Happle R (1980) Klinik und Genetik der Ichthyosis vulgaris-Gruppe. Fortschr Med 98:1809-1815
24. Traupe H, Müller-Migl CR, Kolde G, Happle R, Kövary PM, Hameister H, Ropers HH (1984) Ichthyosis vulgaris with hypogenitalism and hypogonadism. Evidence for different genotypes by lipoprotein electrophoresis and steroid sulfatase testing. Clin Genet 25:42-51
25. Yesudian P, Srinivas K (1977) Ichthyosis with unusual hair shaft abnormalities in siblings. Br J Dermatol 96:199-203

7 Therapy

7.1 Topical Therapy

7.1.1 Introduction

Topical treatment modalities are still the backbone of successful therapy in the various cornification disorders. Because of a certain disillusionment regarding the safety of systemic long-term therapy with retinoids, topical preparations have regained much of their former importance. One should not forget, however, that many of the topical treatment modalities now in everyday use have never undergone a thorough and critical evaluation process, but have been handed down by previous generations of dermatologists or dermatology schools. The assertion that, for instance, long-term treatment with salicylic acid is safe lacks a scientific basis.

Unfortunately, topical therapy of the ichthyoses and other cornification disorders is a neglected research subject. Much of our current therapeutic practice is based on traditions, subjective beliefs, and personal clinical experience ("impressions"), while hard data are scarce. Ideally, one would imagine that certain groups of ichthyosis sharing similar pathophysiologic characteristics (e.g., transepidermal water loss, scale lipid composition, epidermal cell turnover) should be treated with topicals especially suited for them. However, this is not (yet?) the case, and all types of cornification disorders are treated in more or less similar ways.

There are two main principles for the local therapy of ichthyoses and related scaling disorders: (a) keratolysis and (b) hydration of the stratum corneum. The two principles are not mutually exclusive, but some agents such as urea and propylene glycol denature proteins and hydrate the stratum corneum at the same time [7, 15]. Salicylic acid, urea, and propylene glycol are considered keratolytics, while sodium chloride and lactic acid exert their main effects by hydration of the epidermis.

7.1.2 Salicylic Acid: a Drug I Do not Use

Sixty years ago, the classical treatment of ichthyosis was frequent bathing and the application of 3%–6% salicylic acid in a petrolatum base [18]. There is no doubt that salicylic acid is effective in removing scales, and it is still widely used in concentrations ranging from 3% to 10% in adult patients with psoriasis on a short-term basis. Despite this, I advise against its use as a regular topical for ichthyosis patients. There is a fundamental difference between psoriasis and the group of ichthyoses: The latter are genetically determined disorders and require lifelong treatment. The epidermal barrier function is markedly impaired both in psoriasis and in the heterogeneous group of ichthyoses. This means that all kinds of agents permeate at a much higher rate through the inflamed and scaly skin than through normal epidermis. It is not unrealistic to assume that up to 20% of the total dose of salicylic acid applied to the skin is absorbed [16]. If a patient is treated from childhood on with a cream containing 5% salicylic acid, then over the years a considerable amount of this substance will be absorbed. An adult ichthyosis patient needs for his skin care approximately 10–20 g of a cream daily. If 20% of salicylic acid is absorbed, then this would amount to a daily systemic intake of 100–200 mg salicylic acid. The systemic burden of such a long-term treatment may be comparable to that of chronic use of analgesics.

While there are no hard data addressing my concern for a possible long-term toxicity of salicylic acid, the data for acute toxicity are controversial. Acute toxicity of salicylic acid was noted by Van Weiss and Lever [26], who treated adults with widespread psoriasis using 3%–6% of topical preparations with four to six applications daily. Acute toxicity in this study was manifested as nausea, tinnitus, dyspnea, and hallucinations. On the other hand, Taylor and Halprin [23] used 6% salicylic acid in a gel base under occlusion in adults with extensive psoriasis. During a follow-up of 5 days they observed no acute toxicity.

In children, **total body treatment** with salicylic acid should be avoided in any case. At least ten children have died of acute percutaneous intoxication with salicylic acid [16]. Rasmussen [16] considers a treatment of up to 25% of the surface to be still safe in children. Some of the problems connected with acute toxicity of salicylic acid in children may have been due to the fact that their physicians were unaware of the multiplying factor and did not properly assess the systemic burden of topical ointments (see Sect. 7.1.4).

7.1.3 Commonly Used Active Substances: Sodium Chloride, Urea, Lactic Acid, and Propylene Glycol

Sodium chloride (NaCl) in a concentration of 5%–10% in aqueous creams is a substance that has been used for many years [10]. It is especially effective if applied directly after a bath or shower when the skin is still a bit wet. This advice is of course also true for urea and lactic acid. A formulation for a 10% NaCl cream is given in Table 33. I myself have not used sodium chloride preparations very much, since several of my patients found them to be not very agreeable on the skin. Apparently, the salt is not completely dissolved or separates after a while, forming crystals that can be felt. Older books suggest that ichthyosis patients take a daily bath in a 3% sodium chloride solution [10]. Though this may be effective, it is also rather unpractical. If one assumes that a normal bathtub contains at least 100 l, then this would mean that every day 3 kg of high-quality salt are needed.

In 1962, Stüttgen [19] introduced **vitamin A acid** (0.1% tretinoin) as a new substance for topical therapy. He was able to show that vitamin A acid has an intense keratolytic effect and that the action of topically applied vitamin A is much

Table 33. Formulation of topical preparations

1. **NaCl ointments**
   NaCl 10.0
   enough distilled water for solubilization
   olive oil
   lanolin to fill up to 100.0

Comment: I never tried this formulation, given by Korting [10]. Or

NaCl	10,0
distilled water	40.0
Unguentum Cordes*	50.0

Comment: This is an acceptable aqueous sodium salt cream.

2. **Urea-containing creams**

Urea	5.0
distilled water	45.0
Unguentum Cordes	50.0

Comment: The strength of urea can be increased to 10% at the cost of water. This cream gives good results or

Urea	2.5
Tween 80	10.0
cetanol	15.0
lanolin	15.0
distilled water	47.5

Comment: This formulation was given by Swanbeck [21]; I haver never tried it myself.

3. **Lactic acid-containing creams**

Lactic acid	5.0
distilled water	45.0
Unguentum Cordes	50.0

Comment: The strength of lactic acid can be increased to 10% at the cost of water. The effectiveness is comparable to that of urea. Or

Lactic acid	5.0
Unguentum emulsificans aqueosum	95.0

Comment: It is important that aqueous emulsifying unguentum is used. Without water the results are disappointing.

4. **Combinations of urea and NaCl**

NaCl	10.0
Urea	5.0
distilled water	40.0
Unguentum Cordes	45.0

Comment: Other combinations are also possible, but I have no experience of my own. In many commercial products combinations of lactic acid with urea are used.

* Unguentum Cordes is a cheap, commercially available base (manufacturer: Ichthyol-Cordes-Gesellschaft, Hermanni and Co., Hamburg, FRG) especially devised for dermatological formulations. It contains polyethylene glycol, fatty acid esters, partial glycerides, lanolin, and paraffin. It is devoid of preserving additives.

weaker than that of the vitamin A acid. Moreover, Stüttgen performed convincing half-side trials demonstrating a clinical effectiveness of vitamin A acid (tretinoin). A major disadvantage of topically applied vitamin A acid is its irritative property [19, 28]. Tretinoin does not seem to be suitable for patients suffering from ichthyotic erythroderma or atopic dermatitis, which is found in many patients with ichthyosis vulgaris. Lower concentrations of tretinoin (0.03%) can be combined with urea and have been shown to be very effective. However, even at this low concentration vitamin A acid can still cause irritations on the skin [28]. In my experience, vitamin A acid alone or in combination with other substances can work well in "intelligent" patients who know how to handle interval therapy (for example treatment for 2 days followed by 3 days' application of a bland ointment as individually required).

In 1968, Swanbeck [21] introduced therapy with **urea**-containing creams. He demonstrated that urea strongly increased the water-binding capacity of scales from psoriatic patients. The good clinical effect of creams containing up to 10% urea on scaly skin conditions was soon confirmed by other groups (reviewed in [15]. A number of pharmaceutical companies developed commercially available urea ointments. Swanbeck [22] also devised a scheme for the optimal use of urea creams (Table 34). The clinical efficacy of urea can be increased if it is combined with sodium chloride or vitamin A acid. Lactic acid (1%) is often used in these commercial products as an additional substance.

In 1974, Van Scott and Yu [24] introduced the use of **lactic acid** and were able to show a good effect of this agent and related α-hydroxy acids. Recently, Buxman et al. [3] drew attention again to this substance and demonstrated that it is very effective when applied as a 12% lotion. Many patients find lotions more agreeable than creams. This kind of application therefore expands our therapeutic arsenal. According to Van Scott and Yu [25], lactic acid reduces the hyperkeratotic states by weakening intercellular bonding and corneocyte cohesion. A similar effect is also discussed for water and retinoids [25].

Baden [1] and Goldsmith [8] found an occlusive treatment with 60% **propylene glycol** to be very effective in scale removal. Propylene glycol without occlusion gave a less optimal improvement. In my personal experience, other creams containing large amounts of water, such as Eucerin cum aqua (similar to Nivea) or unguentum emulsificans aquosum also produce excellent results, if applied over night and under occlusion with plastic dressing. However, it is not feasible to place the entire body under occlusion, and such a treatment is hardly acceptable for patients on a long-term basis. Nevertheless, the astonishing effect of pure **water** demonstrates that, irrespective of specific substances, marked hydration of the epidermis is a major factor involved in normalization of the diseased skin. The water content of the epidermis is probably involved in regulation of the epidermal lipid metabolism. The experience that patients suffering from X-linked recessive ichthyosis usually show marked improvement of their skin con-

Table 34. Optimal scheme for urea treatment of ichthyosis according to Swanbeck [22]

1. Bath
2. Dry 5–15 min
3. Apply urea cream in excess without scrubbing
4. Wait 10–15 min
5. Wipe off excess cream
6. Repeat daily for 1 week
7. Thereafter, apply urea cream daily in sufficient amount

dition during the summer confirms this notion. Apart from affecting physical properties, hydration of the stratum corneum may have a number of further effects, such as restoring the activity of enzymes involved in cornification. These enzymes usually require water and the water content decreases in the outer part of the stratum corneum.

Very recently, Schrader and Bielfeldt [17] reported that adenosine triphosphate (ATP) disodium salt significantly smoothes rough skin in very low concentrations (0.005%–0.05%). Clinical trials with ichthyotic patients have not been performed yet, but ATP may become a powerful agent in the management of hyperkeratotic skin, if the astonishing results communicated by this group hold true. The ATP concentrations used in the experiments were so low that the effect of this drug cannot be explained by an influence on the physicochemical properties of the stratum corneum; a direct biochemical effect would be more likely.

So far, I myself have treated most of my patients either with urea or lactic acid (Table 33). Most often I use a concentration of 5%, since in my experience a higher percentage of urea or lactic acid may cause irritation or a stinging feeling. If patients tolerate the urea or lactic acid creams well, their strength can of course be increased. In my experience the effects of urea and lactic acid are comparable (Fig. 76). In West Germany, Unguentum Cordes is a commercially available product that can be used as a base. It is cheap and delivered with

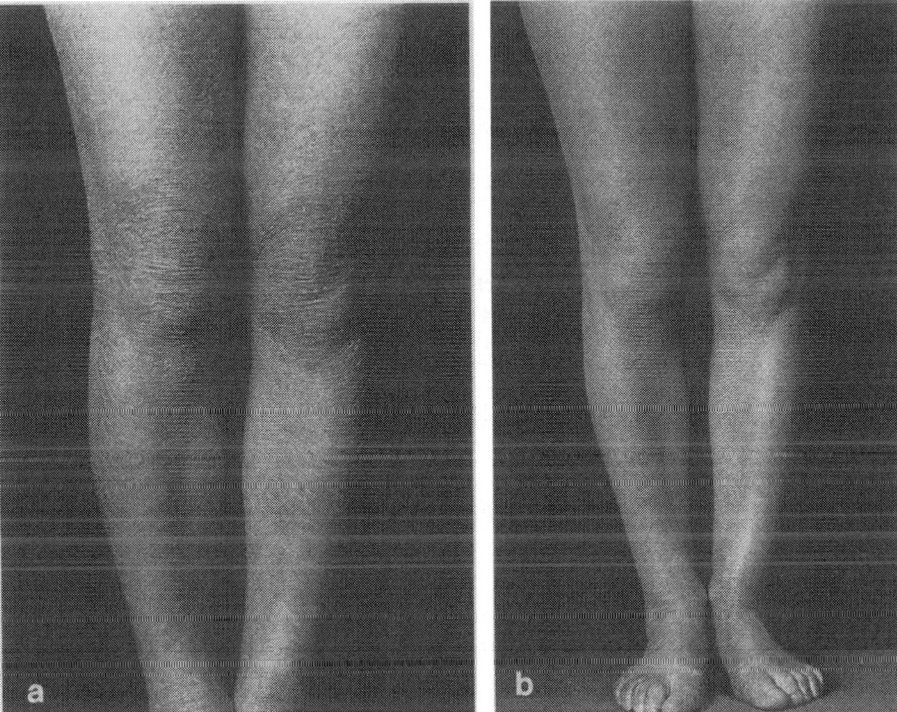

Fig. 76a, b. Comparative half-side trial of 5% urea *(right side)* and 5% lactic acid *(left side)* in a patient with autosomal dominant lamellar ichthyosis: **a** untreated; **b** after 4 weeks. There is no difference in the extent of scaling between the two sides

constant quality. I find this latter aspect of particular importance. There are a number of so-called official ointments which are contained and listed in the pharmacopeias of various countries (e.g., **Deutsches Arzneimittelbuch**). Despite their official character, the consistency of these ointments can differ from one pharmacy to the other and is not predictable. Unfortunately, even if one always uses the same base and the same standard formulations, there is no guarantee that the final results will be the same if these ointments are prepared in different pharmacies. This is, of course, a general disadvantage of formulated ointments. On the other hand, they are usually much cheaper.

As far as Unguentum Cordes is concerned, it is rather messy if applied directly on the skin. However, up to 50% of water can be incorporated into this base without problems, turning it into an agreeable soft cream. Some formulations I have tried are listed in Table 33.

Lykkesfeldt and Hoyer [12] reported a remarkable innovation for topical treatment of patients with X-linked recessive ichthyosis. In an open prospective half-side trial they applied creams containing either 10% cholesterol or 10% urea to the skin of 20 XRI patients. In 18 of their patients there was a good response to the cholesterol cream, and 13 considered the cholesterol cream to be superior to the urea cream. This paper is often quoted because it fits in with modern pathophysiologic concepts concerning scaling in X-linked recessive ichthyosis [13]. However, a more recent study, also from Denmark, failed to confirm any effectiveness of cholesterol in X-linked recessive ichthyosis. Ibsen and Brandrup [9] used the same "inert" cream base (Dansk Laegemiddel Standard) that had been employed by Lykkesfeldt and Hoyer and found that a 10% cholesterol preparation was not superior to its base.

7.1.4 Therapeutic Pitfalls in the Management of Children

There is one major therapeutic pitfall into which physicians caring for children may easily get trapped: the ratio between cutaneous surface area and weight. This ratio is a major determinant for the totally absorbed dose and thus can have

Table 35. Relationship between age, body weight, and body surface, with ratios of body surface to total weight and multiplying factor for a comparable systemic burden in an adult

Age	Weight (kg)	Body surface (cm^2)	Ratio (cm^2/kg)	Multiplying factor[a]
Newborn	3.4	2100	617.6	2.4
½ year	7.5	3500	466.7	1.8
1 year	9.3	4100	440.9	1.7
4 years	15.5	6500	419.4	1.6
10 years	30.5	10500	344.3	1.3
Adult	70.0	18100	258.6	1.0

[a] The multiplying factor is best explained with an example: The absorbed dose/kg body weight of a 10% urea cream in a newborn equals that of a 24% urea cream in an adult. (Data adapted from Stüttgen [20])

serious repercussions on systemic side effects. Some of the problems occurring in children treated with "adult" concentrations of urea or salicylic acid [2, 5] are not primarily caused by the substances, but are due to the physician's ignorance of the above-mentioned ratio and its therapeutic consequences. It is well known that body proportions of children are different from those of adults. 66% of the total body surface of a newborn infant is concentrated on the extremities, while the trunk and the head make up only 34% of the total surface [20]. Therefore, the total surface of a newborn in relation to its weight is significant (factor 2.4 to 2.7) larger than in adults (Table 35). This means that the biologic availability of any substance in an infant is at least 2.4 times greater than in an adult [16, 20, 27]. In other words, if an infant is treated with a 10% urea cream, the systemic burden (absorbed dose/kg/body weight) of this cream is the same as that of urea cream with the strength of 24% in an adult. Moreover, one should not forget that the epidermal barrier function of children (and adults, too) with cornification disorders usually is significantly disturbed and allows for a much faster permeation. Finally, having good intentions, some concerned mothers or nurses will overdo the treatment and, for example, apply a certain cream each time the diaper is changed, i.e., eight times a day instead of twice a day. When such unfortunate mistakes and the ignorance of basic aspects of topical therapy coincide, it is easy to understand that therapeutic disasters can develop. For adult patients, no dermatologist would seriously suggest a whole-body treatment with a urea cream of 25% strength. When treating children one should be aware of the multiplying factor to better assess the possible systemic burden.

Contrary to a widespread belief, the skin of a **mature** infant is not more tender than that of adults [14, 16, 20]. Hence, the local effectiveness of a 10% cream will be more or less similar to that in adults. However, there are some exceptions to this rule. Permeation of arachidonic acid, linoleic acid, and linolenic acid in identical concentrations is ten times greater in newborns than in adults [14]. This has, of course, repercussions on lipophilic drugs (e.g., lindane treatment for scabies). As a general rule, I advise treating newborns with bland ointments only and avoiding active substances such as urea or salicylic acid. In most cases bland ointments will significantly smoothen the skin and give satisfactory results.

Occasionally, children with genetic cornification disorders may contract other diseases, such as scabies. Similar considerations apply in these situations. Very recently, Friedman [4] reported a severe neurotoxic reaction in a 3-year-old boy with erythrodermic lamellar ichthyosis following a single whole-body application of 1% lindane (gamma-benzene hexachloride). In this boy a tenfold increase in the lindane blood level was measured even 72 h after this one application. At least in children with severe genetic cornification disorders, lindane certainly is not the drug of choice for the treatment of scabies. It may be replaced by a 10% crotamiton cream. Since crotamiton is less active than lindane, I advice using it for at least 5 days and to repeat the treatment after 1 week for another course of 5 days. In Europe crotamiton was quite popular for some time in the treatment of atopic dermatitis, and its toxicity, even after long-term use, seems to be very low.

At least in West Germany, certain dyes, such as gentian violet (Pyoktanin) or clioquinol (Vioform) to prevent or treat bacterial skin infections, are very popular. The possible toxicity of these very effective local agents is also a matter of debate. Under optimal absorption conditions these dyes may have toxic effects, for example via the induction of methemoglobin [20]. Widespread use of such dyes should be avoided in children with ichthyosis.

Apart from the pitfalls of topical therapy discussed above, there are some general problems concerning skin care of newborns with cornification disorders. Episodes of hypernatremic dehydration and hypothermia are problems encountered in some children with severe ichthyotic erythroderma [6]. In our own experience, such events are frequent and even typical of children with the Comèl-Netherton syndrome, but they can occur in other conditions, too [6]. Hypernatremia is caused by the imperceptible, increased transepidermal water loss that is associated with a severely inflamed skin lacking a proper epidermal barrier function. Therefore, in these children special attention has to be given to fluid balance and to temperature regulation. Hypothermia and sudden drops of body weight from one day to the next day should be alarming signs [6]. Apparently, episodes of hypernatremia cannot always be avoided in these children, even by physicians aware of these problems. Nevertheless, it helps, of course, if physicians and nurses of the neonatal care units are informed of these problems well in advance. A practical measure may be to place these children in incubators kept at 33 °C and to attach a humidifier to the incubators [11].

References

1. Baden HP, Alper JL (1973) A keratolytic gel containing salicylic acid in propylene glycol. J Invest Dermatol 61:330–333
2. Beverley DW, Wheeler D (1986) High plasma urea concentrations in collodion babies. Arch Dis Child 61:696–698
3. Buxman M, Hickman J, Ragsdale W, Stretcher G, Krochmal L, Wehr RF (1986) Therapeutic activity of lactate 12% lotion in the treatment of ichthyosis. Active versus vehicle and active versus a petrolatum cream. J Am Acad Dermatol 15:1253–1258
4. Friedman SH (1987) Lindane neurotoxic reaction in nonbullous congenital ichthyosiform erythroderma. Arch Dermatol 123:1056–1058
5. Garty BZ (1986) High plasma urea concentration in babies with lamellar ichthyosis. Arch Dis Child 61:1245–1246
6. Garty BZ, Wiseman Y, Metzker A, Reisner SH, Nitzan M (1985) Hypernatremic dehydration and hypothermia in congenital lamellar ichthyosis. Pediatr Dermatol 3:65–68
7. Goldsmith LA (1978) Propylene glycol. Int J Dermatol 17:703–705
8. Goldsmith LA, Baden HP (1972) Management and treatment of ichthyosis. N Engl J Med 286:821–823
9. Ibsen HH, Brandrup F (1984) Topical cholesterol treatment of recessive X-linked ichthyosis. Lancet 2:645
10. Korting GW (1974) Therapie der Hautkrankheiten. Ein Lehrbuch für die Praxis, 3rd edn. Schattauer, Stuttgart, pp 111–116
11. Lawlor F, Peiris S (1985) Harlequin fetus successfully treated with etretinate. Br J Dermatol 112:585–590
12. Lykkesfeldt G, Hoyer H (1983) Topical cholesterol treatment of recessive X-linked ichthyosis. Lancet 2:1337–1338
13. Maloney ME, Williams ML, Epstein EH, Law MYL, Fritsch PO, Elias PM (1984) Lipids in the pathogenesis of ichthyosis: topical cholesterol sulfate-induced scaling in hairless mice. J Invest Dermatol 83:252–256

14. Maibach H, Boisits E (eds) (1982) Neonatal skin structure and function. Dekker, New York
15. Müller KH, Pflugshaupt C (1979) Harnstoff in der Dermatologie. Literaturübersicht. Zentralbl Haut-Geschlechtskr 142:157–168
16. Rasmussen JE (1979) Percutaneous absorption in children. In: Dobson RL (ed) Year book of dermatology 1979. Year Book Medical, Chicago, pp 15–38
17. Schrader K, Bielfeldt S (1988) Die Beeinflussung der Hautfeuchtigkeit und Hautglätte durch den "Biokatalysator" Adenosintriphosphat (ATP). Ärztl Kosmet 18:372–378
18. Siemens HW (1928) Zur Differentialdiagnose und Prognose der überlebenden Fälle von Ichthyosis congenita. Arch Dermatol Syph (Berl) 156:624–655
19. Stüttgen G (1962) Zur Lokalbehandlung von Keratosen mit Vitamin-A-Säure. Dermatologica 124:65–80
20. Stüttgen G (1987) Eczema therapy and permeability of infantile skin for topical preparations. In: Happle R, Grosshans E (eds) Pediatric dermatology. Advances in diagnosis and treatment. Springer, Berlin Heidelberg New York Tokyo
21. Swanbeck G (1968) A new treatment of ichthyosis and other hyperkeratotic conditions. Acta Derm Venereol (Stockh) 48:123–127
22. Swanbeck G (1978) The effect of urea on the skin with special reference to the treatment of ichthyosis. In: Marks R, Dykes PJ (eds) The ichthyoses. MTP, Lancaster, pp 163–166
23. Taylor JR, Halprin K (1975) Percutaneous absorption of salicylic acid. Arch Dermatol 106:740–743
24. Van Scott EJ, Yu RJ (1974) Control of keratinization with α-hydroxy acids and related compounds. I. Topical treatment of ichthyotic disorders. Arch Dermatol 110:586–590
25. Van Scott EJ, Yu RJ (1984) Hyperkeratinization, corneocyte cohesion, and alpha-hydroxy acids. J Am Acad Dermatol 11:867–879
26. Van Weiss DF, Lever WF (1964) Percutaneous salicylic acid intoxication in psoriasis. Arch Dermatol 90:614–619
27. Wester RC, Noonan PK, Cole MP, Maibach HI (1977) Percutaneous absorption of testosterone in the newborn rhesus monkey. Comparison to the adult. Pediatr Res 11:737–739
28. Würsch TG (1980) Topische Behandlung von vulgären Ichthyosen mit Carbamid und Vitamin-A-Säure-haltigen Externa. Schweiz Rundsch Med Prax 69:1060–1063

7.2 Systemic Therapy

7.2.1 Retinoids

7.2.1.1 Historical Aspects

Retinoids are powerful substances providing an effective therapy for almost all keratinization defects and many other related scaling disorders [1, 6, 8, 40, 47]. The beneficial effect of vitamin A [27] and vitamin A acid [44] in the treatment of cornification disorders has been known for many years. As discussed in Sect. 7.1, topical therapy with vitamin A acid was severely hampered by its irritating property [44]. On the other hand, systemic treatment with vitamin A requires high doses and produces unacceptable side effects, now commonly referred to as hypervitaminosis A. The signs of hypervitaminosis A are increased brain pressure and considerable liver and skeletal toxicity. These possible side effects prevented the general use of vitamin A in cornification disorders. In the mid-1970s, Werner Bollag [3], working at the Hoffmann-La Roche laboratories in Switzerland, organized a program to synthesize analogues of vitamin A. Over a thousand compounds were developed and screened. By chemical modification of the retinoid acid molecule, less toxic retinoids such as etretinate, isotretinoin, and - very recently - acitretin, the first metabolite of etretinate, were obtained.

The molecular mechanisms underlying the action of retinoids have been intensively studied but are not yet fully understood. Retinoids affect the expression of genes by specific activation and repression processes [5]. More than 40 different genes and products are known whose expression is influenced by retinoids [5]. Following etretinate therapy, the levels of glucose-6-phosphate dehydrogenase and succinic dehydrogenase in the epidermis of ichthyosis patients were lowered and reached the level found in normal subjects, whereas nonspecific esterase activities were increased [33]. Retinoids exert their effects on gene expression in the nucleus via a cellular retinoic acid receptor which belongs to the family of the steroid/thyroid receptor family [11, 35].

Retinoids have revolutionized pharmacotherapy in dermatology. Their impact on our speciality is comparable to that of glucocorticoids. Today, we know more about retinoids including their possible side effects than about many classical dermatologicals. A recent review [8], dealing only with etretinate, listed more than 250 relevant references. As a consequence of the considerable attention retinoids have received over the past 10 years, most dermatologists are familiar with the pros and cons of these substances. Therefore, this chapter will focus on only a few aspects of retinoid treatment.

Special emphasis will be given to etretinate and its side effects, since I consider this substance to be superior to isotretinoin as far as long-term treatment of patients with ichthyosis is concerned [47, 48]. In addition, problems relating to the treatment of children are covered in some detail.

7.2.1.2 Clinical Efficacy

Retinoids have been employed with good or excellent results in many types of ichthyosis [1, 16, 24, 34, 46]. The advent of retinoid therapy was a major therapeutic breakthrough in this field. For the first time, many patients were able to lead an almost normal life. There are, however, a number of possible side effects. Because of risk/benefit considerations, not all patients with ichthyosis or related scaling disorders should be given retinoids. In my opinion, the use of retinoids should be restricted to patients with severe keratinization disorders. I advise excluding patients with autosomal dominant ichthyosis vulgaris and X-linked recessive ichthyosis from retinoid therapy because their skin affliction is usually too mild [47, 48].

The clinical effect of retinoids is somewhat dependent on the type of ichthyosis treated. The most striking and dramatic effect of a retinoid has been reported by Lawlor and Peiris [22] in a case of **harlequin fetus** (see Sect. 4.1). Because of the availability of etretinate therapy and because of the advances in neonatal care, these most severely afflicted children now have a good chance of surviving. Similar to collodion babies, these small patients progress to lamellar ichthyosis with a background erythema and fine scaling, once the critical neonatal stage is lived through [21]. This means that retinoid therapy can be withdrawn after a few months.

Very rewarding results are obtained with etretinate in patients with the **Sjögren-Larsson syndrome** [18, 47], as far as the skin condition is concerned. Frequently, these patients are also relieved from their severe pruritus by the retinoid treatment. Surprisingly, the good results can be maintained with a rather low dose of etretinate (0.25 mg/kg body weight).

In the various types of **lamellar ichthyosis** the response to etretinate is good to excellent. Initially, a dramatic improvement is mostly observed, especially in the NELI phenotype (Fig. 77). To achieve this excellent result, comparatively high doses (1.0–1.3 mg/kg body weight) of etretinate are needed. In our experience, such a high dose of etretinate cannot be maintained over a long time. After about 4–6 months these patients develop erosive skin lesions and one is forced to decrease the dosage. Inevitably, the skin condition becomes worse under this lower dosage (usually 0.5 0.7 mg/kg) but the results are still satisfactory (Fig. 78). We have observed this phenomenon in several patients with lamellar ichthyosis [48]. It may reflect the peculiar elimination kinetics of etretinate, which has a half-life of 100 days. As a general rule, a steady state – i.e., a level where plasma concentrations no longer rise when the same dosis is maintained – will develop only after 3–4 half-lives. For etretinate, this means that it will take almost a year to achieve a steady state. In other words, the actual plasma levels of

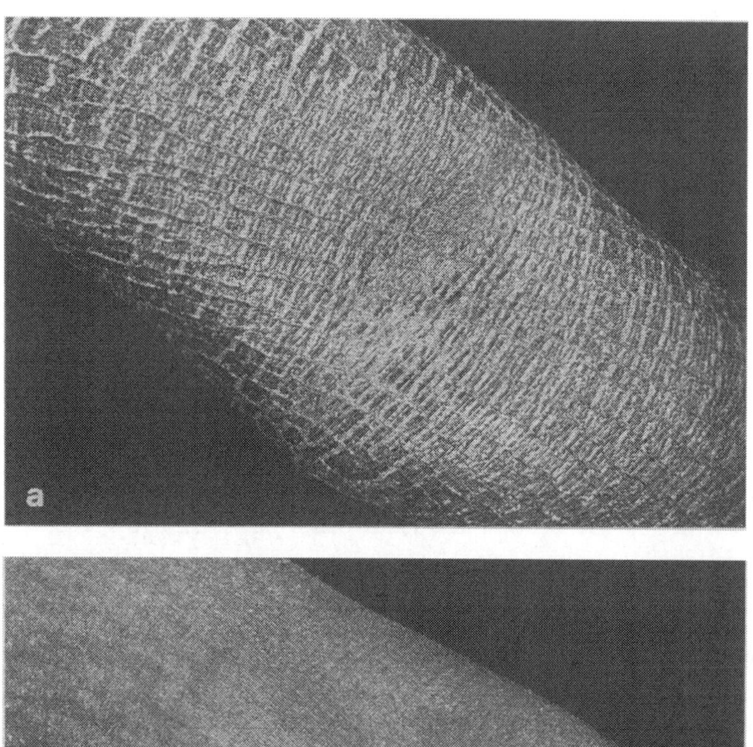

Fig. 77a, b. Effect of etretinate in a 20-year-old woman with lamellar ichthyosis (NELI type C). **a** Before treatment; **b** after 8 weeks of etretinate therapy

etretinate after half a year of treatment are bound to be about twice as high as those at the beginning of therapy.

The elimination kinetics of **acitretin,** the first metabolite of etretinate, are much shorter, since this substance is not stored in the adipose tissue. In my own limited experience with acitretin I have not observed the problem of overdosage becoming manifest after only several months.

Patients with **bullous ichthyotic erythroderma** can profit from retinoid therapy, but in this disorder it is especially important to carefully select the dosage. It is

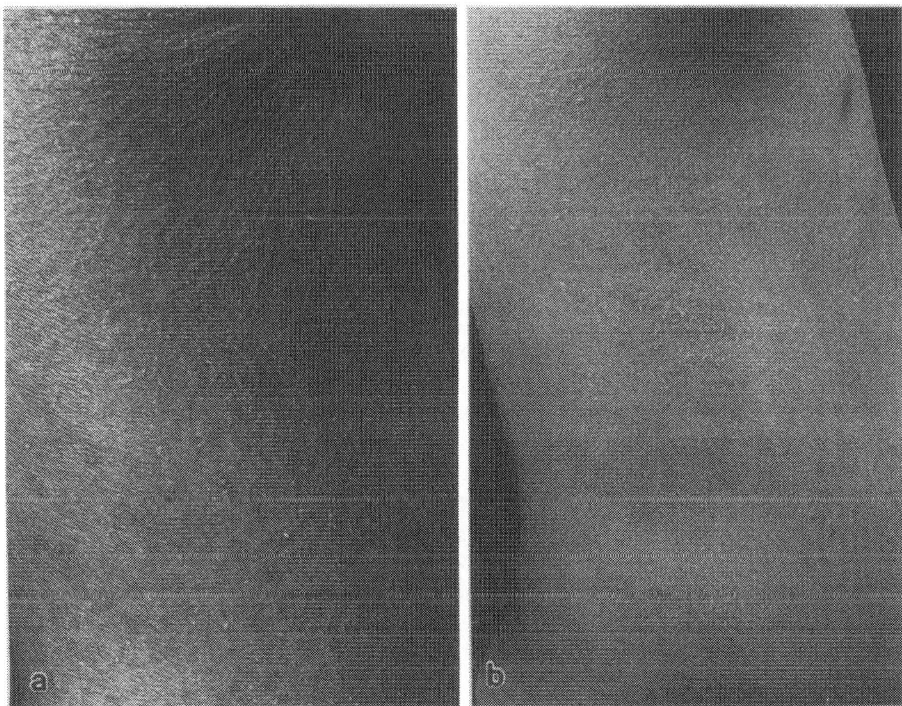

Fig. 78a, b. Lamellar ichthyosis (NELI type A) in a 9-year-old boy. **a** Prominent hyperkeratoses despite treatment with urea ointment; **b** effect of etretinate after 10 weeks. Previous conventional treatment continued. (From [47])

advisable to begin with small doses (0.25 mg/kg body weight) and to slowly increase the dosage until an optimum has been found [2, 41]. Histologically, these patients show the features of epidermolytic hyperkeratosis. This is the reason why they tolerate only comparatively small doses of retinoids. High doses provoke a marked exacerbation of blistering [2, 41].

Similar considerations, as far as the dosage selection is concerned, apply to the **Comèl-Netherton syndrome** (Fig. 79). When a "normal" initial dose of 0.5–0.7 mg/kg body weight is given, these patients may likewise show a dramatic deterioration of their skin condition. Under a low dosage, they usually do very well.

7.2.1.3 Toxicologic Aspects

There are a number of harmless side effects [40] patients will notice and about which they have to be informed well in advance [40]. Almost all patients develop dry lips under etretinate. This cheilitis can be treated with a bland ointment. A diffuse, usually mild hair loss, may be a problem in some patients, especially females who are on long-term therapy with etretinate. However, this hair loss is completely reversed after withdrawal of the substance. An overdosage of etreti-

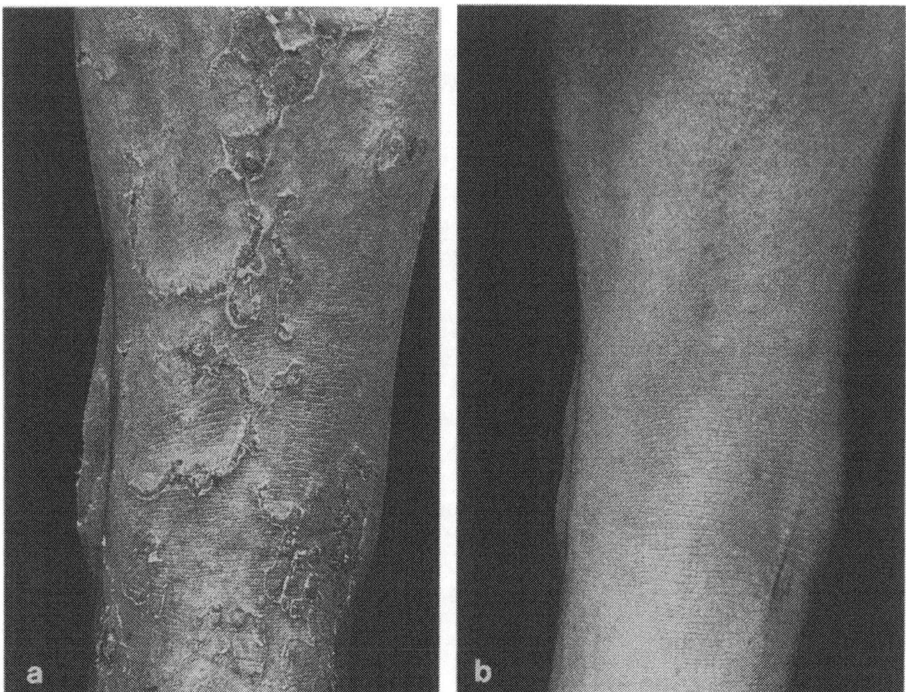

Fig. 79a, b. Comèl-Netherton syndrome in a 12-year-old boy. **a** Typical aspect of ichthyosis linearis circumflexa; **b** effect of 10 weeks of etretinate. (From [47])

nate produces erosions, and the skin can become fragile, especially on palms and soles and on the lower parts of the extremities. According to the literature [29, 45], at the beginning of retinoid therapy quite a number of patients develop a dermatitis, mimicking an eczema craquelé or psoriasis. Though I have seen eczema craquelé as a side effect of isotretinoin therapy, I cannot remember a single instance of true retinoid dermatitis in my patients with cornification disorders. It is conceivable that patients with psoriasis are more prone to develop so-called retinoid dermatitis. Moreover, psoriasis patients treated with etretinate often show an initial expansion of the total affected surface area. This phenomenon is not well known and may account for some retinoid dermatitis cases.

Apart from the harmless mucocutaneous side effects, a number of serious unwanted effects have to be considered. Both isotretinoin [10, 38] and etretinate [15] are known teratogens. As a consequence, female teenagers and women of childbearing age must not become pregnant while being treated. For etretinate, an interval of 2 years after withdrawal of the drug is stipulated because of the slow elimination of the substance. Very recently, a severe embryopathy of the vitamin A type was reported in an infant conceived 1 year after termination of maternal etretinate application [20]. As discussed above, acitretin and isotretinoin are eliminated much faster. A pregnancy-free interval of 8 weeks to 3 months seems to be sufficient. In the United States isotretinoin has earned itself a bad name because of the high number of pregnancies occurring during or after treatment with this teratogen [10, 38]. This problem cannot be blamed on the drug, however, but is mainly caused by the unsafe distribution system and uncontrolled sales over the counter. In Europe, the overall experience with the teratogenic potential of retinoids has been much less dramatic and only a few such pregnancies have occurred [15]. Fortunately, retinoids are not mutagenic. They do not induce chromosome breaks [14] or mutations as measured by the Ames test [17].

In patients with preexisting liver disease retinoids can be toxic [32], and disturbances of lipid metabolism may occur in predisposed patients [13, 26]. These side effects usually are reversible and dosage dependent. In a very few patients, acute toxic hepatitis occurred under etretinate therapy; this appears to be an idiosyncratic reaction that cannot be predicted from the results of intermittent plasma controls of transaminases or even liver biopsies [8]. Combinations of retinoids with methotrexate are better avoided, since this combination may potentiate possible liver toxicity [8].

During the past 10 years a considerable number of patients with severe cornification disorders have received prolonged retinoid therapy, often over many years. Etretinate was first introduced and therefore mostly used in Europe, while isotretinoin was first available in the United States and therefore more often given there. The overall experience with long-term administration of these substances has been encouraging as far as liver and kidney functions and lipid metabolism are concerned [48].

However, there is growing concern about the **skeletal toxicity** of retinoids after long-term therapy. It is evident that isotretinoin can cause disseminated

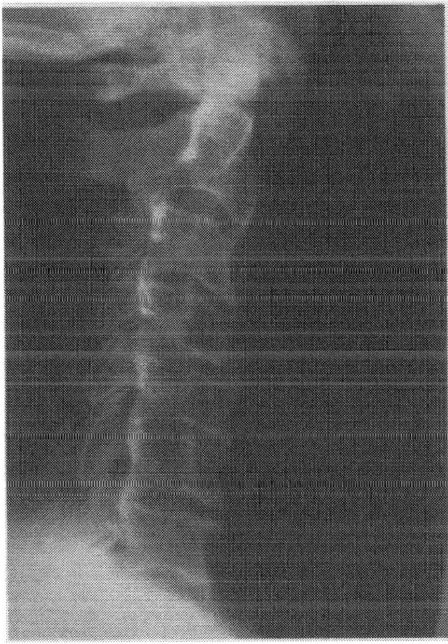

Fig. 80. DISH syndrome showing involvement of the cervical spine in a 51-year-old patient treated continuously for 11 years with etretinate. Note pronounced calcification of the anterior and posterior ligaments. (From [30], courtesy of Dr. Montag, Münster)

retinoid-induced skeletal hyperostosis, and the acronym "DISH" syndrome has been coined for this unwanted effect [9, 36]. Similar bone alterations such as calcification of the anterior spinal ligament, vertebral hyperostosis, hyperostotic bridging of vertebral bodies (Fig. 80), extraspinal calcifications (Fig. 81), periosteal thickening, and periosteal bone resorption were observed under prolonged etretinate therapy [4, 7, 25, 30, 42, 50]. In comparison with isotretinoin, etretinate-induced skeletal changes seem to evolve with a longer latency period and tend to be milder [25, 48]. This is one of the reasons why I suggest using etretinate rather than isotretinoin for ichthyosis patients. The clinical significance of etretinate-induced bone alterations and the incidence of these alterations are still a matter of debate. While some groups [7, 25, 43] observed skeletal toxicity in up to 90% of their patients, others find that these side effects occur much less frequently [12, 30, 39, 50]. These differences are most likely due to a different composition of the patient groups with regard to age, diagnosis, and duration of etretinate exposure. Both isotretinoin and etretinate were reported to produce premature closure of the epiphyseal line [28, 37], but it has to be stressed that this adverse reaction is exceptional.

Retinoid therapy may be associated with subtle retinal changes affecting night vision, dark adaptation, and color sense [49]. Weber and associates [49] reported on four patients who had been under long-term therapy with etretinate and showed alterations of the color sense originating in the blue-yellow spectrum and extending to the red-green spectrum. The patient who had received the highest cumulative dose also had an increased threshold of rod sensitivity at dark adaptation in the Goldman-Weekers test [49].

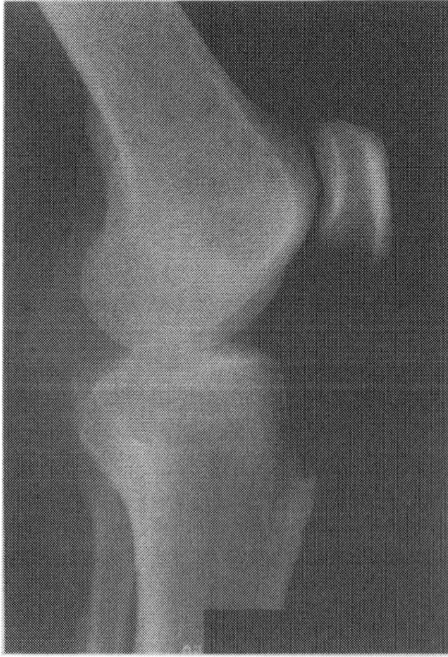

Fig. 81. DISH syndrome with extraspinal involvement after 11 years of etretinate (same patient as in Fig. 80). Note calcification of the insertion of the ligamentum patellae. (From [30], courtesy of Dr. Montag, Münster)

7.2.1.4 *Measures to Minimize and Control Side Effects of Retinoid Therapy*

A number of measures are advisable to minimize the inherent risks of long-term retinoid administration (Table 36). All patients should be given a good emollient program concurrent to the retinoid administration to keep the required dosage of etretinate as low as possible. In this context it is important to remember, however, that children require higher doses than adults to achieve the same effect [47, 48]. This is due to the larger surface/weight ratio already discussed in Sect. 7.1. Extensive radiographic examinations at intervals of 1 year are adivsable in children [43, 46–48], while in adults the radiographic program may be less extensive. According to a recent study [50], bone scintigraphy is too insensitive to monitor possible skeletal alterations. In children, growth curves should be plotted and length and weight recorded at least every 3 months. If possible, data about growth prior to retinoid treatment should be obtained. When evaluating growth curves of children under retinoid treatment, one has to keep in mind that delayed growth is a typical feature of some syndromes (e.g., in the Comèl-Netherton syndrome).

Routine laboratory investigations (blood cell count, liver cell function, kidney function, lipids) should be performed at the beginning of the treatment at rather short intervals (2–4 weeks), while later the intervals can be extended to 8 weeks (to 3 months). Because of very recent reports indicating a possible effect of etretinate on night vision, ophthalmologic controls prior to initiating a therapy and at intervals of 1 year are also advisable.

The problem of teratogenicity is best prevented by a frank discussion of this aspect before initiation of treatment. The need for active contraception for a period of 2 years even after withdrawal of etretinate should be made clear. We

Table 36. Recommended measures to control unwanted effects of long-term therapy with etretinate

1. Inclusion of only severly affected patients for this therapy
2. Informing the patient extensively about the pros and cons, emphasizing the need for contraception in female patients for a period of 2 years after withdrawal
3. Concurrent sufficient topical therapy to keep total retinoid dose low
4. Routine laboratory examinations prior to therapy, and at regular intervals (every 8 weeks)
5. Radiographic controls (lateral views of the cervical, thoracic, and lumbar spine) before starting treatment and thereafter at yearly intervals
6. Ophthalmologic controls including tests for night vision and color sense, before therapy and afterwards at yearly intervals
7. Special precautions in children:
   a) Plotting of growth and weight curves during treatment
   b) More extensive radiographic controls including lateral and frontal views of the elbows, knees, and hand bones
   c) Usually, no prolonged treatment of children under 7 years of age

usually hand out a pamphlet informing about general aspects of the substance including side effects, and ask female patients to sign a statement that they have been made aware of these problems. Pregnancy tests should be performed at regular intervals, as well.

Lay persons and sometimes also physicians confuse teratogenicity and mutagenicity. They ask whether similar precautions apply if a man is treated and the couple wants to have a child. This is not the case. There is no reason for concern in such a situation. Because of the possible skeletal side effects, some colleagues now advocate retinoid holidays as a means of minimizing these unwanted effects [12, 39]. They suggest treating only in the winterime and not in the summer when, due to the more humid climate, many patients with ichthyosis improve a little bit. I think this advice is inconclusive and does not reassure the patient in his decision for therapy. If one follows this philosophy as a regular plan, much of the relief that can be given to patients with severe ichthyosis will be lost. The most important measure to minimize and control side effects is a restrictive selection of patients who are offered retinoid therapy. Their condition should be so severe that they cannot be treated satisfactorily with classical topical means.

Considering the possible side effects associated with long-term administration of retinoids, the question arises whether our patients with ichthyosis, and in particular affected children, should be treated at all. There is no final or general answer to this question, and it has to be discussed anew in each case. Patients have to be properly informed about the possible risks and have to be asked if they are willing to take them. Still, even if the situation is explained in some detail, it is difficult for them to have a realistic picture of the significance of the possible side effects. Often they will ask for our personal view on this matter. Generally, I encourage the patients to take etretinate if they are severely affected and are willing to come for regular checkups. Likewise, I think that it is justifiable to treat children if they suffer from a disfiguring cornification disorder. The skin condition often has dramatic repercussions on the psychosocial development of these children. Many of our patients lack self-confidence or even show considerable psychic alterations due to their skin disease. There is no such thing as absolute safety in medicine. In my opinion, the prospect of leading an almost normal life justifies this treatment in both children and adults.

7.2.2 Other Systemic Treatment Modalities

A phytol-free diet and plasma-exchange therapy have proven very successful in the care of patients with Refsum's disease. Treatment of this condition is discussed in Sect. 3.1.6. Several types of ichthyosis represent hyperproliferative disorders. The increased rate of epidermal cell turnover can be inhibited by cytostatic drugs such as methotrexate or cyclophosphamide [19], but continued use of such cytostatic drugs is not possible. As a general rule, such drugs have no place in the treatment of the ichthyoses. An exception to this rule may be photochemotherapy (PUVA), which is, of course, much less toxic than cyclophosphamide and seems to be especially beneficial in the Comèl-Netherton syndrome [23, 31]. Hintner et al. [16] reported that the combination of etretinate with photochemotherapy (Re-PUVA) may be the therapy of choice in those patients who are difficult to treat with etretinate alone. Systemic glucocorticoids were once popular in the management of collodion baby, but their value has never been established and I see no reason to use them.

So far, no specific systemic treatment modalities are available for the heterogeneous group of ichthyoses. In the near future, the primary biochemical defect will be established in at least some of these disorders. It can be expected that this will result in a better understanding of the underlying pathophysiologic mechanisms, and that new therapeutic approaches will become available.

References

1. Baden HP, Buxman MM, Weinstein GD, Yoder FW (1982) Treatment of ichthyosis with isotretinoin. J Am Acad Dermatol 6:716–720
2. Blanchet-Bardon C, Anton-Lamprecht I, Schnyder UW (1977) Erythrodermie congénitale ichthyosiforme bulleuse. Contrôle ultrastructurale du traitement par l'éther éthylique d'un dérivé aromatique de l'acide rétinoique. Ann Dermatol Venereol 104:648–653
3. Bollag W (1983) The development of retinoids in experimental and clinical oncology and dermatology. J Am Acad Dermatol 9:797–805
4. Cerio R, Wells RS, Mac Donald DM (1987) Calcifying arthropathy of the hip and diffuse hyperostosis associated with etretinate. Clin Exp Dermatol 12:129–131
5. Chytil F, Sherman DR (1987) How do retinoids work? Dermatologica 175 [Suppl 1]:8–12
6. Di Giovanna JJ, Peck GL (1983) Oral synthetic retinoid treatment in children. Pediatr Dermatol 1:77–88
7. Di Giovanna JJ, Helfgott RK, Gerber LH, Peck GB (1986) Extraspinal tendon and ligament calcification associated with long-term therapy with etretinate. N Engl J Med 315:1177–1182
8. Ellis CN, Voorhees JJ (1987) Etretinate therapy. J Am Acad Dermatol 16:267–291
9. Ellis CN, Madison KC, Pennes DR, Martel W, Voorhees JJ (1984) Isotretinoin therapy is associated with early skeletal radiographic changes. J Am Acad Dermatol 10:1024–1029
10. Feinhoff PM, Lammer EJ (1984) Craniofacial features of isotretinoin embryopathy. J Pediatr 105:595
11. Giguere V, Ong ES, Seguj P, Evans RM (1987) Identification of a receptor for the morphogen retinoic acid. Nature 330:624–629
12. Glover MT, Peters AM, Atherton DJ (1987) Surveillance for skeletal toxicity of children treated with etretinate. Br J Dermatol 116:609–614
13. Gollnick H, Luley C, Schwartzkopff W, Orfanos CE (1982) Veränderungen von Serumlipidfraktionen als Nebenwirkung oraler Retinoide. Z Hautkr 57:1255–1267
14. Happle R, Niedworok A (1981) Cytogenetic studies in patients treated with oral retinoid Ro 10-9359. In: Orfanos CE, Braun-Falco O, Farber EM, Grupper C, Polano MK, Schuppli R (eds) Retinoids. Advances in basic research and therapy. Proceedings of the International Dermatology Symposium Oct. 13–15 1980, Berlin. Springer, Berlin Heidelberg New York, pp 61–65
15. Happle R, Traupe H, Bounameaux Y, Fisch T (1984) Teratogene Wirkung von Etretinat beim Menschen. Dtsch Med Wochenschr 109:1476–1480
16. Hintner H, Jaschke E, Fritsch P (1980) Netherton-Syndrom: Abwehrschwäche, generalisierte Verrukose und Karzinogenese. Hautarzt 31:428–432
17. Hummler H, Schüpbach ME (1981) Studies in reproductive toxicology and mutagenicity with Ro 10-9359. In: Orfanos CE, Braun-Falco O, Farber EM, Grupper C, Polano MK, Schuppli R (eds) Retinoids. Advances in basic research and therapy. Proc Int Dermatol Symp Oct. 13–15 1980, Berlin. Springer, Berlin Heidelberg New York, pp 49–59
18. Jagell S, Lidén S (1982) Treatment of the ichthyosis of the Sjögren-Larsson syndrome with etretinate (Tigason). Acta Derm Venereol (Stockh) 63:89–91

19. Klein E, Hahn GM, Solomon JA et al. (1979) Explorations of antimitotic agents in the treatment of a congenital disease, ichthyosis linearis circumflexa. J Surg Oncol 11:85–88
20. Lammer E (1988) Embryopathy in an infant conceived one year after termination of maternal etretinate. Lancet 2:1080–1081
21. Lawlor F (1987) Harlequin baby: inheritance and prognosis. Br J Dermatol 117:528
22. Lawlor F, Peiris S (1985) Harlequin fetus successfully treated with etretinate. Br J Dermatol 112:585–590
23. Manabe M, Yoskiike T, Negi M, Ogawa H (1983) Successful therapy of ichthyosis linearis circumflexa with PUVA. J Am Acad Dermatol 8:905–907
24. Marks R, Finlay AY, Holt PJA (1981) Severe disorders of keratinization. Effects of treatment with Tigason (etretinate). Br J Dermatol 104:667–673
25. Melnik B, Blück S, Jungblut RM, Goerz G (1987) Retrospective radiographic study of skeletal changes after long-term etretinate therapy. Br J Dermatol 116:207–212
26. Melnik B, Bros U, Plewig G (1987) Evaluation of the atherogenic risk of isotretinoin and etretinate-induced alterations of lipoprotein cholesterol metabolism. J Invest Dermatol 88 [Suppl]:39s–43s
27. Miescher G (1954) Behandlung der Ichthyosis mit Vitamin A. Dermatologica 108:300–303
28. Milstone LM, McGuire J, Ablow RC (1982) Premature epiphyseal closure in a child receiving oral 13-**cis**-retinoic acid. J Am Acad Dermatol 7:663–666
29. Molin L, Thomsen K, Volden G, Wantzin GL (1985) Retinoid dermatitis mimicking progression in mycosis fungoides: a report from the Scandinavian mycosis fungoides group. Acta Derm Venereol (Stockh) 65:69–71
30. Montag M, Reiser M, Hamm H, Traupe H, Vogt HJ (1988) Skelettveränderungen nach Langzeitbehandlung mit Retinoiden. Radiologe 28:320–325
31. Nagata T (1980) Netherton's syndrome which responded to photochemotherapy. Dermatologica 161:51–60
32. Orfanos CE, Mahrle G, Goerz G, Happle R, Hofbauer M, Landes E, Schimpf A (1979) Laboratory investigations in patients with generalized psoriasis under oral retinoid treatment. A multicenter study of computerized data. Dermatologica 159:62–70
33. Pearse AD, Gaskell SA, Marks R (1986) The effects of an aromatic retinoid (etretinate) on epidermal cell production and metabolism in normal ichthyotic patients. Br J Dermatol 114:285–294
34. Pehamberger H, Esca SA, Holubar K (1979) Behandlung hyperkeratotischer Dermatosen mit einem oralen, aromatischem Retinoid (Ro 10-9359). Z Hautkr 55:68–78
35. Petkovic M, Brand NJ, Krust A, Chambon P (1987) A human retinoic acid receptor which belongs to the family of nuclear receptors. Nature 330:444–446
36. Pittsley RA, Yoder FW (1983) Skeletal toxicity associated with long-term administration of 13-**cis**-retinoic acid for refractory ichthyosis. N Engl J Med 308:1012–1014
37. Prendiville J, Bingham EA, Burrows D (1986) Premature epiphyseal closure - a complication of etretinate therapy in children. J Am Acad Dermatol 15:1259–1262
38. Rosa FW (1983) Teratogenicity of isotretinoin. Lancet 2:513–514
39. Ruiz-Maldonado R, Tamayo L (1987) Retinoids in disorders of keratinization: their use in children. Dermatologica 175:125–132
40. Schimpf A (1976) Zur systemischen Anwendung eines aromatischen Vitamin-A-Säure-Derivates (Ro 10-9359) bei Psoriasis und Keratosen. Z Hautkr 51:265–274
41. Schnyder UW, Vogel A (1980) Zur Behandlung der Erythrodermia congenitalis ichthyosiformis bullosa mit aromatischen Retinoiden. Aktuel Dermatol 6:133–136
42. Sillevis-Smit JH, de Mari F (1984) A serious side effect of etretinate (Tigason). Clin Exp Dermatol 9:554–556
43. Halkier-Sørensen L, Laurberg G, Andresen J (1987) Bone changes in children on long-term treatment with etretinate. J Am Acad Dermatol 16:999–1006
44. Stüttgen G (1962) Zur Lokalbehandlung von Keratosen mit Vitamin A-Säure. Dermatologica 124:65–80
45. Taïeb A, Maleville J (1985) Retinoid dermatitis mimicking "eczéma craquelé". Acta Derm Venereol (Stockh) 65:570

46. Tamayo L, Ruiz-Maldonado R (1981) Long-term follow-up of 30 children under oral retinoid Ro 10-9359. In: Orfanos CE, Braun-Falco O, Farber EM, Grupper CH, Polano MK, Schuppli R (eds) Retinoids. Advances in basic research and therapy. Proc Int Dermatol Symp Oct 13-15 1980, Berlin. Springer, Berlin Heidelberg New York, pp 41-47
47. Traupe H, Happle R (1985) Etretinate therapy in children with severe keratinization defects. Eur J Pediatr 143:166-169
48. Traupe H, Hamm H (1987) Langzeittherapie von Ichthyosen und anderen Verhornungsstörungen mit Retinoiden. In: Meigel W (ed) Langzeittherapie mit Retinoiden. Editiones Roche, Basel, pp 29-46
49. Weber U, Melnik B, Goerz G, Michaelis L (1988) Abnormal retinal function associated with long-term etretinate? Lancet 1:235-236
50. Wilson DJ, Kay V, Charig M, Hughes DG, Creasy TS (1988) Skeletal hyperostosis and extraosseous calcification in a patient receiving long-term etretinate (Tigason). Br J Dermatol 119:597-607

8 Subject Index

a

b

c

d

e

f

k

l

U

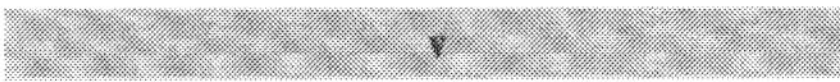

W

X

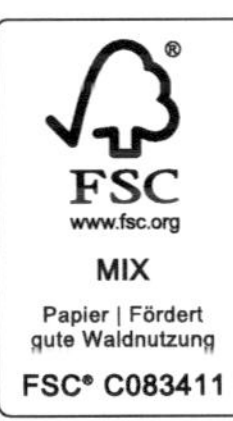

Zeitfracht Medien GmbH
Ferdinand-Jühlke-Straße 7
99095 Erfurt, Deutschland
produktsicherheit@kolibri360.de